MW01178949

# Infection Prevention and Control in Healthcare, Part I: Facility Planning and Management

*Editors*

KEITH S. KAYE
SORABH DHAR

## INFECTIOUS DISEASE CLINICS OF NORTH AMERICA

www.id.theclinics.com

*Consulting Editor*
HELEN W. BOUCHER

September 2016 • Volume 30 • Number 3

**ELSEVIER**

1600 John F. Kennedy Boulevard • Suite 1800 • Philadelphia, Pennsylvania, 19103-2899.
http://www.theclinics.com

**INFECTIOUS DISEASE CLINICS OF NORTH AMERICA Volume 30, Number 3**
**September 2016 ISSN 0891–5520, ISBN-13: 978-0-323-46258-7**

Editor: Kerry Holland
Developmental Editor: Donald Mumford

*Infectious Disease Clinics of North America* (ISSN 0891–5520) is published in March, June, September, and December by Elsevier Inc., 360 Park Avenue South, New York, NY 10010-1710. Periodicals postage paid at New York, NY and additional mailing offices. Subscription prices are $295.00 per year for US individuals, $560.00 per year for US institutions, $100.00 per year for US students, $350.00 per year for Canadian individuals, $699.00 per year for Canadian institutions, $420.00 per year for international individuals, $699.00 per year for international institutions, and $200.00 per year for Canadian and international students. To receive student rate, orders must be accompanied by name of affiliated institution, date of term, and the *signature* of program/residency coordinator on institution letterhead. Orders will be billed at individual rate until proof of status is received. Foreign air speed delivery is included in all *Clinics* subscription prices. All prices are subject to change without notice. **POSTMASTER**: Send address changes to *Infectious Disease Clinics of North America,* Elsevier Health Sciences Division, Subcription Customer Service, 3251 Riverport Lane, Maryland Heights, MO 63043. **Customer Service: 1-800-654-2452 (US). From outside of the US and Canada, call 1-314-447-8871. Fax: 1-314-447-8029. E-mail: JournalsCustomerService-usa@elsevier.com (print support) or JournalsOnlineSupport-usa@elsevier.com (online support).**

*Infectious Disease Clinics of North America* is also published in Spanish by Editorial Inter-Médica, Junin 917, 1$^{er}$ A 1113, Buenos Aires, Argentina.

*Reprints*. For copies of 100 or more, of articles in this publication, please contact the Commercial Reprints Department, Elsevier Inc., 360 Park Avenue South, New York, New York 10010-1710. Tel. 212-633-3874, Fax: 212-633-3820, E-mail: reprints@elsevier.com.

*Infectious Disease Clinics of North America* is covered in *MEDLINE/PubMed (Index Medicus), Current Contents/ Clinical Medicine, Science Citation Alert, SCISEARCH,* and *Research Alert.*

Printed in the United States of America.

# Contributors

## CONSULTING EDITOR

**HELEN W. BOUCHER, MD, FIDSA, FACP**
Director, Infectious Diseases Fellowship Program, Division of Geographic Medicine and Infectious Diseases, Tufts Medical Center, Associate Professor of Medicine, Tufts University School of Medicine, Boston, Massachusetts

## EDITORS

**KEITH S. KAYE, MD, MPH**
Professor of Medicine, Corporate Vice President of Quality and Patient Safety, Corporate Medical Director, Department of Hospital Epidemiology, Infection Prevention and Antimicrobial Stewardship, Detroit Medical Center; Department of Medicine, Wayne State University, Detroit, Michigan

**SORABH DHAR, MD**
Associate Professor of Medicine, Department of Hospital Epidemiology and Infection Prevention, Detroit Medical Center; Department of Medicine, Detroit Receiving Hospital and Rehabilitation Institute of Michigan, Wayne State University; Director of Infection Prevention, Epidemiology, and Antimicrobial Stewardship, Department of Hospital Epidemiology and Infection Prevention, John D Dingell VA Medical Center, Detroit, Michigan

## AUTHORS

**MEREDITH AMBROSE, MHA**
Health Systems Specialist, National Infectious Diseases Service, Specialty Care Services, Patient Care Services, Veterans Health Administration, Department of Veterans Affairs (VA), Washington, DC

**ANA CECILIA BARDOSSY, MD**
Clinical Study Coordinator, Division of Infectious Disease, Henry Ford Health System, Detroit, Michigan

**MAUREEN K. BOLON, MD, MS**
Associate Professor of Medicine, Division of Infectious Diseases, Department of Medicine, Northwestern University Feinberg School of Medicine, Chicago, Illinois

**PHILIP C. CARLING, MD**
Director of Infectious Diseases, Department of Infectious Diseases, Carney Hospital; Professor of Clinical Medicine, Boston University School of Medicine, Boston, Massachusetts

**MARCO CASSONE, MD, PhD**
Research Associate, Division of Geriatric Medicine, University of Michigan Medical School, Ann Arbor, Michigan

**EVELYN COOK, RN, CIC**
Duke Infection Control Outreach Network, Duke University Medical Center, Durham, North Carolina

**SORABH DHAR, MD**
Associate Professor of Medicine, Department of Hospital Epidemiology and Infection Prevention, Detroit Medical Center; Department of Medicine, Detroit Receiving Hospital and Rehabilitation Institute of Michigan, Wayne State University; Director of Infection Prevention, Epidemiology, and Antimicrobial Stewardship, Department of Hospital Epidemiology and Infection Prevention, John D Dingell VA Medical Center, Detroit, Michigan

**ELAINE FLANAGAN, RN, BSN, MSA, CIC**
Regional Director Epidemiology, Quality and Patient Safety, Detroit Medical Center Healthcare System, Detroit, Michigan

**SHANTINI D. GAMAGE, PhD, MPH**
Epidemiologist, National Infectious Diseases Service, Specialty Care Services, Patient Care Services, Veterans Health Administration, Department of Veterans Affairs (VA), Washington, DC; Volunteer Assistant Professor, Division of Infectious Diseases, Department of Internal Medicine, University of Cincinnati College of Medicine, Cincinnati, Ohio

**KEITH S. KAYE, MD, MPH**
Professor of Medicine, Corporate Vice President of Quality and Patient Safety, Corporate Medical Director, Department of Hospital Epidemiology, Infection Prevention and Antimicrobial Stewardship, Detroit Medical Center; Department of Medicine, Wayne State University, Detroit, Michigan

**STEPHEN M. KRALOVIC, MD, MPH**
Medical Epidemiologist, National Infectious Diseases Service, Specialty Care Services, Patient Care Services, Veterans Health Administration, Department of Veterans Affairs (VA), Washington, DC; Associate Professor, Division of Infectious Diseases, Department of Internal Medicine, University of Cincinnati College of Medicine; Hospital Epidemiologist/Staff Infectious Diseases Physician, Cincinnati VA Medical Center, Cincinnati, Ohio

**KERRY L. LaPLANTE, PharmD, FCCP**
Professor of Pharmacy, University of Rhode Island, Kingston, Rhode Island; Adjunct Professor of Medicine, Brown University; Director of the Rhode Island Infectious Diseases Research Program (RIID), Infectious Diseases Pharmacotherapy Specialist, Providence Veterans Medical Center, Providence, Rhode Island

**MICHAEL Y. LIN, MD, MPH**
Associate Professor, Department of Medicine, Rush University Medical Center, Chicago, Illinois

**LONA MODY, MD, MSc**
Amanda Sanford Hickey Collegiate Professor of Internal Medicine; Associate Division Chief; Division of Geriatric Medicine, University of Michigan Medical School; Geriatrics Research, Education and Clinical Center; Associate Director, Veterans Affairs Ann Arbor Healthcare System, Ann Arbor, Michigan

**ANA MONTOYA, MD**
Assistant Professor, Division of Geriatric Medicine, University of Michigan Medical School, Ann Arbor, Michigan

**JEROD L. NAGEL, PharmD**
Clinical Pharmacist, Infectious Diseases, University of Michigan Health System, Ann Arbor, Michigan

**MARY ODEN, RN, MHS-CL**
Corporate Director, Infection Prevention, Clinical Operations, Tenet Health, Dallas, Texas

**RUSSELL N. OLMSTED, MPH, CIC**
Director of Infection Prevention and Control, Unified Clinical Organization, Trinity Health, Livonia, Michigan

**TRISH M. PERL, MD, MSc**
Professor of Medicine, Pathology and Epidemiology, Bloomberg School of Public Health, Johns Hopkins School of Medicine, Baltimore, Maryland

**JASON M. POGUE, PharmD**
Clinical Pharmacist, Infectious Diseases, Sinai-Grace Hospital, Detroit Medical Center, Clinical Assistant Professor of Medicine, Wayne State University School of Medicine, Detroit, Michigan

**GARY A. ROSELLE, MD**
Director, National Infectious Diseases Service, Specialty Care Services, Patient Care Services, Veterans Health Administration, Department of Veterans Affairs (VA), Washington, DC; Professor of Medicine, Division of Infectious Diseases, Department of Internal Medicine, University of Cincinnati College of Medicine; Cincinnati VA Medical Center, Cincinnati, Ohio

**WILLIAM A. RUTALA, PhD, MPH**
Hospital Epidemiology, University of North Carolina Health Care System; Division of Infectious Diseases, University of North Carolina School of Medicine, Chapel Hill, North Carolina

**GEETA SOOD, MD**
Assistant Professor of Medicine, Division of Infectious Diseases, Johns Hopkins University School of Medicine, Hospital Epidemiologist, Johns Hopkins Bayview Medical Center, Baltimore, Maryland

**WILLIAM E. TRICK, MD**
Professor, Department of Medicine, Rush University Medical Center; Department of Medicine, Cook County Health and Hospitals System, Chicago, Illinois

**DAVID J. WEBER, MD, MPH**
Hospital Epidemiology, University of North Carolina Health Care System; Division of Infectious Diseases, University of North Carolina School of Medicine, Chapel Hill, North Carolina

**JOHN ZERVOS, JD**
Manager, Division of Infectious Disease, The Global Health Initiative, Henry Ford Health System, Detroit, Michigan

**MARCUS ZERVOS, MD**
Division Head, Division of Infectious Disease, Henry Ford Health System; Professor, Wayne State University School of Medicine, Detroit, Michigan

# Contents

**Preface: Infection Prevention and Control in Healthcare, Part I: Facility Planning and Management**

Keith S. Kaye and Sorabh Dhar

xiii

**Building a Successful Infection Prevention Program: Key Components, Processes, and Economics**

Sorabh Dhar, Evelyn Cook, Mary Oden, and Keith S. Kaye

567

Infection control is the discipline responsible for preventing health care-associated infections (HAIs) and has grown from an anonymous field, to a highly visible, multidisciplinary field of incredible importance. There has been increasing focus on prevention rather than control of HAIs. Infection prevention programs (IPPs) have enormous scope that spans multiple disciplines. Infection control and the prevention and elimination of HAIs can no longer be compartmentalized. This article discusses the structure and responsibilities of an IPP, the regulatory pressures and opportunities that these programs face, and how to build and manage a successful program.

**Hand Hygiene: An Update**

Maureen K. Bolon

591

The medical field has long recognized the importance of hand hygiene in preventing health care–associated infections, yet studies indicate that this important task is performed only 40% of the time. Health care workers cite several barriers to optimal performance of hand hygiene, but the time required to perform this task is foremost among them. Introduction of alcohol-based hand rubs, bundled interventions, and incorporation of technologies designed to monitor and promote hand hygiene all represent promising advances in this field.

**Disinfection and Sterilization in Health Care Facilities: An Overview and Current Issues**

William A. Rutala and David J. Weber

609

When properly used, disinfection and sterilization can ensure the safe use of invasive and noninvasive medical devices. The method of disinfection and sterilization depends on the intended use of the medical device: critical items (contact sterile tissue) must be sterilized before use; semicritical items (contact mucous membranes or nonintact skin) must be high-level disinfected; and noncritical items (contact intact skin) should receive low-level disinfection. Cleaning should always precede high-level disinfection and sterilization. Current disinfection and sterilization guidelines must be strictly followed.

**Optimizing Health Care Environmental Hygiene**                          639

Philip C. Carling

This article presents a review and perspectives on aspects of optimizing health care environmental hygiene. The topics covered include the epidemiology of environmental surface contamination, a discussion of cleaning health care patient area surfaces, an overview of disinfecting health care surfaces, an overview of challenges in monitoring cleaning versus cleanliness, a description of an integrated approach to environmental hygiene and hand hygiene as interrelated disciplines, and an overview of the research opportunities and challenges related to health care environmental hygiene.

**Outbreaks in Health Care Settings**                          661

Geeta Sood and Trish M. Perl

Outbreaks and pseudo-outbreaks in health care settings can be complex and should be evaluated systematically using epidemiologic tools. Laboratory testing is an important part of an outbreak evaluation. Health care personnel, equipment, supplies, water, ventilation systems, and the hospital environment have been associated with health care outbreaks. Settings including the neonatal intensive care unit, endoscopy, oncology, and transplant units are areas that have specific issues which impact the approach to outbreak investigation and control. Certain organisms have a predilection for health care settings because of the illnesses of patients, the procedures performed, and the care provided.

**Water Safety and *Legionella* in Health Care: Priorities, Policy, and Practice**                          689

Shantini D. Gamage, Meredith Ambrose, Stephen M. Kralovic, and Gary A. Roselle

Health care facility water distribution systems have been implicated in the transmission of pathogens such as Legionella and nontuberculous mycobacteria to building occupants. These pathogens are natural inhabitants of water at low numbers and can amplify in premise plumbing water, especially if conditions are conducive to their growth. Because patients and residents in health care facilities are often at heightened risk for opportunistic infections, a multidisciplinary proactive approach to water safety is important to balance the various water priorities in health care and prevent water-associated infections in building occupants.

**Prevention by Design: Construction and Renovation of Health Care Facilities for Patient Safety and Infection Prevention**                          713

Russell N. Olmsted

The built environment supports the safe care of patients in health care facilities. Infection preventionists and health care epidemiologists have expertise in prevention and control of health care–associated infections (HAIs) and assist with designing and constructing facilities to prevent HAIs. However, design elements are often missing from initial concepts. In addition, there is a large body of evidence that implicates construction and renovation as being associated with clusters of HAIs, many of which are life threatening for select patient populations. This article summarizes known risks and prevention strategies within a framework for patient safety.

**Occupational Health Update: Focus on Preventing the Acquisition of Infections with Pre-exposure Prophylaxis and Postexposure Prophylaxis**    729

David J. Weber and William A. Rutala

Health care personnel are commonly exposed to infectious agents via sharp injuries (eg, human immunodeficiency virus, hepatitis B virus, and hepatitis C virus), direct patient care (eg, pertussis and meningococcus), and the contaminated environment (eg, *Clostridium difficile*). An effective occupational program is a key aspect of preventing acquisition of an infection by offering the following: (1) education of health care personnel regarding proper handling of sharps, early identification and isolation of potentially infectious patients, and hand hygiene; (2) assuring immunity to vaccine-preventable diseases; and, (3) immediate availability of a medical evaluation after a nonprotected exposure to an infectious disease.

**Informatics in Infection Control**    759

Michael Y. Lin and William E. Trick

Informatics tools are becoming integral to routine infection control activities. Informatics has the potential to improve infection control outcomes in surveillance, prevention, and connections with public health. Surveillance activities include fully or semiautomated surveillance of infections, surveillance of device use, and hospital/ward outbreak investigation. Prevention activities include awareness of multidrug-resistant organism carriage on admission, enhanced interfacility communication, identifying inappropriate infection precautions, reducing device use, and antimicrobial stewardship. Public health activities include electronic communicable disease reporting, syndromic surveillance, and regional outbreak detection. The challenge for infection control personnel is in translating the knowledge gained from electronic surveillance systems into action.

**Antimicrobial Stewardship for the Infection Control Practitioner**    771

Jerod L. Nagel, Keith S. Kaye, Kerry L. LaPlante, and Jason M. Pogue

Antibiotic misuse is a serious patient safety concern and a national public health priority. Years of indiscriminant antibiotic use has promoted selection for antibiotic resistant bacteria and *Clostridium difficile*. This crisis has led to clinicians being faced with managing untreatable infections, often in the most vulnerable patient populations. This review summarizes the goals of antimicrobial stewardship programs, the essential members needed to initiate a program, various antimicrobial stewardship strategies, the role of the infection control practitioner in stewardship, barriers to its implementation and maintenance, approaches to measure the impact of a program, and the steps needed to initiate a program.

**Infection Control in Alternative Health Care Settings: An Update**    785

Elaine Flanagan, Marco Cassone, Ana Montoya, and Lona Mody

With changing health care delivery, patients receive care at various settings including acute care hospitals, nursing homes, outpatient primary care and specialty clinics, and at home, exposing them to pathogens in various settings. Various health care settings face unique challenges, requiring individualized infection control programs. Infection control programs in nursing homes should address surveillance for infections and antimicrobial resistance, outbreak investigation and control plan for epidemics, isolation precautions, hand hygiene, staff education, and employee and resident health programs.

**Preventing Hospital-acquired Infections in Low-income and Middle-income Countries: Impact, Gaps, and Opportunities**   805

Ana Cecilia Bardossy, John Zervos, and Marcus Zervos

In low-income and middle-income countries (LMIC) health care–associated infections (HAIs) are a serious concern. Many factors contribute to the impact in LMIC, including lack of infrastructure, inconsistent surveillance, deficiency in trained personnel and infection control programs, and poverty- related factors. In LMIC the risk of HAIs may be up to 25% of hospitalized patients. Building infection control capacity in LMIC is possible where strategies are tailored to the specific needs of LMIC. Strategies must start with simple, cost-effective measures then expand to include more complicated measures. Goals for short-term, medium-term, and long-term actions should be planned and resources prioritized.

**Index**   819

# INFECTIOUS DISEASE CLINICS OF NORTH AMERICA

**FORTHCOMING ISSUES**

*December 2016*
**Infection Prevention and Control in Healthcare, Part II: Clinical Management of Infections**
Keith S. Kaye and Sorabh Dhar, *Editors*

*March 2017*
**Legionnaire's Disease**
Cheston B. Cunha and Burke A. Cunha, *Editors*

*June 2017*
**Bone and Joint Infections**
Steven K. Schmitt, *Editor*

**RECENT ISSUES**

*June 2016*
**Antibacterial Resistance: Challenges and Opportunities**
Richard R. Watkins and Robert A. Bonomo, *Editors*

*March 2016*
**Fungal Infections**
Luis Ostrosky-Zeichner and Jack D. Sobel, *Editors*

*December 2015*
**Pediatric Infectious Disease: Part II**
Mary Anne Jackson and Angela L. Myers, *Editors*

# Preface

# Infection Prevention and Control in Healthcare, Part I: Facility Planning and Management

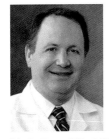 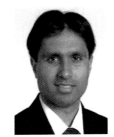

Keith S. Kaye, MD, MPH    Sorabh Dhar, MD
*Editors*

Infection Prevention and Control has grown and changed significantly since it first became nationally recognized in the early 1970s. Initially, Infection Control was focused on occupational health and infection surveillance in the hospital. More recently, there has been a growing emphasis on prevention and process in the hospital and also in a multitude of other types of health care settings. Over the past several years, there has been increasing recognition of the quality and cost implications associated with health care–associated infections and the value of infection control. Now more than ever, infection prevention has been thrust into the spotlight with regards to patient safety, financial accountability, and regulatory readiness. While individual textbooks, articles, and other resources are available to address specific questions and issues pertaining to infection prevention and control, this issue (as well as the subsequent one) of *Infectious Diseases Clinics of North America* serves as an inclusive, relatively concise and focused primer on Infection Control.

This issue focuses on facility planning and infrastructure necessary to support a comprehensive, effective infection prevention program. A multitude of topics are covered, including hand hygiene, environmental hygiene, sterilization and disinfection, water safety, occupational health, informatics, construction, outbreak investigation, antimicrobial stewardship, and infection prevention in alternative and resource limited settings.

This issue is intended to serve as a useful reference and primer for infection prevention and control, particularly with regards to facility planning and infrastructure. We want to thank the authors who have contributed valuable time and effort to this issue.

Infect Dis Clin N Am 30 (2016) xiii–xiv
http://dx.doi.org/10.1016/j.idc.2016.06.001
0891-5520/16/$ – see front matter © 2016 Published by Elsevier Inc.

**id.theclinics.com**

We hope that you will enjoy it and find it to be a wonderful resource for helping to build and sustain an effective infection prevention and control program.

Keith S. Kaye, MD, MPH
University Health Center
4201 Saint Antoine
Suite 2B, Box 331
Detroit, MI 48201, USA

Sorabh Dhar, MD
Harper University Hospital
5 Hudson
3990 John R Street
Detroit, MI 48201, USA

E-mail addresses:
KKaye@dmc.org (K.S. Kaye)
sdhar@med.wayne.edu (S. Dhar)

# Building a Successful Infection Prevention Program

## Key Components, Processes, and Economics

Sorabh Dhar, MD[a,b,c,d,*], Evelyn Cook, RN, CIC[e],
Mary Oden, RN, MHS-CL[f], Keith S. Kaye, MD, MPH[a,b,g]

KEYWORDS

- Infection prevention • Infection control • Hospital epidemiology
- Hospital-acquired infections

KEY POINTS

- Infection prevention and hospital epidemiology programs are responsible for monitoring and preventing health care–associated infections in hospitals.
- Infection prevention programs have been shaped by a complex landscape of health care safety, regulatory, reporting, and payment requirements.
- The infection prevention committee is a multidisciplinary team that includes clinical and nonclinical members who meet to review findings, make recommendations, and meet requirements.
- Knowledge of surveillance for infections and the ability to make a business case/economic model are essential components of a successful program.

## THE EMERGENCE AND DEVELOPMENT OF REGULATION AND REQUIREMENTS OF INFECTION PREVENTION AND CONTROL

Multistate prevalence surveys of health care-associated infections (HAIs) conducted by the Centers for Disease Control and Prevention (CDC) have provided estimates that 721,800 HAIs occurred in US acute care hospitals in 2011 and accounted for

The authors have nothing to disclose.
[a] Department of Hospital Epidemiology and Infection Prevention, Detroit Medical Center, Detroit, MI, USA; [b] Department of Medicine, Wayne State University, Detroit, MI, USA; [c] Department of Hospital Epidemiology and Infection Prevention, John D Dingell VA Medical Center, Detroit, MI, USA; [d] Harper University Hospital, 5 Hudson, 3990 John R, Detroit, MI 48201, USA; [e] Duke Infection Control Outreach Network, Duke University Medical Center, 1610 Sycamore Street, Durham, NC 27707, USA; [f] Infection Prevention, Clinical Operations, Tenet Health, 1443 Ross Avenue Suite 1400, Dallas, TX 75202, USA; [g] University Health Center, 4201 Saint Antoine, Suite 2B, Box 331, Detroit, MI 48201, USA
* Corresponding author. Harper University Hospital, 5 Hudson, 3990 John R, Detroit, MI 48201.
E-mail address: sdhar@med.wayne.edu

Infect Dis Clin N Am 30 (2016) 567–589
http://dx.doi.org/10.1016/j.idc.2016.04.009
0891-5520/16/$ – see front matter © 2016 Elsevier Inc. All rights reserved.

id.theclinics.com

75,000 associated deaths.[1] Approximately 1 in 25 patients hospitalized in the United States will develop an HAI every day. The most common types of HAIs were device-associated infections (25.6%), pneumonias (21.8%), surgical site infections (SSIs; 21.8%), and gastrointestinal infections (17.1%).[2] Total annual costs resulting from HAIs have been estimated at $9.8 billion in 2009.[3] It has also been estimated that 55% to 75% of these HAIs are preventable, translating into potential savings of up to $5.5 billion and, more important, improved patient outcomes. As a result, HAI prevention is a national priority resulting in a significant evolution of infection prevention and control.[4]

Infection prevention programs (IPP), now a standard in health care, saw their inception in the1970s and 1980s after studies (such as the CDC's Study on the Efficacy of Nosocomial Infection Control [SENIC]) showed a 32% reduction in HAIs in hospitals with established programs compared with the 18% increases in infection in hospitals without.[5] This coincided with the development of the National Nosocomial Infection Surveillance System for voluntary reporting of surveillance data in 1970 and the incorporation of requirements for surveillance into the Joint Commission Accreditation for Healthcare Organizations (now called The Joint Commission [TJC]) standards for hospital accreditation in 1976. Since this time, there have been several groups that have had direct influence on the development of IPP ranging from professional societies (such as the Society for Healthcare Epidemiology of America [SHEA] and the Association of Processionals in Infection Control and Epidemiology [APIC]), government agencies (such as the CDC, Occupational Safety and Health Administration, and Department of Health and Human Services), nonprofit organizations, accreditation bodies, and payers (such as the Centers for Medicare and Medicaid Services [CMS]).[6] This complex landscape for infection prevention has led to the development of quality initiatives, legislative reforms, shifts in payment for HAIs, and an increased demand for transparency through public reporting of HAI data.[7]

IPPs have focused on 2 major goals: (1) the protection of the health care worker and (2) patient safety initiatives. Regulatory oversight of hospital infections dramatically increased in the late 1980s and early 1990s as the result of health care worker safety concerns, pertaining to the risk of occupational exposure to human immunodeficiency virus and hepatitis B virus. In 1991, the Occupational Safety and Health Administration released Standard 29 CFR Bloodborne Pathogens-1910.1030, which concluded that blood-borne pathogen exposure could be minimized or eliminated by a combination of administrative, engineering, and work practice controls (such as personal protective equipment, training, and vaccines).[8] This was followed by additional legislative mandates aimed at increasing respiratory protection (use of respirators requiring fit testing) for workers at significant risk of incurring *Mycobacterium tuberculosis* infection (which today is regulated by Occupational Safety and Health Administration standards). Components of this program include the appropriate use of and the medical clearance to wear a respirator.[9,10] Over the past several decades, infection prevention and control professionals have been charged with ensuring compliance of these and similar health care worker safety initiatives (as seen in the recent preparedness efforts for highly communicable diseases, such as Ebola).

The prevention of HAIs gained much public attention with the publication of several studies that categorized these infections as avoidable and preventable, and have helped to shape current prevention initiatives. The Institute of Medicine's 1999 report "To Err is Human: Building a Safer Healthcare System" and the subsequent 2003 report "Transforming Healthcare Quality" focused on HAI prevention as one of its priority areas for national action.[11] Subsequently, several organizations have advocated for or required HAI prevention and reduction initiatives. For example, in 2005 the Institute for Healthcare Improvement targeted 3 major categories of infections (SSIs, central line–associated bloodstream infections [CLABSI], and ventilator-associated pneumonia) in their initial "Saving 100,000 Lives Campaign."[12] In December 2006, the Institute for Healthcare Improvement launched a second campaign, "The 5 Million Lives Campaign," which focused on hand hygiene and a reduction in infections from methicillin-resistant *Staphylococcus aureus* (MRSA).[13] In 2008, the US Department of Health and Human Services released its national action plan to prevent HAIs, which provided a road map for the reduction of CLABSI, catheter-associated infections (CAUTIs), SSIs, and *Clostridium difficile* infection in various health care settings.[4] This national action plan was updated in April 2013 and provides a detailed account of the progress that has been made in HAI reduction as well as further opportunities.[1] Such initiatives have successfully solicited hospital administration to participate in their campaigns and to commit resources to reduce HAIs.

Health care reform in the first decade of this century (such as the Deficit Reduction Act of 2005 and the Affordable Care Act of 2010) and the categorizing of HAIs as preventable, have led to a paradigm shift in the reporting of and reimbursement related to these infections. Beginning October 1, 2007, the Department of Health and Human Services CMS, in consultation with the CDC, began to select hospital-acquired conditions (HACs) to target for reduction. These conditions had to meet the following criteria: (a) be high cost, high volume or both, (b) require a higher paying diagnosis related group when present as a secondary diagnosis, and (c) could reasonably have been prevented if optimal health care practices had been followed. If not present on admission, such HACs would not be reimbursed to hospitals. Initially, CAUTIs, CLABSIs, and SSIs after coronary artery bypass graft surgery were chosen, followed in 2009 by additional SSIs occurring after orthopedic procedures (spinal fusion and surgeries of the shoulder and elbow), bariatric surgery for obesity, and, in 2013, by infections complicating cardiac implantable electronic device placement.

In 2011, with an increasing need for transparency for both consumers and stakeholders, CMS required reporting of hospital specific HAI data using the preexisting CDC National Healthcare Safety Network (NHSN) for hospitals to qualify for full reimbursement and such reporting continues today. Data being reported includes CLABSI and CAUTI in adult and pediatric critical care units, medical units, surgical units, and medical/surgical units; SSI (after colon and abdominal hysterectomy surgery), LabID events (MRSA bacteremia and *C difficile* infection), health care worker influenza immunization, and ventilator-associated events in long-term acute care. These reporting requirements encompass inpatient and outpatient facilities, acute care, and long-term acute care, as well as specialized centers (such as outpatient hemodialysis, cancer facilities, inpatient psychiatry, and inpatient rehabilitation) to various degrees with respect to specific reporting requirements.[14] These data are used as metrics by the CMS to determine hospital payments under value-based purchasing and HAC programs. Data used by CMS to determine hospital payments are publicly available to consumers.[15] In addition to federal requirements for mandatory reporting, individual states have initiated state specific requirements, which in most cases exceed those of the federal government.

Similarly, accreditation organizations such as TJC have been influential in guiding the course of infection prevention. Initially formed in 1976 to promote health care reform based on patient outcomes, TJC has issued various sentinel event alerts, standards, and patient safety goals that hospitals must meet to become accredited and eligible for Medicare reimbursement.[16] For instance, in 2003 TJC issued an infection control–related sentinel event alert recommending that hospitals comply with the CDC's new hand hygiene guidelines and also mandated that hospitals evaluate all cases of death and major permanent loss of function attributed to HAIs as sentinel events.[17] Subsequently, in 2004 these recommendations became a part of the National Patient Safety Goals,[18] which were further broadened by 2012 to include a focus on reducing the risks associated with multidrug-resistant organisms (MDROs), CLABSIs, SSIs, and CAUTIs.[19] These regulations and standards have helped to guide the development, scope, policies, and willingness of hospital leadership to fund and support IPPs.

As a result of these changes in reporting and reimbursement, there has been significant pressure to achieve "zero rates" of HAIs. Despite not reaching the 2013 goals for HAI reductions, the CDC's HAI Progress Report describes significant reductions in the rates of CLABSI (46%), SSI (19%), MRSA bacteremia (8%), and hospital-onset *C difficile* infection (10%), but reported an increase in CAUTIs (6%).[20] Although not all HAIs are preventable, APIC and other experts agree that a primary goal of infection prevention should be the elimination of all preventable infections. The focus should be on "getting to zero" HAIs by optimizing processes pertaining to the prevention of HAIs.

In summary, this is an exciting but challenging time for infection prevention and control. The past decade has witnessed changes in the way that hospital-associated infections are viewed—from passive acceptance to the stout view of preventability, leading to policy changes, transparency, and increased collaboration among various agencies at federal and state levels.[21] IPPs remain in the crossfire of regulatory bodies and payers such as TJC and CMS, manifested by increasing regulatory requirements and hospital efforts to meet the elusive goals of "zero infections." As such, these programs have a unique opportunity to impact and reshape the way that health care is delivered, and to create a safer environment for patients and health care workers.

## INFECTION PREVENTION AND CONTROL PROGRAM
### Mission, Vision, and Values

Infection prevention and control programs will vary according to the size and scope of the organization for which they work. However, there are 3 essential and fundamental concepts to all programs: mission statement, vision, and core values.

The mission statement is a reflection of the primary goals of the organization or needs that should be addressed by infection prevention. TJC standards require health care organizations to identify risks for acquiring and transmitting infections.[22] This standard explicitly describes the mission of IPPs and their link to the organization's primary mission, for example, provision of safe, quality patient care. A typical mission statement for any IPP may be: *"Our facility maintains an organized, effective hospital-wide program designed to systematically identify and reduce the risk of acquiring and transmitting infections among patients, visitors, and healthcare workers. This program involves the collaboration of many programs and services within the hospital and is designed to meet the intent of the Joint Commission standards."*

Although the mission statement describes the "why," the vision statement describes future goals for the organizations. Organizational leaders have historically used strategic planning sessions to gather input from primary stakeholders to help determine an organization's vision and goals. Infection prevention departments can use a similar approach and invite key stakeholders, such as critical care and surgical staff, to participate. The visions or goals should be included in the infection prevention plan. As an example, a program's vision or goal may be that no patient in the critical care unit will acquire ventilator-associated pneumonia.

The next component integral to a successful IPP is core values. A core value statement describes "how" the program functions on a daily basis and may serve as the blueprint for the program. Core values, or objectives, identify how the department will reach established goals and achieve the vision of the program. For example, a core value might be: The Institute for Healthcare Improvement ventilator-associated pneumonia bundle will be implemented and compliance with all bundle elements will be monitored and reported to the appropriate stakeholders.

### Infection Prevention and Control Committee

The SENIC project found that 4 components of "highly effective" infection prevention surveillance programs were: (1) surveillance with feedback to health care workers, (2) an intense infection control program including best practices with sterilization, disinfection, asepsis and handling of medical devices, (3) an infection prevention nurse to supervise the program, and (4) a physician epidemiologist or microbiologist with special skill in infection prevention.

The preventionists, physician epidemiologist, a data analyst, and administrative assistant form the central infection prevention team and are the core components of the larger, multidisciplinary infection prevention and control committee (IPCC). These core members are responsible for conducting surveillance, helping the organization maintain regulatory compliance and carrying out key programs geared toward HAI prevention. Typically, this core group meets routinely for work meetings (eg, weekly), reviews data, identifies issues, and develops and oversees quality improvement programs. This core group develops agendas for larger IPCC meetings and brings proposals forth to the IPCC for approval and feedback.

The organization's governing body typically delegates authority and responsibility for the IPP to the IPCC. The IPCC is the central decision and policymaking body whose primary purpose is to advocate for infection prevention and control[23] and should have the authority to take immediate action in the event that patient, visitor, or health care worker safety is endangered with regard to infection prevention, which is often found in a formal infection control hospital authority statement. In the majority of health care organizations, the IPCC is designated as a "medical staff" committee and has reporting obligations to both the hospital and medical staff leadership. The chairperson should be a physician who has knowledge and/or a special interest in infection prevention.

The IPCC is multidisciplinary, with representation from a variety of specialties and services. At a minimum, members should include infection prevention, administration, nursing, medical staff, microbiology, employee/occupational health, surgical services, environmental services, and pharmacy. Other disciplines within the organization should be considered ad hoc members and be invited to attend the committee meeting based on agenda items and need. The IPCC should meet on a regular basis (such as monthly or quarterly) as determined by the complexity and needs of the facility with a predetermined time and location.

Before the IPCC meeting, the core or central infection prevention team should meet to review surveillance findings, address any unusual events, and achieve consensus among team members on proposed actions or recommendations. A meeting agenda should be circulated to IPCC members before the meeting with action and/or approval items so designated. It is imperative that complete and accurate minutes of the committee's discussion, actions, and recommendations be recorded for each meeting and reported to all appropriate stakeholders, based on the organizational infrastructure. These minutes are often extremely useful for documentation of responsibility and "ownership" of particular projects and problems. All IPCC minutes should be marked as "peer review and/or confidential." See **Box 1** for a summary of the responsibilities of the IPCC members.

## KEY MEMBERS OF THE INFECTION PREVENTION TEAM AND/OR PROGRAM
### Hospital Physician Epidemiologist or Medical Director of Infection Prevention

Hospital epidemiologists are typically physicians, often specializing in infectious diseases with expertise in the field of infection prevention and act as watchman for the modern health care system.[24,25] They provide oversight for infection control in larger health care facilities. Some hospitals, such as smaller community hospitals, might not have a fully trained physician epidemiologist or infectious diseases physicians on staff, so other members of the medical staff (eg, the hospital pathologist) might serve as the medical director of infection prevention and chairperson of the IPCC. Medical staff leadership is essential to achieve infection prevention goals and objectives. **Box 2** summarizes the major responsibilities of the hospital epidemiologist.

The physicians assuming the role of hospital epidemiologist have preferably received training from senior epidemiologists in longstanding programs; however, frequently a physician might find themselves in this position without training, out of necessity. Contrary to infection preventionists, there is no formal certification process for the hospital epidemiologist. Recently, SHEA published guidance to highlight the roles and necessary skills for a physician to run an effective IPCC. The roles of the hospital epidemiologist are many and might include that of an epidemiologist, subject matter expert, quality and performance improvement leader, regulatory/public health liaison, health care administrator, clinician educator, outcomes assessment evaluator, and researcher. These diverse areas highlight the multifaceted components and the increasing needs, demands, and complexities of IPPs, and represent the core competencies that are vital in this demanding field.[25]

### Data Programmer and Analyst

Data programmers and analysts are essential for the development and maintenance of databases used in infection prevention. These individuals collaborate with the infection prevention department regarding database structure and organization of data

---

**Box 1**
**Primary responsibilities for Infection Prevention/Control Committee**

1. Identify strategies designed to reduce or eliminate risk of acquiring a hospital-acquired and/or health care-associated infection.
2. Review findings related to hospital-acquired and health care-associated infections.
3. Review findings related to outbreak investigations.
4. Review relevant infection prevention and control guidelines.
5. Review findings related to monitoring of antibiotic resistant organisms (infection and/or colonization).
6. Make recommendations and take action based on findings from activities described.
7. Address issues related to emerging and reemerging communicable diseases.
8. Make recommendations for new procedures, policies, and/or activities as appropriate.
9. Participate in the review and revision of the infection prevention/control risk assessment and program as warranted to improve outcomes.
10. Approve all hospital wide infection prevention/control policies.

---

**Box 2**
**Primary responsibilities of the hospital physician epidemiologist or medical director of infection prevention**

- Provide medical and technical advice and support within the department, as well as within the health care facility.
- In collaboration with the infection preventionist(s), establish long- and short-term goals for the department.
- Provide expertise in regard to health care-associated infections, emerging communicable diseases, postexposure management, isolation precaution(s), as well as construction and environmental issues/concerns.
- Oversee development of programs designed to prevent and/or reduce the transmission of epidemiologically important microorganisms within the facility (ie, antibiotic resistant organisms) and/or other projects with which the department may be involved.
- Participate in and oversee analysis of surveillance findings and development of interventional strategies.
- Assist with preparation of data and policy revisions for presentation to the IPCC.
- Serve as the liaison between the infection prevention department, other members of the medical staff and often with external agencies (state health departments, free press).
- Represent infection prevention in quality meetings and efforts.
- Communicate infection control/prevention data to the IPCC, members of the medical staff, quality of care team(s), and other internal committees/teams as appropriate.

*Abbreviation:* IPCC, Infection Prevention and Control Committee.

---

related to the infection prevention activities and assist in preparing visual presentation of that data (ie, graphs, tables, etc). These persons should be able to manipulate existing databases or the electronic medical records to retrieve baseline data that often are necessary to define a problem, set baseline benchmarks, and also assist in ensuring that the desired outcomes data are collected. They are also critical in ensuring that local hospital electronic data are distributed to the appropriate committees or hospital leaders, as well as ensuring a rapid and consistent submission of data to national databases (such as the NHSN).

## Administrative Assistant

Effective administrative assistants possess the essential qualities needed to enhance the effectiveness and productivity of IPPs. They should be highly skilled in organizing and scheduling appointments and/or meetings for the hospital epidemiologist and/or the infection preventionists. These individuals often serve as the "gatekeeper" and organizer for the infection prevention department and assist in eliminating unnecessary interruptions and unscheduled appointments.

## Infection Preventionist

Authority for daily oversight and management of the IPP is typically delegated to the infection preventionist. Based on the size and complexity of the facility, this individual may perform other key functions in addition to infection prevention. Some of the functions more commonly assigned to the infection preventionist include employee health and nursing education. Infection preventionists predominately have backgrounds in nursing, medical technology, microbiology, and/or public health.[23] Additional certification in infection prevention may either be required or preferred, depending on the institution. Clinical experience, managerial experience, and good communication skills are also prerequisites for an infection preventionist position. Daily responsibilities are multifaceted and require strong organizational skills. **Box 3** lists some of the major responsibilities of infection preventionists in the hospital. Infection preventionists must also have the ability to lead and manage a multitude of diverse health care workers. Recognizing the difference in leadership and management and how they apply to specific situations is essential to implementing change.

Leadership is the art of influencing behavior and most facilities have "informal" leaders within each department. These local leaders often have the ability to influence the behavior of others they work with. Infection preventionists should recruit these individuals to be infection prevention champions.

Management is achieving desired results through efficient utilization of human and material resources.[26] **Box 4** depicts various management styles and characteristics. An infection preventionist should exhibit good management skills when working with individuals within their own department or who work on units for which the infection preventionist is responsible.

## Meeting Management

Meetings consume an enormous amount of human resources, and when executed suboptimally, often do not achieve desired goals. The infection prevention/control committee is only one of many multidisciplinary groups whose activities involve infection prevention. Infection preventionists can facilitate efficient, effective meetings by using key strategies. **Box 5** list various strategies for conducting effective and efficient meetings.

## Infection Prevention Staffing

Staffing for infection prevention is an ongoing challenge for most programs. There continues to be a lack of strong recommendations from recognized experts in the field, such as the CDC.

---

**Box 3**
**Primary responsibilities of the infection preventionists**

- Application of epidemiologic principles in the performance of surveillance activities, including data collection and analysis as directed by the infection prevention/control plan and risk assessment.

- Assist with product evaluation.

- Develop and present educational programs designed for employee and patient education.

- Consult with internal and external customers on issues related to infection prevention.

- Review hospital and department specific infection prevention policies and procedures.

- Conduct outbreak investigations.

- Conduct infection control risk assessment for all construction activities.

- Report infection prevention surveillance findings to the IPCC, hospital leadership, specific hospital departments and committees, public health department (local and state and referring/receiving health care facilities as appropriate).

- Assist other departments by serving as a resource for continuous compliance with federal/state (eg, OSHA, Design for Safety [DFS]) and accreditation (eg, The Joint Commission) standards as they pertain to infection prevention and control activities.

*Abbreviations:* IPCC, Infection Prevention and Control Committee; OSHA, Occupational Safety and Health Administration.

| Box 4 |
| --- |
| **Management styles and their characteristics** |

*Autocratic*

The infection preventionist solves problems independently and without input or advice from others. This style may be necessary when patient and or employee safety is at risk and decisions must be made quickly.

*Consultative*

The infection preventionist shares problems with peers and solicit their ideas before making a decision. Infection preventionists use this approach most often.

*Democratic*

Finally, the democratic style is when the infection preventionist shares problems with the group and together they make decisions as a team. Multidisciplinary teams often use this style.

In the early 1970s, the CDC's SENIC recommended that hospitals have at least 1 full-time equivalent infection control professional for every 250 occupied beds.[27] Later in the 1990s, participation in the National Nosocomial Infection Surveillance System required 1 infection control professional full-time equivalent for the first 100 beds and then 1 full-time equivalent for each additional 250 beds.[28] In 2002, APIC initiated the DELPHI project on staffing. This project noted that staffing recommendations should consider not only the number of occupied beds, but also the scope of the program, complexity of the health care organization, patient characteristics, and the unique needs of the facility, and recommended a ratio of 0.8 to 1.0 infection preventionists per 100 occupied beds.[23] One US state has incorporated staffing requirements into their acute care licensure rules. This state requirement uses a formula that incorporates inpatient and outpatient volume, reimbursement information, and case mix index.

Despite various recommendations and need for increased infection preventionist staffing, many organizations have understaffed programs. As the roles of IPPs have increased in scope and complexity, the traditional ratios may not be sufficient to provide the necessary staffing needs of an institution. Alternative staffing ratios have been proposed. For example, 1 proposal counts 1 bed in the intensive care unit as the equivalent of 2 acute care beds, and a long-term care bed as one-half of an acute care bed; and counts a hemodialysis facility as the equivalent of 50 acute care beds and an ambulatory clinic the equivalent of 10 acute care beds.[29] These adjusted calculations may capture workload more accurately and should be factored into business models when developing or expanding programs. Although not substitutes for trained preventionists, adjuncts to the infection preventionist such as electronic surveillance systems, unit-based nurse liaisons, and nurse advisors can help to facilitate the work of preventionists and should also be factored into staffing calculations and needs. Despite the obvious benefits of automated surveillance systems, in 1 study, only one-third of programs reported having electronic systems in place.[30] Unfortunately, the increases in demands on infection prevention and control has not led to a proportional increase in infection control staffing, with reports indicating that only 18% of programs have received increased support after the implementation of the CMS Inpatient Prospective Payment System.[7]

### Budget

Budget preparation is an essential component of any efficient program. Infection preventionists may have total responsibility for budget preparation or in some institutions may be responsible for providing input. Chief executive officers will often use budget

---

**Box 5**
**Strategies for conducting effective, efficient meetings**

1. Be prepared.
   All items included on the agenda should be reviewed in advance. Surveillance data should be evaluated for accuracy and completeness and presented in a visual, easy to understand format. Items requiring approval should be distributed in advance.

2. Have an agenda.
   The agenda should be distributed before the meeting. Most institutions distribute the agenda no less than 1 week before the meeting to give members an opportunity to review and be prepared to discuss issues.

3. Start and end on time.
   This simple concept demonstrates respect for members' time and work schedule. When meetings do not begin and end on time, members become disengaged and often times will stop attending.

4. Meet only when necessary.
   Base your frequency of meetings on your facility's activities and needs. Meeting schedules vary from monthly to quarterly. Selecting the appropriate frequency will also help with number 2 (starting and ending on time). Some individual states have included a specific requirement for the frequency of IPCC meetings. Be sure that you are aware of what your state requirements are and that your schedule is in compliance.

5. Include all issues and solicit input relevant to all committee members.
   Members want to be part of the team; when they do not feel included, they will be less likely to offer new ideas and input.

6. Stay on target.
   Stick to the agenda items as outlined. Some facilities actually time the agenda with an estimated allotment for each discussion or activity. Issues that cannot be resolved or generate more discussion than anticipated can be tabled or deferred until the next meeting.

7. Capture action items.
   The Joint Commission will expect to see closure to action items. The minutes should reflect approval, rejection or deferral of action items and the supporting rationale.

8. Get feedback.
   An effective way of improving the flow and productivity of meeting is to request feedback from the members. It is generally more successful if this is included as an agenda item and feedback is solicited immediately after the meeting. Feedback can also be obtained through written or verbal communication after the meeting as well.

9. A secret "ninth" key.
   Having the meeting at meal time will typically improve attendance and providing food is an inexpensive way to demonstrate appreciation for the committee member's time.

*Abbreviation:* IPCC, Infection Prevention and Control Committee.

---

variances as the financial metric for the IPP. Basic components of any budget include labor, capital, and miscellaneous expenses. Elements of each are described in **Box 6**. The cost of HAIs has become an integral component of financial planning for organizations. Decreased reimbursement and nonpayment for certain conditions has forced hospital administration to confront the financial impact of HAIs, a topic that will be discussed in much greater detail later in this paper.

### Surveillance

Surveillance is defined as the "ongoing systematic collection, analysis and interpretation of health data essential to the planning, implementation and evaluation of public

---

**Box 6**
**Budget: major components**

Labor expenses
   Includes staffing expenses for infection preventionists, clerical support, data entry/analyst support, hospital epidemiologist or IPCC physician chair support. Consideration should also be given to the labor expenses required in the event that an outbreak investigation would be necessary.

Capital expenses
   Most organizations have a minimum cost that items must incur before qualifying as a capital expense. These are "big ticket" items and requests requiring capital expenses should be well thought out and have supportive rationale.

Expenses
   All other expenses fall into this category and typically include education, travel, journals, professional memberships, and so on.

*Abbreviation:* IPCC, Infection Prevention and Control Committee.

---

health practice, closely integrated with the timely dissemination of these data to those who need to know."[31] Studies in the United States reported that infection preventionists spent the greatest percentage of time (mean 44.5%) on surveillance activities.[28] **Table 1** lists the percentage of time spent on each work task as reported by preventionists. The type of surveillance activities conducted will be influenced by:

- Organizational demographics (critical access center vs community hospital vs academic medical center);
- Community demographics (urban or rural);
- Types of procedures and services provided;
- Infection prevention risk assessment; and
- Annual evaluation of the infection prevention plan and goals.

The CDC and TJC recommend surveillance be focused on high-risk, high-volume activities.[32] Surveillance for HAIs should be performed by screening a variety of data sources such as admissions/discharge records, pharmacy databases, patient charts, vital signs records, and laboratory, radiology, and pathology reports. Often, effective surveillance requires the application of clinical criteria to laboratory-based

---

**Table 1**
**Activities reported by infection preventionists regarding how they spent their time**

| Activity | Median | Mean | SD | Minimum | Maximum |
|---|---|---|---|---|---|
| Collecting analyzing and interpreting data on the occurrence of infections | 49.0 | 44.5 | 14.3 | 7 | 80 |
| Policy development and meetings | 14.0 | 15.0 | 8.8 | 0 | 55 |
| Daily isolation issues | 10.0 | 12.9 | 9.0 | 0 | 50 |
| Teaching infection prevention and control policies and procedures | 10.0 | 13.0 | 6.2 | 1 | 35 |
| Other (eg, product evaluation, employee health, and emergency preparedness) | 5.0 | 8.8 | 8.2 | 0 | 60 |
| Activities related to outbreaks | 5.0 | 6.1 | 4.8 | 0 | 40 |

Data are presented as percent of time.
*From* Stone PW, Dick A, Pogorzelska M, et al. Staffing and structure of infection prevention and control programs. Am J Infect Control 2009;37(5):354; with permission.

surveillance data. Automated surveillance technologies allow for a paperless method of analyzing, documenting, categorizing, and uploading HAI data into national databases (such as the NHSN).

Concurrent surveillance, conducted while the patient is still in the hospital, is preferred to retrospective surveillance. Retrospective surveillance should only be used when patients are discharged before all the pertinent data can be obtained during hospital admission.[33] NHSN definitions for HAIs are used for infection prevention surveillance and must be applied consistently to ensure valid comparisons between health care organizations. Infection preventionists should consult with the physician epidemiologist if clinical questions or judgment are needed to interpret patient data appropriately. Given the increased focus on HAIs and their financial implications, many infection preventionists are working routinely with physician epidemiologists to evaluate HAIs such as CLABSI, CAUTI, and SSI and to identify areas for improvement.

There are various types of surveillance philosophies and methodologies. Unfortunately, many of the surveillance strategies are labor and resource intensive, and are limited as a result of poor intrarater reliability.[1] Total or whole house surveillance is the collection of infection prevention data throughout an entire facility. All HAIs are identified, analyzed, and reported. If this methodology is chosen, care should be taken not to report only an overall "hospital rate of infection." Rates should be reported separately for specific HAIs and may be stratified by service and/or department. Typically, this type of whole house surveillance is conducted for invasive infections such as CLABSI, CAUTI, *C difficile* infection, and MDROs.

Focused or targeted surveillance is surveillance conducted only in a particular type of unit or part of an organization where high-risk and/or high-volume activities occur with regard to HAI. Rather than identifying every infection in the hospital, an infection preventionist program might focus efforts to detect device-related infections toward the critical care areas or burn units and/or hematology wards. Rates are then calculated and reported by unit and/or service. In the 1990s, the CDC shifted the National Nosocomial Infection Surveillance System away from whole house surveillance, toward "targeted" surveillance for certain types of HAI, such as CAUTI.[34] However, in light of recent policies and reimbursements, the pendulum has shifted and hospitals now often perform housewide surveillance for a variety of infections.

A combination surveillance strategy is used by many programs. This strategy uses a combination of targeted and modified total house surveillance. Many programs monitor targeted events in defined populations while also monitoring selected events house wide.[34]

Regardless of the type of surveillance methodology used, data must be collected, analyzed, and presented using a consistent and standardized approach. Data that are not reliable or valid are ineffectual and will not engender confidence in the IPP.

Surveillance priorities should include the following: device-associated infections (CLABSI, CAUTI, and ventilator-associated events), infections associated with procedures (SSIs), and infections related to epidemiologically important microorganisms (MDROs). Surveillance data pertaining to HAI are usually presented as rates; however, the NHSN has shifted to using standardized infection ratios for reporting HAIs. In HAI data analysis, the standardized infection ratio compares the actual number of HAIs with the predicted number based on the baseline US experience.[35]

When calculating meaningful infection rates, it is important to select the most appropriate and accurate denominator. Whenever possible, the denominator should reflect the "exposure risk," that is, the number of surgical procedures and the number of device-days or number of patient-days on a given unit or in the hospital.

Examples of numerators, denominators and rate calculation are shown below:

- Device-associated infections: rate of infections per 1000 device-days (number of device-associated infections/number of device-days) × 1000.
- SSIs: rate of SSI per 100 procedures (number of SSIs/number of surgical procedures) × 100.
- Multidrug-resistant organism infections: rate of infection per 1000 patient-days (number of infections/patient days/number of patient-days) × 1000.
- Standardized infection ratio = observed HAIs/expected HAIs.

Other surveillance methodologies include the use of "active surveillance" for certain populations and/or pathogens. Active surveillance is a process to identify proactively the reservoir of an organism in asymptomatically colonized patients. Diagnostic testing is generally performed by culturing the body site, which most commonly serves as reservoirs for a specific organism, that is, culturing the nares for MRSA and the perirectal area for vancomycin-resistant *enterococci* or carbapenem-resistant Enterobacteriaceae. Cultures are generally performed on high-risk patients at the time of admission to the facility or before surgery. In some cases, active surveillance cultures might be repeated after hospital admission, on a routine basis (typically weekly) during the hospitalization, until a positive result is recovered or the patient is discharged. Active surveillance may provide the opportunity for proactive interventions, such as placing a patient on contact isolation based on surveillance culture results. Active surveillance data should be trended and reported to the IPCC and to the various hospital departments or units.

In May of 2009, APIC issued a position paper in support of using automated surveillance technologies as an essential part of the infection prevention and control activities.[36] Automated surveillance can be defined as the process of obtaining useful information for infection prevention surveillance from hospital databases through the systematic application of medical informatics and computer science technologies.[36] These automated technologies can either be developed by the hospital data programmers or purchased through third party vendors, including the makers of electronic medical records. Automated surveillance can increase the ability of infection preventionist programs to conduct broader surveillance programs, to rapidly identify HAIs and trends in infections and, most important, to free up time spent on surveillance. The use of automated surveillance can decrease infection preventionist effort spent on surveillance by up to 61%, which allows infection preventionists to reallocate their efforts and spend less time entering and mining data and more time rounding, educating, analyzing, and implementing programs.[30]

## Outbreak Investigation

Outbreaks of both infectious and noninfectious adverse events can occur in any health care setting and pose a threat to patient safety. An outbreak is defined as an increased occurrence of a disease and/or infection above the usual or expected frequency. In some cases, even a single case may constitute an outbreak (eg, smallpox). Outbreaks are usually identified when there is an increase in rates or numbers of infections from the "endemic" infection rate, which is defined as the usual or expected occurrence of a disease and/or infection. An endemic infection rate represents a baseline or background rate, which may fluctuate slightly from month to month.[37]

The ultimate goal of any outbreak investigation is to identify factors contributing to the outbreak and to stop or reduce the risk for further occurrences.[37] One of the key components for investigating an outbreak is developing a case definition, which details specific criteria for identifying a case. Initially, this may be a broad definition that is refined as the investigation proceeds and a specific agent or diagnosis is confirmed. **Box 7** lists the components of an outbreak investigation. This topic is covered in greater detail in the "Outbreak Investigations" (see Sood G, Perl TM: Outbreaks in Healthcare Settings, in this issue).

---

**Box 7**
**Primary components of an outbreak investigation**

- Establish or verify the diagnosis of reported cases
  - Identify agent if possible. Describe the initial magnitude of the problem and what brought the problem to the attention of the infection control/employee health department(s)
  - Confirm laboratory or other clinical findings.
  - Review microbiology/laboratory records to confirm increased frequency of certain pathogens.
  - Consult with staff to identify lapses in infection control techniques.
- Confirm that an outbreak exists.
  - Develop a case definition to estimate the magnitude of the problem.
  - Compare the current incidence with usual or baseline incidence (endemic rate).
  - Formulate a line listing tailored to the illness and population affected.
- Search for additional cases.
  - Notify laboratories, physicians, and/or other personnel to immediately report additional cases.
  - Search for other cases by retrospective review, laboratory reports, and so on.
  - Continue to add cases to the line list as they are identified.
- Characterize cases by person, place and time.
  - *Person*: Includes patient characteristics such as age, disease, exposures, treatments, and risk factors.
  - *Place*: Consider patient location, that is, hall, unit, or room. Check and confirm status of air exchange, pattern of flow, and other environmental issues as they relate to the outbreak.
  - *Time*: Identify the exact period of the outbreak by going back to the first case or indication of an outbreak. Identify the probable period of exposure based on the diagnosis. Plot data on an epidemic curve.
- Take immediate control measures, if indicated.
  - Institute control measures such as increased attention to hand hygiene and/or additional use of personal protective equipment.
  - Confiscate specific suspected products if identified (ie, patient care item).
- Formulate tentative hypothesis (best guess).
  - Review data to determine common host factors and exposures.
  - Determine nature of organism and base a hypothesis on source or reservoir, mode of transmission or exposure risk factors.
- Institute preliminary control measures.
  - Institute control measures based on what is known about the outbreak.
  - Consider whether outside assistance is needed.
- Monitor and evaluate effectiveness of the control measures.
  - Monitor compliance with control measures.
  - Evaluate effectiveness of the control measures in controlling the outbreak.
  - Consider additional measures if outbreak continues.
- Communicate and document findings.
  - Date of report.
  - Reported to.
  - Reported by.
  - Findings.
  - Future recommendations.

### Quality Improvement: Role of the Infection Preventionist

The process of measuring quality of care and reporting the findings is not a new concept. Florence Nightingale collected mortality data and related it to the lack of sanitary conditions.[38] In the early 20th century, Dr Ernest Codman proposed to his surgeon colleagues that they measure their SSI rates and disclose them to the public.[39] Performance improvement encompasses all of the systems, projects, and team activities an organization implements to achieve its goals. These goals include the prevention of HAIs for patients, visitors, and staff.[40]

Using a multidisciplinary team approach, systems should be designed to monitor processes as well as outcomes. Direct patient care staff should be included as partners and team members and be provided with training regarding quality concepts and team building skills. A mechanism to ensure feedback of data to appropriate disciplines in a timely manner should be incorporated. IPPs should design systems and processes to ensure timely feedback of infection prevention data to all disciplines as appropriate. Feedback should include outcome measures, infection rates, and process measures, such as compliance with hand hygiene or compliance with the central line insertion bundle. Surveillance activities and feedback of data provide value only when findings are used as a mechanism to improve the quality of care that is provided to patients.

### ECONOMICS AND BUSINESS PLAN

Society as a whole would clearly benefit from a reduced incidence of HAIs and transmission of MDROs within health care institutions. Unfortunately, there are currently no direct reimbursement programs related to hospital-based infection prevention and control. Hospitals are required by regulatory bodies to have an IPP, but the funding is often based on their administrators' subjective discretions. Therefore, for IPPs to achieve desirable goals, 1 critical role of hospital epidemiologists and infection preventionists is to convince administrators of the beneficial impact of investing in infection control activities, and demonstrate that these activities will ultimately lead to improved patient care and reduced hospital costs.[41] In 1 report, IPPs were demonstrated to be much more cost effective than many other commonly applied health care practices such as Pap smear screening to prevent cervical cancer, mammography screening to prevent breast cancer, and cholesterol screening programs in high-risk populations. In this report, infection control was estimated to be extremely cost effective, requiring only $2000 to $8000 per year of life saved.[42] Unfortunately, hospital administrators are faced routinely with demands to reduce costs and are subjected to continuous inspection and monitoring of their financial expenses and balances.[43] Because IPPs are typically categorized as cost centers and not as revenue generators, they are often identified as potential areas for budget cuts.[44] In fact, many infection control programs have faced downsizing in recent years.[41,45,46] This downsizing has occurred during a period where the roles and responsibilities of hospital epidemiologists have continuously and rapidly increased. Apart from traditional infection control activities, programs and infection preventionists often have responsibilities related to antimicrobial stewardship programs, patient safety, employee health, and emergency preparedness.[41]

The best way for infection control programs to obtain adequate funding from hospital leadership is to construct a business case and to assess and demonstrate the cost effectiveness of an IPP or intervention. The business case for infection control should incorporate all the various components of the institutional infection control program. Guidelines published by SHEA provide guidance regarding constructing a business case for infection control that can assist hospital epidemiologists in justifying and expanding their programs.[41] These guidelines also provide references and tools to assist IPPs in developing a business plan to support a specific intervention.[41] There are multiple other published economic analyses and data that can be used to support business cases for a wide range of infection control interventions and practices.[41,43,44,47–74] Using data such as published costs of HAIs and MDROs are often key ingredients to justifying interventions to decrease the incidence of hospital infections. Although published costs and cost-effectiveness analyses have limitations regarding applicability and generalizability, hospital epidemiologists and infection preventionists can still use these analyses to make persuasive cases for hospital support.

The value-based purchasing and HAC programs have tied HAIs directly to CMS reimbursement. Value-based purchasing and HACs should be also be used as components of business plans for programs. Preparation of a successful business plan takes planning and, when possible, input from financial professionals. It is important to make an honest assessment of the infection control situation at your institution. Most hospital epidemiologists and infection preventionists want to increase the resources available for infection control activities, but it is important to avoid overestimating potential benefits and the rapidity with which benefits might be achieved or underestimating staff costs and efforts required for success.[41] Overestimation of efficacy in an initial analysis may provide resources in the short term, but will undermine efforts and necessary trust for success in the long term.[41] The SHEA guidelines outline a 9-step approach for completing a business case analysis, so that all crucial components can be assessed and included.[41] Some key components include identifying the right audience and key stakeholders to support and approve a business proposal and to meet with key leaders and administrators early in the process, and to get feedback and input to help effectively frame the business case before a formal presentation. Whenever possible, the infection control team should seek input and support from business and financial leaders in the organization. These 10 steps include the following.

1. Frame the problem and develop a hypothesis about potential solutions.
2. Meet with key administrators before initiation of the proposal to obtain agreement that the issue is of institutional interest, gain leadership support, and identify critical individuals and departments who may be affected by the proposal and whose needs should be included in the business case analysis.[41]
3. Determine the annual cost using local institutional budgets or surveys available online.[75]
4. Determine what costs can be avoided through reduced infection rates using local data, CMS resources and medical literature available on various infection control cost-savings subjects.[76–104]
5. Determine the costs associated with the infections of interest at your hospital. Attributable costs are preferable to overall costs, and variable costs preferable to fixed costs. In infection prevention, the greatest opportunity to improve hospital profits comes from reducing excess durations of stay; therefore, some argue that this should be the main component for cost reduction calculations.[105]
6. Calculate the financial impact of the program or intervention by adding the estimated cost savings or additional profits and subtracting the costs of the upfront development and implementation.
7. Estimate the impact of reduction of certain HAIs on reimbursement from CMS.
8. Include additional financial or health benefits including reduction in morbidity and mortality, reduced legal costs, and enhanced reputation for the institution. To try

to capture as many indirect benefits as possible, mathematical models might be used.[106]

9. Make the case for your business case: communicate the findings effectively to critical stakeholders at the institution and present at an executive level meeting.
10. Prospectively collect cost and outcome data once the program is implemented.

In the era of limited resources, IPPs and initiatives are subject to continuous threats and budget reductions. Hospital epidemiologists should be familiar with the basics involved with preparing a business case and try to establish relationships with financial experts and administrators who can provide advice and assist in business case preparation. Although most infection control professionals do not have formal economic or business training, fiscal analysis and responsibility has become a critical part of hospital epidemiology. The role of effective business plans and cost justifications will continue to grow in importance for infection control programs. Despite limitations, the medical literature provides economic data that can assist the hospital epidemiologist and infection preventionists in constructing a business plan for establishing and maintaining an infection control program.

## SUMMARY

IPPs have seen much evolution in terms of scope of activities and complexity since their inception in the 1970s. They play the lead role in HAI surveillance, reporting, and prevention. Successful programs consist of a multidisciplinary team led by a hospital epidemiologist and managed by infection preventionists. Knowledge of the economics of HAIs and the ability to make a business plan is now essential to the success of programs. Although the landscape of payers and consumers continues to evolve, increasing regulatory and reimbursement demands pertaining to HAIs are aligning with many of the core values and priorities of infection prevention.

## REFERENCES

1. National Action Plan to Prevent Health-care Associated Infections: Road Map to Elimination April 2013. Available at: http://health.gov/hcq/prevent-hai-action-plan.asp. Accessed March 11, 2016.
2. Magill SS, Edwards JR, Bamberg W, et al. Multistate point-prevalence survey of health care-associated infections. N Engl J Med 2014;370(13):1198–208.
3. Zimlichman E, Henderson D, Tamir O, et al. Health care-associated infections: a meta-analysis of costs and financial impact on the US health care system. JAMA Intern Med 2013;173(22):2039–46.
4. Yokoe DS, Anderson DJ, Berenholtz SM, et al. A compendium of strategies to prevent healthcare-associated infections in acute care hospitals: 2014 updates. Infect Control Hosp Epidemiol 2014;35(8):967–77.
5. Haley RW, Culver DH, White JW, et al. The efficacy of infection surveillance and control programs in preventing nosocomial infections in US hospitals. Am J Epidemiol 1985;121(2):182–205.
6. Edmond M, Eickhoff TC. Who is steering the ship? External influences on infection control programs. Clin Infect Dis 2008;46(11):1746–50.
7. Septimus E, Yokoe DS, Weinstein RA, et al. Maintaining the momentum of change: the role of the 2014 updates to the compendium in preventing healthcare-associated infections. Infect Control Hosp Epidemiol 2014; 35(Suppl 2):S6–9.

8. Final Rule on Occupational Exposure to Bloodborne Pathogen. Federal Regist 1991;56:64004. Standard 1910.10301991.

9. Henshaw JL. Occupational exposure to tuberculosis. Fed Regist 2003;68: 75767–75. Standard 1910; 12/31/2003: OSHA.

10. Centers for Disease Control and Prevention, Hospital Infection Control Practices Advisory Committee. Guideline for isolation precautions: preventing transmission of infectious agents in healthcare settings. Atlanta (GA): Centers for Disease Control and Prevention; Hospital Infection Control Practices Advisory Committee; 2007.

11. Yokoe DS, Mermel LA, Anderson DJ, et al. A compendium of strategies to prevent healthcare-associated infections in acute care hospitals. Infect Control Hosp Epidemiol 2008;29(Suppl 1):S12–21.

12. Institute for Healthcare Improvement (IHI). Saving 100,000 lives campaign. 2008. Available at: www.ihi.org/IHI/Programs/Campaign/. Accessed March 11, 2016.

13. Institute for Healthcare Improvement (IHI). Protecting 5 million lives from harm. 2006. Available at: www.ihi.org/IHI/Programs/Campaign/. Accessed March 11, 2016.

14. Centers for Disease Control and Prevention, National Healthcare Safety Network. Healthcare Facility HAI Reporting Requirements to CMS via NHSN– Current or Proposed Requirements. Available at: www.cdc.gov/nhsn/pdfs/cms/cms-reporting-requirements.pdf. Accessed February 5, 2016.

15. Centers for Medicare and Medicaid Services (CMS). Medicare.gov: hospital compare. Available at: www.medicare.gov/hospitalcompare/search.html. Accessed February 1, 2016.

16. Sydnor ER, Perl TM. Hospital epidemiology and infection control in acute-care settings. Clin Microbiol Rev 2011;24(1):141–73.

17. The Joint Commission. Infection control related sentinel events. 2003. Available at: www.jointcommission.org/SentinelEvents/SentinelEventAlert/sea_28.htm. Accessed January 22, 2003.

18. The Joint Commission. National Patient Safety Goals 2004. 2004. Available at: www.jointcommission.org/PatientSafety/NationalPatientSafetyGoals/2004_npsgs.htm. Accessed March 11, 2016.

19. The Joint Commission. Hospital accreditation program: 2009 National Patient Safety Goals. Reduce the risk of healthcare associated infections. Oakbrook Terrace (IL): The Joint Commission; 2009. p. 11–7. Available at: http://www.jointcommission.org/PatientSafety/NationalPatientSafetyGoals/09_npsgs.htm. Accessed March 11, 2016.

20. Centers for Disease Control and Prevention. Healthcare associated infections progress report. Available at: www.cdc.gov/hai/pdfs/stateplans/factsheets/us.pdf. Accessed February 1, 2016.

21. Srinivasan A, Craig M, Cardo D. The power of policy change, federal collaboration, and state coordination in healthcare-associated infection prevention. Clin Infect Dis 2012;55(3):426–31.

22. The Joint Commission. 5 Sure-Fire Methods. Identifying Risks for Infections. 2010. The Source, February, Volume 8, Issue 2. Available at: https://www.jointcommission.org/assets/1/18/5_sure-fire_methods.pdf. Accessed June 16, 2016.

23. Friedman C. Infection prevention and control programs. In: Carrico R, editor. APIC text of infection control and epidemiology, vol. 1, 3rd edition. Washington, DC: APIC; 2009. p. 1–4.

24. Strausbaugh LJ. Anxiety on the watchtower: the hospital epidemiologist and emerging infectious diseases. Curr Infect Dis Rep 2003;5(6):451–3.
25. Kaye KS, Anderson DJ, Cook E, et al. Guidance for infection prevention and healthcare epidemiology programs: healthcare epidemiologist skills and competencies. Infect Control Hosp Epidemiol 2015;36(4):369–80.
26. Nutty C. Project management and communication. Certification study guide. 3rd edition. Washington, DC: APIC; 2007.
27. Haley RW, Quade D, Freeman HE, et al, The SENIC Project. Study on the Efficacy of Nosocomial Infection Control (SENIC Project). Summary of study design. Am J Epidemiol 1980;111(5):472–85.
28. Stone PW, Dick A, Pogorzelska M, et al. Staffing and structure of infection prevention and control programs. Am J Infect Control 2009;37(5):351–7.
29. Gase KA, Babcock HM. Is accounting for acute care beds enough? A proposal for measuring infection prevention personnel resources. Am J Infect Control 2015;43(2):165–6.
30. Grota PG, Stone PW, Jordan S, et al. Electronic surveillance systems in infection prevention: organizational support, program characteristics, and user satisfaction. Am J Infect Control 2010;38(7):509–14.
31. Gaynes R, Richards C, Edwards J, et al. Feeding back surveillance data to prevent hospital-acquired infections. Emerg Infect Dis 2001;7(2):295–8.
32. Hospital interpretive guidelines, vol. 42. Washington (DC): Department of Health & Human Services (DHHS); Centers for Medicare and Medicaid; 2008. CFR 482.42 (a)(2). Available at: http://www.cms.gov/manuals/downloads/som107ap_a_hospitals.pdf. Accessed June 16, 2016.
33. Patient safety component protocol. Atlanta (GA): National Healthcare Safety Network (NHSN) Manual; 2008. Available at: http://www.dhcs.ca.gov/provgovpart/initiatives/nqi/Documents/NHSNManPSPCurr.pdf. Accessed June 16, 2016.
34. Arias KM. Surveillance. In: Carrico R, editor. APIC text of infection control and epidemiology, vol. 1, 3rd edition. Washington, DC: APIC; 2009. p. 3–5.
35. Centers for Disease Control and Prevention. National Healthcare-Associated Infections Standardized Infection Ratio Report; January – December 2010. Available at: www.cdc.gov/HAI/pdfs/SIR/national-SIR-Report_03_29_2012.pdf. Accessed March 11, 2016.
36. Greene L, Cain TA, Khoury R. APIC position paper: the importance of surveillance technologies in the prevention of healthcare-associated infections. Am J Infect Control 2009;37(6):510–3.
37. Srinivasan A. Outbreak investigation. In: Carrico R, editor. APIC text of infection control and epidemiology, vol. 1, 3rd edition. Washington, DC: APIC; 2009. p. 1–4.
38. McDonald L. Florence Nightingale and the early origins of evidence-based nursing. Evid Based Nurs 2001;4(3):68–9.
39. Shahian DM, Edwards FH, Jacobs JP, et al. Public reporting of cardiac surgery performance: Part 1–history, rationale, consequences. Ann Thorac Surg 2011;92(3 Suppl):S2–11.
40. Murphy DM, Hanchett M, Olmsted RN, et al. Competency in infection prevention: a conceptual approach to guide current and future practice. Am J Infect Control 2012;40(4):296–303.
41. Perencevich EN, Stone PW, Wright SB, et al. Raising standards while watching the bottom line: making a business case for infection control. Infect Control Hosp Epidemiol 2007;28(10):1121–33.

42. Fraser VJ, Olsen MA. The business of health care epidemiology: creating a vision for service excellence. Am J Infect Control 2002;30(2):77–85.
43. Maragakis LL, Perencevich EN, Cosgrove SE. Clinical and economic burden of antimicrobial resistance. Expert Rev Anti Infect Ther 2008;6(5):751–63.
44. Murphy DM. From expert data collectors to interventionists: changing the focus for infection control professionals. Am J Infect Control 2002;30(2):120–32.
45. Burke JP. Infection control - a problem for patient safety. N Engl J Med 2003; 348(7):651–6.
46. Calfee DP, Farr BM. Infection control and cost control in the era of managed care. Infect Control Hosp Epidemiol 2002;23(7):407–10.
47. Freedberg KA, Paltiel AD. Cost effectiveness of prophylaxis for opportunistic infections in AIDS. An overview and methodological discussion. Pharmacoeconomics 1998;14(2):165–74.
48. Davey P, Craig AM, Hau C, et al. Cost-effectiveness of prophylactic nasal mupirocin in patients undergoing peritoneal dialysis based on a randomized, placebo-controlled trial. J Antimicrob Chemother 1999;43(1):105–12.
49. Richter A, Brandeau ML, Owens DK. An analysis of optimal resource allocation for prevention of infection with human immunodeficiency virus (HIV) in injection drug users and non-users. Med Decis Making 1999;19(2):167–79.
50. Reid RJ. A benefit-cost analysis of syringe exchange programs. J Health Soc Policy 2000;11(4):41–57.
51. Walker D, Fox-Rushby JA. Economic evaluation of communicable disease interventions in developing countries: a critical review of the published literature. Health Econ 2000;9(8):681–98.
52. Wilkinson D, Floyd K, Gilks CF. National and provincial estimated costs and cost effectiveness of a programme to reduce mother-to-child HIV transmission in South Africa. S Afr Med J 2000;90(8):794–8.
53. Lelekis M, Gould IM. Sequential antibiotic therapy for cost containment in the hospital setting: why not? J Hosp Infect 2001;48(4):249–57.
54. Akalin HE. Surgical prophylaxis: the evolution of guidelines in an era of cost containment. J Hosp Infect 2002;50(Suppl A):S3–7.
55. Floyd K, Blanc L, Raviglione M, et al. Resources required for global tuberculosis control. Science 2002;295(5562):2040–1.
56. Hutton G, Wyss K, N'Diekhor Y. Prioritization of prevention activities to combat the spread of HIV/AIDS in resource constrained settings: a cost-effectiveness analysis from Chad, Central Africa. Int J Health Plann Manage 2003;18(2): 117–36.
57. Kampf G. The six golden rules to improve compliance in hand hygiene. J Hosp Infect 2004;56(Suppl 2):S3–5.
58. Currie CS, Floyd K, Williams BG, et al. Cost, affordability and cost-effectiveness of strategies to control tuberculosis in countries with high HIV prevalence. BMC Public Health 2005;5:130.
59. Muniyandi M, Ramachandran R, Balasubramanian R. An economic commentary on the occurrence and control of HIV/AIDS in developing countries: special reference to India. Expert Opin Pharmacother 2006;7(18):2447–54.
60. Wilson AP, Hodgson B, Liu M, et al. Reduction in wound infection rates by wound surveillance with postdischarge follow-up and feedback. Br J Surg 2006;93(5):630–8.
61. Anderson DJ, Kirkland KB, Kaye KS, et al. Underresourced hospital infection control and prevention programs: penny wise, pound foolish? Infect Control Hosp Epidemiol 2007;28(7):767–73.

62. Graves N, Halton K, Lairson D. Economics and preventing hospital-acquired infection: broadening the perspective. Infect Control Hosp Epidemiol 2007; 28(2):178–84.

63. Perencevich EN, Thom KA. Commentary: preventing Clostridium difficile-associated disease: is it time to pay the piper? Infect Control Hosp Epidemiol 2008;29(9):829–31.

64. Kaye KS. The financial impact of antibiotic resistance. In: Soule BM, Weber S, editors. What every health care executive should know: the cost of antibiotic resistance. Oakbrook Terrace (IL): Joint Commission Resources; 2009. p. 29–42.

65. Ju MH, Ko CY, Hall BL, et al. A comparison of 2 surgical site infection monitoring systems. JAMA Surg 2015;150(1):51–7.

66. Lee KK, Berenholtz SM, Hobson DB, et al. Building a business case for colorectal surgery quality improvement. Dis Colon Rectum 2013;56(11):1298–303.

67. van Limburg M, Wentzel J, Sanderman R, et al. Business modeling to implement an eHealth portal for infection control: a reflection on co-creation with stakeholders. JMIR Res Protoc 2015;4(3):e104.

68. Branch-Elliman W, Wright SB, Howell MD. Determining the ideal strategy for ventilator-associated pneumonia prevention. Cost-benefit analysis. Am J Respir Crit Care Med 2015;192(1):57–63.

69. Dick AW, Perencevich EN, Pogorzelska-Maziarz M, et al. A decade of investment in infection prevention: a cost-effectiveness analysis. Am J Infect Control 2015;43(1):4–9.

70. Gidengil CA, Gay C, Huang SS, et al. Cost-effectiveness of strategies to prevent methicillin-resistant *Staphylococcus aureus* transmission and infection in an intensive care unit. Infect Control Hosp Epidemiol 2015;36(1):17–27.

71. Goldsack JC, DeRitter C, Power M, et al. Clinical, patient experience and cost impacts of performing active surveillance on known methicillin-resistant Staphylococcus aureus positive patients admitted to medical-surgical units. Am J Infect Control 2014;42(10):1039–43.

72. Kollef MH. Ventilator-associated pneumonia prevention. Is it worth it? Am J Respir Crit Care Med 2015;192(1):5–7.

73. McKinnell JA, Bartsch SM, Lee BY, et al. Cost-benefit analysis from the hospital perspective of universal active screening followed by contact precautions for methicillin-resistant Staphylococcus aureus carriers. Infect Control Hosp Epidemiol 2015;36(1):2–13.

74. Murthy A, De Angelis G, Pittet D, et al. Cost-effectiveness of universal MRSA screening on admission to surgery. Clin Microbiol Infect 2010;16(12):1747–53.

75. Association for Professional in Infection Control and Epidemiology. APIC Member Salary and Career Survey. 2006. Available at: www.apic.org/Content/NavigationMenu/MemberServices/2006SalarySurveyResults/2006_Salary_Survey.htm. Accessed September 1, 2006.

76. Coskun D, Aytac J, Aydinli A, et al. Mortality rate, length of stay and extra cost of sternal surgical site infections following coronary artery bypass grafting in a private medical centre in Turkey. J Hosp Infect 2005;60(2):176–9.

77. Rello J, Ollendorf DA, Oster G, et al. Epidemiology and outcomes of ventilator-associated pneumonia in a large US database. Chest 2002;122(6):2115–21.

78. Carmeli Y, Troillet N, Karchmer AW, et al. Health and economic outcomes of antibiotic resistance in Pseudomonas aeruginosa. Arch Intern Med 1999;159(10): 1127–32.

79. Carmeli Y, Eliopoulos G, Mozaffari E, et al. Health and economic outcomes of vancomycin-resistant enterococci. Arch Intern Med 2002;162(19):2223–8.

80. Cosgrove SE, Kaye KS, Eliopoulous GM, et al. Health and economic outcomes of the emergence of third-generation cephalosporin resistance in Enterobacter species. Arch Intern Med 2002;162(2):185–90.

81. Cosgrove SE, Carmeli Y. The impact of antimicrobial resistance on health and economic outcomes. Clin Infect Dis 2003;36(11):1433–7.

82. Engemann JJ, Carmeli Y, Cosgrove SE, et al. Adverse clinical and economic outcomes attributable to methicillin resistance among patients with Staphylococcus aureus surgical site infection. Clin Infect Dis 2003;36(5):592–8.

83. Cosgrove SE, Qi Y, Kaye KS, et al. The impact of methicillin resistance in Staphylococcus aureus bacteremia on patient outcomes: mortality, length of stay, and hospital charges. Infect Control Hosp Epidemiol 2005;26(2):166–74.

84. Schwaber MJ, Navon-Venezia S, Kaye KS, et al. Clinical and economic impact of bacteremia with extended- spectrum-beta-lactamase-producing Enterobacteriaceae. Antimicrob Agents Chemother 2006;50(4):1257–62.

85. Giske CG, Monnet DL, Cars O, et al. Clinical and economic impact of common multidrug-resistant gram-negative bacilli. Antimicrob Agents Chemother 2008; 52(3):813–21.

86. Warren DK, Shukla SJ, Olsen MA, et al. Outcome and attributable cost of ventilator-associated pneumonia among intensive care unit patients in a suburban medical center. Crit Care Med 2003;31(5):1312–7.

87. Hugonnet S, Eggimann P, Borst F, et al. Impact of ventilator-associated pneumonia on resource utilization and patient outcome. Infect Control Hosp Epidemiol 2004;25(12):1090–6.

88. Blot SI, Depuydt P, Annemans L, et al. Clinical and economic outcomes in critically ill patients with nosocomial catheter-related bloodstream infections. Clin Infect Dis 2005;41(11):1591–8.

89. Coello R, Charlett A, Wilson J, et al. Adverse impact of surgical site infections in English hospitals. J Hosp Infect 2005;60(2):93–103.

90. Hollenbeak CS, Murphy DM, Koenig S, et al. The clinical and economic impact of deep chest surgical site infections following coronary artery bypass graft surgery. Chest 2000;118(2):397–402.

91. Tambyah PA, Knasinski V, Maki DG. The direct costs of nosocomial catheter-associated urinary tract infection in the era of managed care. Infect Control Hosp Epidemiol 2002;23(1):27–31.

92. Lai KK, Fontecchio SA. Use of silver-hydrogel urinary catheters on the incidence of catheter-associated urinary tract infections in hospitalized patients. Am J Infect Control 2002;30(4):221–5.

93. Maslikowska JA, Walker SA, Elligsen M, et al. Impact of infection with extended-spectrum beta-lactamase-producing Escherichia coli or Klebsiella species on outcome and hospitalization costs. J Hosp Infect 2016;92(1):33–41.

94. Goudie A, Dynan L, Brady PW, et al. Attributable cost and length of stay for central line-associated bloodstream infections. Pediatrics 2014;133(6):e1525–32.

95. Farbman L, Avni T, Rubinovitch B, et al. Cost-benefit of infection control interventions targeting methicillin-resistant Staphylococcus aureus in hospitals: systematic review. Clin Microbiol Infect 2013;19(12):E582–93.

96. Roberts RR, Scott RD 2nd, Hota B, et al. Costs attributable to healthcare-acquired infection in hospitalized adults and a comparison of economic methods. Med Care 2010;48(11):1026–35.

97. Masterton RG. Evaluating the cost-effectiveness of strategies to prevent vascular access device infections. Br J Nurs 2014;23(14 Suppl):S15–9.

98. Verlee K, Berriel-Cass D, Buck K, et al. Cost of isolation: daily cost of isolation determined and cost avoidance demonstrated from the overuse of personal protective equipment in an acute care facility. Am J Infect Control 2014;42(4): 448–9.

99. Stevenson KB, Balada-Llasat JM, Bauer K, et al. The economics of antimicrobial stewardship: the current state of the art and applying the business case model. Infect Control Hosp Epidemiol 2012;33(4):389–97.

100. Fukuda H, Lee J, Imanaka Y. Costs of hospital-acquired infection and transferability of the estimates: a systematic review. Infection 2011;39(3):185–99.

101. Kang J, Smith KJ, Bryce CL, et al. Economic analysis of universal active surveillance screening for methicillin-resistant Staphylococcus aureus: perspective matters. Infect Control Hosp Epidemiol 2015;36(1):14–6.

102. Hospital-Acquired Condition Reduction Program (HACRP) 2015. Available at: www.medicare.gov/hospitalcompare/HAC-reduction-program.html. Accessed March 11, 2016.

103. Centers for Disease Control and Prevention. National and state healthcare associated infections progress Report. 2015. Available at: http://www.cdc.gov/hai/surveillance/progress-report/. Accessed June 16, 2016.

104. Dudeck MA, Edwards JR, Allen-Bridson K, et al. National Healthcare Safety Network report, data summary for 2013, Device-associated Module. Am J Infect Control 2015;43(3):206–21.

105. Ward WJ Jr, Spragens L, Smithson K. Building the business case for clinical quality. Healthc Financ Manage 2006;60(12):92–8.

106. Perencevich EN, Fisman DN, Lipsitch M, et al. Projected benefits of active surveillance for vancomycin-resistant enterococci in intensive care units. Clin Infect Dis 2004;38(8):1108–15.

# Hand Hygiene: An Update

Maureen K. Bolon, MD, MS

## KEYWORDS

- Hand hygiene • Handwashing • Alcohol-based hand rub
- Health care-associated infections

## KEY POINTS

- Hand hygiene by health care workers is a key factor in preventing health care–associated infections, yet hand hygiene occurs only 40% of the time.
- Alcohol-based hand rubs offer excellent antimicrobial killing, while facilitating hand hygiene with their ease of use.
- New technologies offer innovative ways to monitor and improve hand hygiene by health care workers, yet costs and limitations remain.

## INTRODUCTION

The crucial role of hand hygiene in the prevention of health care–associated infection was initially established independently by Oliver Wendell Holmes and Ignaz Semmelweis in the 1840s.[1] Semmelweis, whose insights predated the germ theory by several decades, is credited with recognizing that the hands of medical staff were contaminated while performing autopsies and consequently were responsible for the transmission of "cadaverous particles" during obstetric examinations, leading to puerperal sepsis and death.[2] He further demonstrated that hand antisepsis with chlorinated lime resulted in a dramatic decrease in maternal mortality. More than a century later, Mortimer and colleagues[3] established the importance of hand hygiene in preventing *Staphylococcus aureus* transmission in a neonatal unit. When cared for by nurses who did not perform hand hygiene, infants in this study were more likely to acquire *S aureus* than those cared for by nurses who performed hand hygiene with hexachlorophene. As was the case in Semmelweis' time, evidence of the benefits of hand hygiene have not translated into universal adoption of the practice. Recent decades have seen major advances in medical science, including in the field of health care epidemiology. Yet, despite these advances and the development of well-accepted guidelines regarding the practice of hand hygiene, rates of hand hygiene performance by health care workers remain disappointingly low.

A version of this article originally appeared in Volume 25, Issue 1 of *Infectious Disease Clinics of North America*.
Disclosures: None.
Division of Infectious Diseases, Department of Medicine, Northwestern University Feinberg School of Medicine, 645 North Michigan Avenue, Suite 900, Chicago, IL 60611, USA
*E-mail address:* m-bolon@northwestern.edu

Infect Dis Clin N Am 30 (2016) 591–607
http://dx.doi.org/10.1016/j.idc.2016.04.007
0891-5520/16/$ – see front matter © 2016 Elsevier Inc. All rights reserved.

id.theclinics.com

## HUMAN SKIN AND SKIN FLORA

Human skin is colonized with bacteria. Counts vary depending on body location; bacterial counts on the hands of health care workers have been reported to range from $3.9 \times 10^4$ to $4.6 \times 10^6$ colony-forming units (CFUs)/cm$^2$.[1] Two classifications of skin flora have been delineated: transient flora and resident flora. Transient flora are those associated most frequently with health care–associated infections and are, therefore, the primary target of hand hygiene within the health care setting. Transient flora reside in the uppermost level of the stratum corneum and are acquired by direct contact with patients or with environmental surfaces associated with patients.[1] These loosely adherent organisms can be transmitted to other patients or to the environment if they are not removed by mechanical friction, the detergent properties of soap and water, or killed by antiseptic agents.[4] Numerous pathogens have been identified among the transient flora of health care workers' hands, including S aureus, Klebsiella pneumoniae, Acinetobacter spp., Enterobacter spp., and Candida spp. Health care workers with skin damage or chronic skin conditions are more likely to be colonized with pathogenic organisms in greater quantities (both the number of different organisms and the bacterial counts), which can make them more likely to transmit infectious pathogens.[5,6] Resident flora are the low-pathogenicity, permanent residents of the deeper layers of the skin.[4,7] These organisms cause infection only when a normal barrier is disrupted, such as with the placement of an intravenous catheter. Resident flora cannot be removed solely by mechanical friction; thus, an antiseptic agent must be used before the performance of invasive procedures. Surgical hand antisepsis is a special case, in that the goal is to reduce resident flora for the duration of the surgical procedure to prevent contamination of the surgical field if a glove becomes punctured or torn.[1]

To interrupt transmission of health care–associated infections spread via health care workers' hands, it is useful to consider the sequence of events necessary for this to occur[1]:

1. Organisms present on the patient's skin or in the proximity of the patient are transferred to the hands of the health care worker;
2. Organisms must be capable of surviving for a short period on the hands of the health care worker;
3. Hand hygiene is inadequate, performed with an inappropriate agent, or omitted entirely; and
4. Contaminated hands of the health care worker must come in direct contact with another patient or with an inanimate object that will come in direct contact with the patient.

The contribution of contact with the immediate patient environment (as opposed to the patient directly) to the contamination of health care workers' hands must be emphasized. Viable organisms are present in the $10^6$ skin squames that humans shed daily; these may proceed to contaminate patient gowns, bed linen, and furniture.[1] Organisms that are resistant to desiccation, such as staphylococci and enterococci, may thereby join transient flora on the hands of health care workers.

Hand hygiene terms are listed in **Table 1**. The antimicrobial activity of the 3 categories of hand hygiene agents (plain soap, alcohol-based hand rub, and antimicrobial soap) are discussed herein. Handwashing with plain soap removes dirt and transient flora via a detergent effect and mechanical friction. The log reduction of hand flora increases with duration of handwashing, but because the duration of handwashing averages from 6 to 24 seconds in observational studies of health care workers, a realistic expectation would be a reduction of 0.6 to 1.1 $\log_{10}$ CFU after a "typical"

**Table 1**
**Hand hygiene terms**

| Term | Definition |
|---|---|
| Plain soap | A detergent-based soap without antimicrobial properties. Action is achieved by physically removing dirt and microorganisms. |
| Alcohol-based hand rub | A waterless, alcohol-containing agent that kills microorganisms, but does not remove soil or organic material physically. |
| Antimicrobial soap | An agent that possesses activity against skin flora. Action is achieved via (1) physical removal of dirt and microorganisms and (2) killing of microorganisms. |
| Hand hygiene | Any method intended to remove or destroy microorganisms on the hands. |
| Handwashing | A method involving the use of water and plain soap to generate a lather, which is then distributed across all surfaces of the hands and rinsed off by water. |
| Hand antisepsis | Hand hygiene using either antimicrobial soap or an alcohol-based hand rub to physically remove and/or kill microorganisms. |
| Surgical scrub or surgical hand rub | Use of either antimicrobial soap or an alcohol-based hand rub to kill transient organisms and reduce resident flora for the duration of a surgical procedure. |

*Adapted from* Boyce JM, Pittet D. Guideline for hand hygiene in health-care settings. Recommendations of the Healthcare Infection Control Practices Advisory Committee and the HICPAC/SHEA/APIC/IDSA Hand Hygiene Task Force. Society for Healthcare Epidemiology of America/Association for Professionals in Infection Control/Infectious Diseases Society of America. MMWR Recomm Rep 2002;51(RR-16):1–45. [quiz: CE41–44]; and Larson EL. APIC guideline for handwashing and hand antisepsis in health care settings. Am J Infect Control 1995;23(4):251–69.

15-second handwashing episode.[1,7] There is some concern that the trauma caused by frequent handwashing may increase counts of skin flora and episodes of transmission by encouraging desquamation of the epithelial layer of skin and shedding of resident flora.[4,5] In contrast to plain soap, alcohol-based hand rubs work by killing the organisms on the skin, rather than physically removing them. The antimicrobial activity of alcohols is attributed to the denaturation of proteins. Although activity varies by compound and concentration, alcohols are active against gram-positive cocci, gram-negative bacilli, *Mycobacterium tuberculosis*, many fungi, and a number of viruses.[1,4] With a 30-second application, alcohol-based hand rubs lead to a bacterial reduction of 3.2 to 5.8 $\log_{10}$ CFUs.[7] Alcohols are considered somewhat less active against non-enveloped viruses, such as hepatitis A virus, rotavirus, enteroviruses, and adenovirus. Alcohols have very poor activity against bacterial spores, such as those of *Clostridium difficile*. The antimicrobial action of antimicrobial soaps also varies by agent. Chlorhexidine, one of the more commonly used agents, is a cationic bisguanide that derives its antimicrobial action by disrupting cell membranes and precipitating cell contents.[4] Chlorhexidine is considered to have good activity against gram-positive cocci and somewhat less activity against gram-negative bacilli, fungi, and viruses. Chlorhexidine has minimal antimycobacterial activity and is not active against spore-forming bacteria. A distinguishing feature of chlorhexidine is its persistent activity on the skin, a property that makes it a good candidate for surgical hand antisepsis. Bacterial reduction of 2.1 to 3 $\log_{10}$ CFU has been observed with shorter applications (<1 minute) of chlorhexidine.[8]

## EVOLUTION OF GUIDELINES

Hand hygiene practices in the United States have been shaped by guidelines issued by the Centers for Disease Control and Prevention (CDC). The earliest guidelines encouraged the use of plain soap and promoted the use of waterless agents only when sinks were not available.[9] In 1995, guidelines were issued by the Association for Professionals in Infection Control.[4] Handwashing with plain soap was advised for general patient care and removing visible soil. Hand antisepsis with antimicrobial soap or alcohol-based hand rub was recommended in the following circumstances: (1) before performance of invasive procedures such as surgery or the placement of intravenous catheters, indwelling urinary catheters, or other invasive devices, (2) when persistent antimicrobial activity is desired, and (3) when the reduction of resident flora is important. Opportunities for handwashing with plain soap and water or hand antisepsis with an alcohol-based hand rub included: before and after patient contact and after contact with a source of microorganisms (body fluids and substances, mucous membranes, nonintact skin, and inanimate objects that are likely to be contaminated). The role of hand antisepsis with either antimicrobial soap or a waterless agent was further expanded in the recommendations issued by the Healthcare Infection Control Practices Advisory Committee.[10,11] In these documents, hand antisepsis was recommended upon exiting the room of a patient with a multidrug-resistant pathogen.

In 2002, the CDC released an updated hand hygiene guideline and, for the first time, endorsed the use of alcohol-based hand rubs for the majority of clinical interactions, provided that hands are not visibly soiled.[1] In addition to the previous recommendation that hand hygiene should be performed before and after patient contact, more comprehensive guidance regarding situations that should prompt hand hygiene was detailed (**Box 1**). After the release of the 2002 CDC guidelines, hand hygiene practices in United States health care facilities changed dramatically as institutions adopted alcohol-based hand rubs, which had been used in Europe for several decades.[12]

Numerous other national and international bodies have issued guidelines for hand hygiene in health care settings. It would be a significant omission not to mention the contribution of the World Health Organization (WHO) to this effort. The WHO First Global Patient Safety Challenge was launched in 2005, a major focus of which was the promotion of hand hygiene practices in the health care setting.[13] As a follow-up, the WHO released hand hygiene guidelines in 2009 with indications for hand hygiene similar to those of the CDC. To assist campaign implementation, the WHO Toolkit was developed with freely available materials. These materials were formulated to be applicable to both developed and developing nations, as well as in poorly resourced settings, and attempt to take into account different cultural or religious influences on hand hygiene practices. The WHO Toolkit also provides a simplified and elegant construct to assist health care workers in recognizing hand hygiene opportunities, termed "Your Five Moments for Hand Hygiene." These are (1) before patient contact, (2) before aseptic task, (3) after body fluid exposure, (4) after patient contact, and (5) after contacts with patient surroundings.[14] Many institutions now use the WHO's 5 Moments as the basis for hand hygiene improvement methods. For the purposes of hand hygiene audits, institutions may choose to focus on hand hygiene opportunities before and after care, which correspond with moment 1 and moments 4 or 5.[15]

## ALCOHOL-BASED HAND RUBS

The reduction in bacterial counts achieved after application of an alcohol-based hand rub varies depending on the alcohol used; n-propanol is more bactericidal than isopranolol, which is more bactericidal than ethanol.[8,16] Efficacy is also related to concentration of the alcohol, with higher concentrations having greater bactericidal effect (up to 95%). Greater flammability limits the use of the higher concentrations of alcohol.

**Box 1**
**Centers for Disease Control and Prevention indications for hand hygiene**

- When hands are visibly dirty or contaminated with proteinaceous material or are visibly soiled with blood or other body fluids, wash hands with either a nonantimicrobial soap and water or an antimicrobial soap and water (categorization of recommendation: IA)

- If hands are not visibly soiled, use an alcohol-based hand rub for routinely decontaminating hands in all other clinical situations described below (categorization of recommendation: IA). Alternatively, wash hands with an antimicrobial soap and water in all clinical situations described below (categorization of recommendation: IB).

- Decontaminate hands before having direct contact with patients (categorization of recommendation: IB).

- Decontaminate hands before donning sterile gloves when inserting an intravascular catheter (categorization of recommendation: IB).

- Decontaminate hands before inserting indwelling urinary catheters, peripheral vascular catheters, or other invasive devices that do not require a surgical procedure (categorization of recommendation: IB).

- Decontaminate hands after contact with a patient's intact skin (categorization of recommendation: IB).

- Decontaminate hands after contact with body fluids or excretions, mucous membranes, nonintact skin, and wound dressings if hands are not visibly soiled (categorization of recommendation: IB).

- Decontaminate hands if moving from a contaminated body site to a clean body site during patient care (categorization of recommendation: II).

- Decontaminate hands after contact with inanimate objects (including medical equipment) in the immediate vicinity of the patient (categorization of recommendation: II).

- Decontaminate hands after removing gloves (categorization of recommendation: IB).

- Before eating and after using a restroom, wash hands with a nonantimicrobial soap and water or with antimicrobial soap and water (categorization of recommendation: IB).

- Antimicrobial-impregnated wipes may be considered as an alternative to washing hands with nonantimicrobial soap and water. Because they are not as effective as alcohol-based hand rubs or washing hands with an antimicrobial soap and water for reducing bacterial counts on the hands of health care workers, they are not a substitute for hand antisepsis (categorization of recommendation: IB).

- Wash hands with nonantimicrobial soap and water or with antimicrobial soap and water if exposure to Bacillus anthracis is suspected or proven (categorization of recommendation: II).

- No recommendation can be made regarding the routine use of non–alcohol-based hand rubs for hand hygiene in health-care settings. Unresolved issue.

Centers for Disease Control and Prevention/Healthcare Infection Control Practices Advisory Committee system for categorizing recommendations:
Category IA. Strongly recommended for implementation and strongly supported by well-designed experimental, clinical, or epidemiologic studies.
Category IB. Strongly recommended for implementation and supported by certain experimental, clinical, or epidemiologic studies and using theoretic rationale.
Category IC. Required for implementation, as mandated by federal or state regulation or standard.
Category II. Suggested for implementation and supported by suggestive clinical or epidemiologic studies or a theoretic rationale.

No recommendation. Unresolved issue. Practices for which insufficient evidence or no consensus regarding efficacy exist.

*From* Boyce JM, Pittet D. Guideline for hand hygiene in health-care settings. Recommendations of the Healthcare Infection Control Practices Advisory Committee and the HICPAC/SHEA/APIC/IDSA Hand Hygiene Task Force. Society for Healthcare Epidemiology of America/Association for Professionals in Infection Control/Infectious Diseases Society of America. MMWR Recomm Rep 2002;51(RR-16):1–45. [quiz: CE41–44].

In the United States, alcohol-based hand rubs are typically composed of 60% to 95% ethanol or isopranolol.[1] Thirteen clinical studies have compared the antibacterial efficacy of alcohol-based hand rub with soap and water for use by health care workers; 12 reported alcohol-based hand rub to be superior to soap and 1 found the products to be equivalent.[15]

Alcohol-based hand rubs are among the best tolerated agents for hand hygiene, in large part because of the addition of emollients.[1,16] From this standpoint, they are superior even to plain soap, the detergent effect of which causes loss of protein and lipids from the stratum corneum layers and consequent drying through water loss.[8] Furthermore, the incidence of allergic reactions owing to alcohols is believed to be nonexistent, although there remains the possibility of allergy to an emollient component.[7,17]

An additional important benefit of alcohol-based hand rubs is the relative time saved in the performance of hand hygiene compared with the use of soap and water. Hand hygiene performance with an alcohol-based hand rub is estimated typically to require one-third the length of time of a handwash procedure. In an oft-cited study, health care workers were timed performing handwashing, including the travel to and from the sink.[18] The average duration of the handwashing procedure was 61.7 seconds (range, 37–84). These same authors modeled the total time required for hand hygiene on an inpatient unit. If health care workers were 100% compliant with hand hygiene requirements, a 12-person team would spend 16 hours per shift performing handwashing, but just 3 hours using an alcohol-based hand rub. Because time constraints are one of the most frequently cited explanations for failure to perform hand hygiene, it is expected that the change from handwashing to alcohol-based hand rub should improve hand hygiene performance. This issue is examined in more detail below.

Given the known inactivity of alcohols against C difficile spores, there was some initial concern that the move away from handwashing to alcohol-based hand rubs would have the unintended consequence of increased C difficile infection rates. Early indications are that this has not occurred. In a study conducted soon after the introduction of alcohol-based hand rub at a large community teaching hospital, Boyce and colleagues[19] reported a 10-fold increase in the use of alcohol-based hand rub from 2000 to 2003 and a commensurate increase in the proportion of hand hygiene episodes using alcohol-based hand rub (from 10% to 85%). Despite this, they noted no increase in C difficile infection over this period. Other authors have failed similarly to demonstrate a correlation between alcohol-based hand rub use and C difficile infection.[20] Current guidelines do not specify deviation from routine hand hygiene practices when caring for individuals with C difficile infection; however, handwashing with soap and water is recommended when caring for patients with C difficile infection during outbreaks or in settings of hyperendemicity.[21] Because patients with C difficile infection should be placed in contact precautions, the use of gloves may be an important factor in preventing transmission regardless of method of hand hygiene. A study by Landelle and colleagues[22] identified use of gloves as an independent factor in reducing health care worker hand contamination by C difficile spores. Recent Society for Healthcare Epidemiology of America practice recommendations continue to support the use of alcohol-based hand rub for C difficile infection except during outbreaks and prioritize the use of gloves to prevent transmission.[15]

## HAND HYGIENE ADHERENCE

The commonly cited figure for health care worker hand hygiene adherence is 40%, which is derived from the average adherence reported in 34 studies performed between

1981 and 2000.[1] Baseline adherence in those studies ranged from 5% to 81%. Although there have been numerous hand hygiene improvement studies published in early part of the 21st century, as of this writing there has not been a comprehensive review that has provided an update to this 40% adherence figure. The expectations of health care worker hand hygiene performance have surely increased, and at one point The Joint Commission, the body that accredits health care organizations in the United States, expected hospitals to achieve greater than 90% hand hygiene compliance.[23] The wording of that standard has since been changed to, "Set goals for improving hand cleaning. Use the goals to improve hand cleaning."[24]

Three methods are most commonly used in the evaluation of health care worker adherence with hand hygiene practices: direct observation of hand hygiene opportunities, measurement of hand hygiene product use, and use of advanced technologies. Each of these methods has advantages and disadvantages in terms of accuracy, reproducibility, and ease of measurement. Obtaining estimates of hand hygiene performance by self-report or querying health care workers on their own performance is known to be highly inaccurate and is specifically not recommended by the Society for Healthcare Epidemiology of America.[15]

Direct observation is considered to be the "gold standard" for assessing hand hygiene compliance.[25,26] This metric is presented generally as the number of hand hygiene episodes divided by the number of hand hygiene opportunities. Direct observation of hand hygiene is the only method that can provide information on when and why hand hygiene lapses occur, which allows focus on individuals or groups of individuals requiring further motivation. Direct observation also allows identification of problems with technique or performance that require further education and reinforcement. However, direct observation is very labor intensive and, as such, it is possible to capture only a minority of hand hygiene episodes that occur. This factor leads to selection bias, particularly if observations are limited to weekday or daytime shifts. Finally, the act of observation can influence the behavior of those being observed and affect the outcome being studied, a phenomenon known as the Hawthorne effect. One group estimated that the Hawthorne effect increased hand hygiene compliance by 55%,[27] which is surely a desirable impact, but not one that is likely to be sustained.

Evaluation of product consumption is an appealing method for determining hand hygiene adherence because of its fairly low cost. A metric of hand hygiene performance can be derived by monitoring volume of product use and dividing by volume dispensed and number of patients to quantify the number of hand hygiene episodes per patient day. Some authors have failed to demonstrate a correlation between hand hygiene adherence as measured by direct observation and product use,[28,29] although 1 group pointed out that in their study direct observations only captured a minority of hand hygiene events (0.4%) and thus may not have accurately represented adherence rates.[29] This methodology may be most useful for following trends of consumption or internal comparisons of use between units.[30] To establish the methods currently being used by health care facilities to monitor hand hygiene adherence, a recent international survey indicated that most facilities were relying on direct observations of hand hygiene opportunities, with less attention given to hand hygiene technique.[31] Product use was monitored as an adjunct. These authors highlighted several areas of concern, including the fact that time devoted to training observers was typically less than 1 hour and most programs did not evaluate interobserver validity.

There has been a rapid expansion of technologies to assist in measuring hand hygiene performance. A number of these technologies are designed both to measure and improve performance. This discussion is limited to measurement of compliance, and use of technology to improve performance is handled in a later section. Broad categories of these technologies include (1) methodologies that facilitate direct observations of hand hygiene performance, such as applications that allow data input into mobile tablets and collation of data into centralized databases; (2) video monitoring of direct observations, (3) electronic counters on hand hygiene product dispensers that often broadcast counts to a centralized database, and (4) automated hand hygiene monitoring networks that can detect when a health care worker enters a patient area, detect when hand hygiene is performed, and may provide an alert or prompt to perform hand hygiene.[32] The primary barrier to video surveillance of hand hygiene performance is cost of installation of the required equipment as well as ongoing costs of reviewing video. There are, additionally, concerns of patient privacy.[32] Monitoring hand hygiene events by tabulating pumps of hand hygiene dispensers has the advantage of being able to capture large numbers of events, but the total number of opportunities remains unknown, as does whether proper technique is being used and whether there are poor performers who require further education. This methodology is also unable to distinguish between product usage by health care workers versus patients or visitors.[30] A significant financial investment is also necessary for wireless technologies that interface with specialized health care worker badges to track health care worker location as well as alcohol sensors or information from electronic dispenser pumps to determine when hand hygiene is performed. Health care workers may not accept these systems owing to concerns about accuracy as well as fear of punitive action.[33] A study by Pineles and colleagues[34] describes some of the limitations of an radiofrequency identification tracking system. Although the accuracy of the system compared with direct observation was good under simulation testing, it was significantly lower in real-life use (88.5% vs 52.4%; $P<.01$). Accounting for the inaccuracy, a large proportion of hand hygiene events were missed, as were room entries and exits. Further investigation identified that functionality was affected by where the radiofrequency identification badge was worn and the position of the health care worker relative to the sensors. The authors concluded that the inaccuracy of the system was responsible for falsely low hand hygiene compliance rates.

## BARRIERS TO HAND HYGIENE

The study of barriers to optimal hand hygiene performance helps to inform interventions intended to improve performance. Barriers and risk factors have been reviewed comprehensively by other authors,[35] a few issues will be highlighted here. With multiple demands on their time, the time required for hand hygiene performance is a frequently mentioned barrier to acceptable hand hygiene adherence. As mentioned, one of the benefits of alcohol-based hand rubs is the time savings in their application. Yet, given the "hands-on" nature of care in a modern hospital, countless hand hygiene opportunities occur throughout the day. One group estimated that, despite the use of an alcohol-based hand rub, 230 minutes per patient per day would need to be devoted to hand hygiene in an intensive care unit (ICU).[36] The inconvenience of hand hygiene owing to inaccessibility of sinks, towels, or product dispensers is another issue that may increase the time to perform hand hygiene and reduce adherence. Although sink accessibility would be anticipated to impact handwashing compliance, 2 groups have reported no effect on hand hygiene adherence when sink accessibility improved after construction of new hospital facilities.[37,38] These findings are refuted by a more recent study of the effect of sequentially introducing alcohol-based hand rub dispensers on hand hygiene performance.[39] The authors noted that the optimal number of dispensers per bed was 2, with no additional benefit seen in hand hygiene performance with the addition of further dispensers. They also observed that dispensers in the hallway were used more frequently than in-room dispensers.

Irritant contact dermatitis is a common occurrence among health care workers with a reported prevalence of 10% to 45%.[5,17] Accordingly, skin irritation and dryness may discourage the performance of hand hygiene, even with alcohol-based products, although true allergies are not felt likely to be owing to alcohols and studies have shown beneficial effects of alcohol-based hand rubs on skin water loss.[7,17,40] For this reason, provision of lotions to reduce the occurrence of dermatitis merits a category IA recommendation in the CDC guidelines.[1] Fortunately, skin care products are not felt to adversely affect the antimicrobial properties of alcohol-based hand rubs.[41]

Glove use by health care workers often occurs in patient care, whether because of standard or contact precautions or because of the performance of invasive procedures. Gloves are not felt to represent an adequate barrier to the contamination that occurs during patient care, hence the recommendation that hand hygiene should be performed after glove removal.[1] There is controversy as to whether the act of wearing gloves stimulates or discourages hand hygiene; studies have demonstrated both outcomes.[42,43] A related issue is whether contact precautions—the use of gowns and gloves by health care workers to prevent transmission of infectious agents—impacts hand hygiene adherence. Whereas an earlier study showed no impact of gown use on hand hygiene rates,[44] a more recent study performed in Switzerland evaluated the effect of eliminating the requirement for glove use for patients on contact precautions.[45] These authors noted a marked increase in hand hygiene (from 52% to 85%; $P<.001$) when gloves were not required. At this point, it seems premature to characterize either glove or gown use as definite barriers to hand hygiene performance.

The professional role of the health care worker has been repeatedly found to be a factor in hand hygiene performance; unfortunately, physicians who have completed their training have been identified as having the lowest hand hygiene adherence rates by several authors.[46,47] Because attending physicians often serve as role models for trainees, students, and other professionals, their poor hand hygiene performance can adversely affect that of their charges. In an observational study of resident hand hygiene practices, hand hygiene adherence increased from 14% to 65% if the senior member of the team practiced hand hygiene.[48] Conversely, if the senior member of the team did not practice hand hygiene, no other member of the team did. Other groups have found that role models have a predominantly negative impact on the hand hygiene of their trainees.[37] In direct surveys of trainees, role modeling has been identified as important in influencing the practice of hand hygiene.[48,49] Pittet and colleagues[50] administered a survey to physicians to explore barriers and motivators of hand hygiene adherence. Among other findings, the belief that one is a role model for other colleagues did influence hand hygiene performance positively, whereas high work load was a risk factor for nonadherence. On a more optimistic note, several strategies have been found to effectively influence physician adoption of alcohol-based hand rubs. The change observed after educational infection control sessions was more dramatic among physicians than any other group, a difference that was postulated to be owing to the fact that physicians are more comfortable changing practice when faced with evidence-based recommendations.[51] An intervention in a critical care unit, which involved physician report cards, regular feedback to chiefs of service, and ranking of hand hygiene performance by service line, increased hand hygiene to levels to greater than 90% and was sustainable for 24 months beyond the original intervention.[52]

## IMPROVING HAND HYGIENE ADHERENCE

At its root, the practice of hand hygiene can be considered a behavior to be encouraged among health care workers. The practice of hand hygiene occurs outside of the health care setting as well, and the variance in practices learned in the home and the expectations within the health care setting explains in part the poor performance of health care workers. Under 1 rubric, there are 2 types of hand hygiene behaviors: inherent and elective. Inherent hand hygiene occurs when hands are perceived as physically dirty, either because of sensation, odor, or contact with an "emotionally dirty area" such as the groin or axilla.[53] Inherent hand hygiene is the predominant form of hand hygiene practiced in the community and elicits maximal adherence in both community and health care settings. Conversely, elective hand hygiene practice comprises all other opportunities, including those that should follow many patient and environmental contacts within the health care setting. Although these contacts do not trigger a self-protective response to perform hand hygiene, elective hand hygiene is desirable to prevent transmission to patients.

In terms of interventions intended to improve hand hygiene adherence, the introduction of alcohol-based hand gel as the preferred agent for hand hygiene has become one of the best studied interventions. Introducing an alcohol-based hand hygiene product would be anticipated to be effective in that it represents an easily accessible or even portable agent that can be applied in less time than handwashing, thus reducing the primary barriers to hand hygiene. Many authors have found that the introduction of an alcohol-based hand rub did improve hand hygiene adherence.[54–58] One of these studies is notable for also demonstrating a reduction in health care–associated infection rates, and is described in more detail below.[55] Conversely, some authors have noted limited or no success in improving hand hygiene rates after the introduction of alcohol-based hand rubs.[59,60] A common theme in failed interventions is the lack of an accompanying educational program or an ineffective educational program to promote the use of these agents.[58,60]

Reporting and feedback of individual- or unit-level performance is a common strategy for motivating practice improvements. One large, multicenter project ascertained hand hygiene performance based on product usage and provided regular feedback on hand hygiene adherence.[61] These authors demonstrated significant improvements in hand hygiene performance both in ICU and non-ICU settings (median percentage change of 63% and 92%, respectively) over a 12-month period.

As the group most likely to benefit from improved health care worker hand hygiene practices, patients may have a role in encouraging hand hygiene. In fact, both the CDC and WHO guidelines recommend that patients be involved in promoting health care worker hand hygiene (category II recommendation in both guidelines).[1,13] Although a phone survey of US households indicated that 80% of those surveyed would ask a health care worker to perform hand hygiene,[62] there are many factors that may thwart this intention. Surveys of patients reveal a potential willingness to mention hand hygiene to health care workers that is not always mirrored by actual execution of a request.[63] More successful strategies have involved positive reinforcement (ie, thanking a health care worker for performing hand hygiene), providing posters or placards for patients to display that encourage hand hygiene, or requests from the health care workers themselves to be asked about hand hygiene.[64,65] Health care workers do seem to be amenable to patient prompting to perform hand hygiene.[63] Concerns remain as to whether this is a realistic expectation for patients who are too ill or intimidated by caregivers to participate, but in some settings this may constitute 1 aspect of an overall safety culture.

It is fairly well-accepted that complex problems like health care–associated infections are best approached with multipronged, bundled solutions. In the same vein, many of the recently published efforts to improve hand hygiene have used an amalgamation of interventions. To give 1 example, a single institution introduced multiple, sequential categories of interventions intended to improve hand hygiene, including leadership/accountability, measurement/feedback, hand sanitizer availability, and education/training.[66] Efforts such as these have been able to achieve levels of hand hygiene compliance approaching 90% or greater and have also been able to improve the performance of numerous health care worker categories, including physicians.[66–69] Furthermore, these efforts have been shown to impact selected health care-associated infection outcomes.[66,67] Such interventions can require significant investment of both resources and effort, but when thoughtfully designed and applied can truly impact the health care culture.

Hand hygiene improvement efforts using technologic enhancements have also demonstrated success. One such report of technology facilitating direct observations by Chen and colleagues[70] used handheld devices to collect events and link to a database via the Internet. By increasing the pool of observers beyond the infection prevention department, the authors were able to increase the number of observations many-fold as well as demonstrate hand hygiene compliance of 86% (compared with 50% before the program). Another study used an electronic network of hand hygiene dispensers and room entry–exit monitors to monitor hand hygiene in an ICU.[71] Hand hygiene performance was monitored in real time and displayed on computer monitors on the unit. This system successfully increased daily hand hygiene events by 24% and led to a 40% increase in the ratio of hand hygiene to room entry/exit events, both of which were significant improvements. Lastly, an example of technological innovation described by Armellino and colleagues[72] involved installing video cameras in an ICU to remotely audit every room entry/exit and determine whether it was associated with a hand hygiene event. Feedback of hand hygiene performance was achieved through monitors on the unit as well as through summary reports to unit leadership. This intervention resulted in a marked improvement in hand hygiene performance (from 10% to 81.6%) that was sustained for more than 1 year. The authors noted that feedback of performance was an integral part of the improvement efforts that supplemented the surveillance by video cameras. They also believe that the improvements would not be sustained if the monitoring and feedback were removed. Given the expense of such an intervention on a single unit, this raises concerns regarding the practicality of wider implementation.

## HEALTH CARE–ASSOCIATED INFECTIONS

Although improving hand hygiene is frequently cited as an important component of preventing health care–associated infections, the evidence basis for this assertion has yet to be established satisfactorily.[73] An updated Cochrane review attempted to synthesize the numerous studies published on the topic, but arrived at no conclusion because only 4 studies were felt adequate for inclusion.[74] It is worthwhile to mention a few select examples of studies that have attempted to answer the question in order to gauge progress on the topic.

An older study that has been extremely influential is the work by Pittet and colleagues,[55] which demonstrated the success of a multicomponent campaign to promote the use of an alcohol-based hand rub at a large hospital in Geneva, Switzerland. The program encouraged hand hygiene through increased accessibility of alcohol-based hand rub at the patient bedside and in individual pocket-sized bottles, a poster campaign that was developed by collaborative groups of health care workers, and strong institutional commitment to the program. Hospital-wide hand hygiene adherence increased from 48% in 1994% to 66% in 1997 (P<.001). Over the same time period, there was a significant reduction in the prevalence of nosocomial infections and methicillin-resistant S aureus transmission. In follow-up studies, these authors have reported sustained hand hygiene and infection outcomes out to 7 years.[75] The success of this program has inspired others to attempt similar campaigns. Additionally, lessons from the Geneva experience have been incorporated into the WHO programs.[13]

Two studies mentioned previously that used multiple interventions demonstrated an impact of improved hand hygiene performance on an infection outcome. The study by Johnson and colleagues[67] reported a 10-fold reduction in central line-associated blood stream infection (4.08 vs 0.42 per 1000 device-days) when hand hygiene improved from 58% to 98%. Of note, a central line bundle was also instituted. Kirkland and colleagues[66] demonstrated improvement in multiple infection outcomes in a 3-year interrupted time series, including rates of health care–associated S aureus, C difficile, and bloodstream infection. Successes have also been seen in pediatric populations. Song and colleagues[76] demonstrated nearly 50% reductions in methicillin-resistant S aureus acquisition at a children's hospital when hand hygiene performance improved from 50.3% to 84%. In contrast, a population-based study of an Ontario initiative to promote hand hygiene failed to demonstrate any association between hand hygiene and the publically reportable outcomes of methicillin-resistant S aureus bacteremia or C difficile infection over 3 years of study.[77]

A common refrain in reviews and editorials is the flawed nature of these types of studies, which must, by necessity, be conducted without a "placebo group" of health care workers who do not wash their hands. As is the nature of many infection control studies, many are uncontrolled or before-and-after studies. Additionally, although multicomponent interventions may be more successful at improving hand hygiene performance, it becomes difficult to tease out which aspect is responsible for a change in infection rates. Furthermore, the occurrence of health care-associated infections is influenced by factors other than hand hygiene, such as outbreaks that may be occurring, antimicrobial use, and environmental cleanliness, making it difficult to isolate the contribution of hand hygiene interventions to changing infection rates. One interesting evaluation of this was a study performed by Barnes and colleagues.[78] These authors attempted to determine the relative contribution of environmental cleanliness and hand hygiene compliance to transmission of multidrug-resistant organisms with a modelling study. They found that a 20% improvement in terminal cleaning was equivalent to a 10% improvement in hand hygiene compliance.

## SUMMARY

Despite the abundance of hand hygiene literature, there remain numerous unanswered questions that should engage future researchers. As an example: what is the optimal level of hand hygiene adherence necessary to improve infectious outcomes? Several modeling studies have explored this issue and seem to reach consensus that there exists a level of adherence beyond which incremental improvements will achieve no further reduction in the transmission of infection, yet it is not clear what the threshold adherence might be and whether it might vary for different organisms or different levels of colonization pressure.[79,80] A further question: what is the most appropriate metric of infection to use as the outcome for hand hygiene intervention studies? Is the failure to establish conclusively improvements in health care–associated infection associated with hand hygiene simply an issue of selecting the wrong outcome? Finally, which intervention or interventions can sustain improvements over time and are cost effective enough to be applied widely? The patients who place themselves in our care deserve answers to these important questions.

## REFERENCES

1. Boyce JM, Pittet D. Guideline for Hand Hygiene in Health-Care Settings. Recommendations of the Healthcare Infection Control Practices Advisory Committee and the HICPAC/SHEA/APIC/IDSA Hand Hygiene Task Force. Society for Healthcare Epidemiology of America/Association for Professionals in Infection Control/Infectious Diseases Society of America. MMWR Recomm Rep 2002;51(RR-16): 1–45 [quiz: CE41–44].
2. Rotter ML. Semmelweis' sesquicentennial: a little-noted anniversary of handwashing. Curr Opin Infect Dis 1998;11(4):457–60.
3. Mortimer EA Jr, Lipsitz PJ, Wolinsky E, et al. Transmission of staphylococci between newborns. Importance of the hands to personnel. Am J Dis Child 1962; 104:289–95.
4. Larson EL. APIC guideline for handwashing and hand antisepsis in health care settings. Am J Infect Control 1995;23(4):251–69.
5. Larson E. Hygiene of the skin: when is clean too clean? Emerg Infect Dis 2001; 7(2):225–30.
6. Rocha LA, Ferreira de Almeida EBL, Gontijo Filho PP. Changes in hands microbiota associated with skin damage because of hand hygiene procedures on the health care workers. Am J Infect Control 2009;37(2):155–9.
7. Widmer AF. Replace hand washing with use of a waterless alcohol hand rub? Clin Infect Dis 2000;31(1):136–43.
8. Kampf G, Kramer A. Epidemiologic background of hand hygiene and evaluation of the most important agents for scrubs and rubs. Clin Microbiol Rev 2004;17(4): 863–93.
9. Garner JS, Favero MS. CDC guidelines for the prevention and control of nosocomial infections. Guideline for handwashing and hospital environmental control, 1985. Supersedes guideline for hospital environmental control published in 1981. Am J Infect Control 1986;14(3):110–29.
10. Hospital Infection Control Practices Advisory Committee (HICPAC). Recommendations for preventing the spread of vancomycin resistance. Infect Control Hosp Epidemiol 1995;16(2):105–13.
11. Garner JS. Guideline for isolation precautions in hospitals. The Hospital Infection Control Practices Advisory Committee. Infect Control Hosp Epidemiol 1996;17(1): 53–80.
12. Mody L, Saint S, Kaufman SR, et al. Adoption of alcohol-based handrub by United States hospitals: a national survey. Infect Control Hosp Epidemiol 2008; 29(12):1177–80.
13. Pittet D, Allegranzi B, Boyce J. The World Health Organization Guidelines on Hand Hygiene in Health Care and their consensus recommendations. Infect Control Hosp Epidemiol 2009;30(7):611–22.
14. Sax H, Allegranzi B, Uckay I, et al. 'My five moments for hand hygiene': a user-centred design approach to understand, train, monitor and report hand hygiene. J Hosp Infect 2007;67(1):9–21.
15. Ellingson K, Haas JP, Aiello AE, et al. Strategies to prevent healthcare-associated infections through hand hygiene. Infect Control Hosp Epidemiol 2014;35(8): 937–60.

16. Rotter ML. Arguments for alcoholic hand disinfection. J Hosp Infect 2001; 48(Suppl A):S4–8.
17. Loffler H, Kampf G. Hand disinfection: how irritant are alcohols? J Hosp Infect 2008;70(Suppl 1):44–8.
18. Voss A, Widmer AF. No time for handwashing!? Handwashing versus alcoholic rub: can we afford 100% compliance? Infect Control Hosp Epidemiol 1997; 18(3):205–8.
19. Boyce JM, Ligi C, Kohan C, et al. Lack of association between the increased incidence of Clostridium difficile-associated disease and the increasing use of alcohol-based hand rubs. Infect Control Hosp Epidemiol 2006;27(5):479–83.
20. Kaier K, Hagist C, Frank U, et al. Two time-series analyses of the impact of antibiotic consumption and alcohol-based hand disinfection on the incidences of nosocomial methicillin-resistant Staphylococcus aureus infection and Clostridium difficile infection. Infect Control Hosp Epidemiol 2009;30(4):346–53.
21. Dubberke ER, Gerding DN, Classen D, et al. Strategies to prevent clostridium difficile infections in acute care hospitals. Infect Control Hosp Epidemiol 2008; 29(Suppl 1):S81–92.
22. Landelle C, Verachten M, Legrand P, et al. Contamination of healthcare workers' hands with Clostridium difficile spores after caring for patients with C. difficile infection. Infect Control Hosp Epidemiol 2014;35(1):10–5.
23. Boyce JM. Update on hand hygiene. Am J Infect Control 2013;41(5 Suppl): S94–6.
24. 2015 Hospital National Patient Safety Goals. 2015. Available at: www.jointcommission.org/assets/1/6/2015_hap_nspg_er.pdf. Accessed January 13, 2016.
25. Boyce JM. Hand hygiene compliance monitoring: current perspectives from the USA. J Hosp Infect 2008;70(Suppl 1):2–7.
26. Haas JP, Larson EL. Measurement of compliance with hand hygiene. J Hosp Infect 2007;66(1):6–14.
27. Eckmanns T, Bessert J, Behnke M, et al. Compliance with antiseptic hand rub use in intensive care units: the Hawthorne effect. Infect Control Hosp Epidemiol 2006; 27(9):931–4.
28. Muller A, Denizot V, Mouillet S, et al. Lack of correlation between consumption of alcohol-based solutions and adherence to guidelines for hand hygiene. J Hosp Infect 2005;59(2):163–4.
29. van de Mortel T, Murgo M. An examination of covert observation and solution audit as tools to measure the success of hand hygiene interventions. Am J Infect Control 2006;34(3):95–9.
30. Boyce JM. Measuring healthcare worker hand hygiene activity: current practices and emerging technologies. Infect Control Hosp Epidemiol 2011;32(10): 1016–28.
31. Braun BI, Kusek L, Larson E. Measuring adherence to hand hygiene guidelines: a field survey for examples of effective practices. Am J Infect Control 2009;37(4): 282–8.
32. Ward MA, Schweizer ML, Polgreen PM, et al. Automated and electronically assisted hand hygiene monitoring systems: a systematic review. Am J Infect Control 2014;42(5):472–8.
33. McGuckin M, Govednik J. A Review of Electronic Hand Hygiene Monitoring: Considerations for Hospital Management in Data Collection, Healthcare Worker Supervision, and Patient Perception. J Healthc Manag 2015;60(5):348–61.

34. Pineles LL, Morgan DJ, Limper HM, et al. Accuracy of a radiofrequency identification (RFID) badge system to monitor hand hygiene behavior during routine clinical activities. Am J Infect Control 2014;42(2):144–7.
35. Pittet D. Compliance with hand disinfection and its impact on hospital-acquired infections. J Hosp Infect 2001;48(Suppl A):S40–6.
36. McArdle FI, Lee RJ, Gibb AP, et al. How much time is needed for hand hygiene in intensive care? A prospective trained observer study of rates of contact between healthcare workers and intensive care patients. J Hosp Infect 2006;62(3):304–10.
37. Lankford MG, Zembower TR, Trick WE, et al. Influence of role models and hospital design on hand hygiene of healthcare workers. Emerg Infect Dis 2003;9(2):217–23.
38. Whitby M, McLaws ML. Handwashing in healthcare workers: accessibility of sink location does not improve compliance. J Hosp Infect 2004;58(4):247–53.
39. Chan BP, Homa K, Kirkland KB. Effect of varying the number and location of alcohol-based hand rub dispensers on usage in a general inpatient medical unit. Infect Control Hosp Epidemiol 2013;34(9):987–9.
40. Graham M, Nixon R, Burrell LJ, et al. Low rates of cutaneous adverse reactions to alcohol-based hand hygiene solution during prolonged use in a large teaching hospital. Antimicrob Agents Chemother 2005;49(10):4404–5.
41. Heeg P. Does hand care ruin hand disinfection? J Hosp Infect 2001;48(Suppl A):S37–9.
42. Franca SR, Marra AR, de Oliveira Figueiredo RA, et al. The effect of contact precautions on hand hygiene compliance. Am J Infect Control 2013;41(6):558–9.
43. Fuller C, Savage J, Besser S, et al. "The dirty hand in the latex glove": a study of hand hygiene compliance when gloves are worn. Infect Control Hosp Epidemiol 2011;32(12):1194–9.
44. Golan Y, Doron S, Griffith J, et al. The impact of gown-use requirement on hand hygiene compliance. Clin Infect Dis 2006;42(3):370–6.
45. Cusini A, Nydegger D, Kaspar T, et al. Improved hand hygiene compliance after eliminating mandatory glove use from contact precautions-Is less more? Am J Infect Control 2015;43:922–7.
46. Duggan JM, Hensley S, Khuder S, et al. Inverse correlation between level of professional education and rate of handwashing compliance in a teaching hospital. Infect Control Hosp Epidemiol 2008;29(6):534–8.
47. Wendt C, Knautz D, von Baum H. Differences in hand hygiene behavior related to the contamination risk of healthcare activities in different groups of healthcare workers. Infect Control Hosp Epidemiol 2004;25(3):203–6.
48. Rome M, Sabel A, Price CS, et al. Hand hygiene compliance. J Hosp Infect 2007;65(2):173.
49. Erasmus V, Brouwer W, van Beeck EF, et al. A qualitative exploration of reasons for poor hand hygiene among hospital workers: lack of positive role models and of convincing evidence that hand hygiene prevents cross-infection. Infect Control Hosp Epidemiol 2009;30(5):415–9.
50. Pittet D, Simon A, Hugonnet S, et al. Hand hygiene among physicians: performance, beliefs, and perceptions. Ann Intern Med 2004;141(1):1–8.
51. Wisniewski MF, Kim S, Trick WE, et al. Effect of education on hand hygiene beliefs and practices: a 5-year program. Infect Control Hosp Epidemiol 2007;28(1):88–91.
52. Reich JA, Goodstein ME, Callahan SE, et al. Physician report cards and rankings yield long-lasting hand hygiene compliance exceeding 90%. Crit Care 2015;19:292.

53. Whitby M, McLaws ML. Methodological difficulties in hand hygiene research. J Hosp Infect 2007;67(2):194–5.
54. Girou E, Oppein F. Handwashing compliance in a French university hospital: new perspective with the introduction of hand-rubbing with a waterless alcohol-based solution. J Hosp Infect 2001;48(Suppl A):S55–7.
55. Pittet D, Hugonnet S, Harbarth S, et al. Effectiveness of a hospital-wide programme to improve compliance with hand hygiene. Infection Control Programme. Lancet 2000;356(9238):1307–12.
56. Randle J, Clarke M, Storr J. Hand hygiene compliance in healthcare workers. J Hosp Infect 2006;64(3):205–9.
57. Souweine B, Lautrette A, Aumeran C, et al. Comparison of acceptability, skin tolerance, and compliance between handwashing and alcohol-based handrub in ICUs: results of a multicentric study. Intensive Care Med 2009;35(7):1216–24.
58. Harbarth S, Pittet D, Grady L, et al. Interventional study to evaluate the impact of an alcohol-based hand gel in improving hand hygiene compliance. Pediatr Infect Dis J 2002;21(6):489–95.
59. Santana SL, Furtado GH, Coutinho AP, et al. Assessment of healthcare professionals' adherence to hand hygiene after alcohol-based hand rub introduction at an intensive care unit in Sao Paulo, Brazil. Infect Control Hosp Epidemiol 2007;28(3):365–7.
60. Whitby M, McLaws ML, Slater K, et al. Three successful interventions in health care workers that improve compliance with hand hygiene: is sustained replication possible? Am J Infect Control 2008;36(5):349–55.
61. McGuckin M, Waterman R, Govednik J. Hand hygiene compliance rates in the United States–a one-year multicenter collaboration using product/volume usage measurement and feedback. Am J Med Qual 2009;24(3):205–13.
62. McGuckin M, Waterman R, Shubin A. Consumer attitudes about health care-acquired infections and hand hygiene. Am J Med Qual 2006;21(5):342–6.
63. Julian KG, Subramanian K, Brumbach A, et al. Attitudes of healthcare workers and patients toward individualized hand hygiene reminders. Infect Control Hosp Epidemiol 2008;29(8):781–2.
64. Lent V, Eckstein EC, Cameron AS, et al. Evaluation of patient participation in a patient empowerment initiative to improve hand hygiene practices in a Veterans Affairs medical center. Am J Infect Control 2009;37(2):117–20.
65. Longtin Y, Sax H, Allegranzi B, et al. Patients' beliefs and perceptions of their participation to increase healthcare worker compliance with hand hygiene. Infect Control Hosp Epidemiol 2009;30(9):830–9.
66. Kirkland KB, Homa KA, Lasky RA, et al. Impact of a hospital-wide hand hygiene initiative on healthcare-associated infections: results of an interrupted time series. BMJ Qual Saf 2012;21(12):1019–26.
67. Johnson L, Grueber S, Schlotzhauer C, et al. A multifactorial action plan improves hand hygiene adherence and significantly reduces central line-associated bloodstream infections. Am J Infect Control 2014;42(11):1146–51.
68. Kowitt B, Jefferson J, Mermel LA. Factors associated with hand hygiene compliance at a tertiary care teaching hospital. Infect Control Hosp Epidemiol 2013;34(11):1146–52.
69. Schweizer ML, Reisinger HS, Ohl M, et al. Searching for an optimal hand hygiene bundle: a meta-analysis. Clin Infect Dis 2014;58(2):248–59.
70. Chen LF, Carriker C, Staheli R, et al. Observing and improving hand hygiene compliance: implementation and refinement of an electronic-assisted

direct-observer hand hygiene audit program. Infect Control Hosp Epidemiol 2013;34(2):207–10.

71. Ellison RT 3rd, Barysauskas CM, Rundensteiner EA, et al. A Prospective Controlled Trial of an Electronic Hand Hygiene Reminder System. Open Forum Infect Dis 2015;2(4):ofv121.

72. Armellino D, Hussain E, Schilling ME, et al. Using high-technology to enforce low-technology safety measures: the use of third-party remote video auditing and real-time feedback in healthcare. Clin Infect Dis 2012;54(1):1–7.

73. Sepkowitz KA. Why doesn't hand hygiene work better? Lancet Infect Dis 2012; 12(2):96–7.

74. Gould DJ, Moralejo D, Drey N, et al. Interventions to improve hand hygiene compliance in patient care. Cochrane Database Syst Rev 2010;(9):CD005186.

75. Pittet D, Sax H, Hugonnet S, et al. Cost implications of successful hand hygiene promotion. Infect Control Hosp Epidemiol 2004;25(3):264–6.

76. Song X, Stockwell DC, Floyd T, et al. Improving hand hygiene compliance in health care workers: Strategies and impact on patient outcomes. Am J Infect Control 2013;41(10):e101–5.

77. DiDiodato G. Has improved hand hygiene compliance reduced the risk of hospital-acquired infections among hospitalized patients in Ontario? Analysis of publicly reported patient safety data from 2008 to 2011. Infect Control Hosp Epidemiol 2013;34(6):605–10.

78. Barnes SL, Morgan DJ, Harris AD, et al. Preventing the transmission of multidrug-resistant organisms: modeling the relative importance of hand hygiene and environmental cleaning interventions. Infect Control Hosp Epidemiol 2014;35(9): 1156–62.

79. Austin DJ, Bonten MJ, Weinstein RA, et al. Vancomycin-resistant enterococci in intensive-care hospital settings: transmission dynamics, persistence, and the impact of infection control programs. Proc Natl Acad Sci U S A 1999;96(12): 6908–13.

80. Beggs CB, Shepherd SJ, Kerr KG. How does healthcare worker hand hygiene behaviour impact upon the transmission of MRSA between patients?: an analysis using a Monte Carlo model. BMC Infect Dis 2009;9:64.

# Disinfection and Sterilization in Health Care Facilities: An Overview and Current Issues

William A. Rutala, PhD, MPH[a,b,*], David J. Weber, MD, MPH[a,b]

KEYWORDS

- Disinfection • Sterilization • Health care facilities

KEY POINTS

- All invasive procedures involve contact by a medical device or surgical instrument with patients' sterile tissue or mucous membrane.
- The level of disinfection or sterilization depends on the intended use of the object: critical (items that contact sterile tissue, such as surgical instrument), semicritical (items that contact mucous membranes, such as endoscopes), and noncritical (items that contact only intact skin, such as stethoscopes) require sterilization, high-level disinfection, or low-level disinfection, respectively.
- Cleaning must precede high-level disinfection and sterilization.
- Failure to properly disinfect devices used in health care (eg, endoscopes) has led to many outbreaks.
- Health care providers should be familiar with current issues, such as the role of the environment in disease transmission, reprocessing semicritical items (eg, endoscopes), and new technologies (eg, hydrogen peroxide mist).

## INTRODUCTION

In the United States in 2010 there were approximately 51.4 million inpatient surgical procedures and an even larger number of invasive medical procedures.[1] In 2009, there were more than 6.9 million gastrointestinal (GI) upper, 11.5 million GI lower, and 228,000 biliary endoscopies performed.[2] Each of these procedures involves contact by a medical device or surgical instrument with patients' sterile tissue or mucous membranes. A major risk of all such procedures is the introduction of pathogenic

Potential Conflicts of Interest: Dr W.A. Rutala is a consultant for Clorox and has received honoraria from 3M. Dr D.J. Weber is a consultant for Clorox and Germitec.
a Hospital Epidemiology, University of North Carolina Health Care System, Chapel Hill, NC 27514, USA; b Division of Infectious Diseases, University of North Carolina School of Medicine, Chapel Hill, NC 27599-7030, USA
* Corresponding author. Hospital Epidemiology, UNC Hospitals, Room 1001, West Wing, Manning Drive, Chapel Hill, NC 27599-7030.
E-mail address: brutala@unch.unc.edu

Infect Dis Clin N Am 30 (2016) 609–637
http://dx.doi.org/10.1016/j.idc.2016.04.002
0891-5520/16/$ – see front matter © 2016 Elsevier Inc. All rights reserved.

microbes, which can lead to infection. Failure to properly disinfect or sterilize equipment may lead to transmission via contaminated medical and surgical devices (eg, carbapenem-resistant *Enterobacteriaceae* [CRE]).[3,4]

Achieving disinfection and sterilization through the use of disinfectants and sterilization practices is essential for ensuring that medical and surgical instruments do not transmit infectious pathogens to patients. Because it is not necessary to sterilize all patient-care items, health care policies must identify whether cleaning, disinfection, or sterilization is indicated based primarily on each item's intended use, manufacturers recommendations, and guidelines.

Multiple studies in many countries have documented lack of compliance with established guidelines for disinfection and sterilization.[5] Failure to comply with scientifically based guidelines has led to numerous outbreaks and patient exposures.[6–8] Because of noncompliance with recommended reprocessing procedures, the Centers for Disease Control and Prevention (CDC) and the Food and Drug Administration (FDA) issued a health advisory alerting health care providers and facilities about the public health need to properly maintain, clean, and disinfect and sterilize reusable medical devices in September 2015.[9] In this article, which is an updated and modified version of earlier articles,[10–14] a pragmatic approach to the judicious selection and proper use of disinfection and sterilization processes is presented, based on well-designed studies assessing the efficacy (via laboratory investigations) and effectiveness (via clinical studies) of disinfection and sterilization procedures.

## A RATIONAL APPROACH TO DISINFECTION AND STERILIZATION

Almost 50 years ago, Earle H. Spaulding[15] devised a rational approach to disinfection and sterilization of patient-care items or equipment. This classification scheme is so clear and logical that it has been retained, refined, and successfully used by infection control professionals and others when planning methods for disinfection or sterilization.[10–14] Spaulding thought that the nature of disinfection could be understood more readily if instruments and items for patient care were divided into 3 categories based on the degree of risk of infection involved in the use of the items. The 3 categories he described were critical, semicritical, and noncritical. This terminology is used by the CDC's "Guidelines for Environmental Infection Control in Healthcare Facilities"[16] and the CDC's "Guideline for Disinfection and Sterilization in Healthcare Facilities."[13] These categories and the methods to achieve sterilization, high-level disinfection, and low-level disinfection are summarized in **Table 1**. Although the scheme remains valid, there are some examples of disinfection studies with prions, viruses, mycobacteria, and protozoa that challenge the current definitions and expectations of high-level disinfection (HLD) and low-level disinfection.[22]

In May 2015, the FDA convened a panel to discuss recent reports and epidemiologic investigations of the transmission of infections associated with the use of duodenoscopes in endoscopic retrograde cholangiopancreatography (ERCP) procedures.[23] After presentations from industry, professional societies, and invited speakers, the panel made several recommendations to include reclassifying duodenoscopes based on the Spaulding classification from semicritical to critical to support the shift from HLD to sterilization.[24] This change could be accomplished by shifting from HLD for duodenoscopes to sterilization and modifying the Spaulding definition of critical items from "objects which enter sterile tissue or the vascular system or through which blood flows should be sterile" to "objects which directly or secondarily (ie, via a mucous membrane such as duodenoscope) enter normally sterile tissue of the vascular system of through which blood flows should be sterile."[24,25] Implementation of this

**Table 1**
Methods for disinfection and sterilization of patient-care items and environmental surfaces

| Process | Level of Microbial Inactivation | Method | Examples (with Processing Times) | Health Care Application (Examples) |
|---|---|---|---|---|
| Sterilization[a] | Destroys all microorganisms, including bacterial spores | High temperature | Steam (~40 min), dry heat (1–6 h depending on temperature) | Heat-tolerant critical (surgical instruments) and semicritical patient-care items |
| | | Low temperature | Ethylene oxide gas (~15 h), HP gas plasma (28–52 min), HP and ozone (46 min), HP vapor (55 min) | Heat-sensitive critical and semicritical patient-care items |
| | | Liquid immersion | Chemical sterilants[b]: >2% glut (~10 h); 1.12% glut with 1.93% phenol (12 h); 7.35% HP with 0.23% PA (3 h); 8.3% HP with 7.0% PA (5 h); 7.5% HP (6 h); 1.0% HP with 0.08% PA (8 h); ≥0.2% PA (12 min at 50°C–56°C) | Heat-sensitive critical and semicritical patient-care items that can be immersed |
| HLD | Destroys all microorganisms except some bacterial spores | Heat automated | Pasteurization (65°C–77°C, 30 min) | Heat-sensitive semicritical items (eg, respiratory therapy equipment) |
| | | Liquid immersion | Chemical sterilants/HLDs[b]: >2% glut (20–90 min at 20°C–25°C); >2% glut (5 min at 35.0°C–37.8°C); 0.55% OPA (12 min at 20°C); 1.12% glut with 1.93% phenol (20 min at 25°C); 7.35% HP with 0.23% PA (15 min at 20°C); 7.5% HP (30 min at 20°C); 1.0% HP with 0.08% PA (25 min); 400–450 ppm chlorine (10 min at 20°C); 2.0% HP (8 min at 20°C); 3.4% glut with 26% isopropanol (10 min at 20°C) | Heat-sensitive semicritical items (eg, GI endoscopes, bronchoscopes, endocavitary probes) |

(continued on next page)

**Table 1**
**(continued)**

| Process | Level of Microbial Inactivation | Method | Examples (with Processing Times) | Health Care Application (Examples) |
|---|---|---|---|---|
| Low-level disinfection | Destroys vegetative bacteria and some fungi and viruses but not mycobacteria or spores | Liquid contact | EPA-registered hospital disinfectant with no tuberculocidal claim (eg, chlorine-based products, phenolics, improved HP, HP plus PA, quaternary ammonium compounds, exposure times at least 1 min) or 70%–90% alcohol | Noncritical patient care item (blood pressure cuff) or surface (bedside table) with no visible blood |

*Abbreviations:* EPA, Environmental Protection Agency; glut, glutaraldehyde; HLD, high-level disinfection; HP, hydrogen peroxide; OPA, ortho-phthalaldehyde; PA, peracetic acid; ppm, parts per million.

[a] Prions (such as Creutzfeldt-Jakob disease) exhibit an unusual resistance to conventional chemical and physical decontamination methods and are not readily inactivated by conventional sterilization procedures.[17]

[b] Consult the FDA-cleared package insert for information about the cleared contact time and temperature, and see reference[18] for discussion why greater than 2% glutaraldehyde products are used at a reduced exposure time (2% glutaraldehyde at 20 minutes, 20°C). Increasing the temperature using an automated endoscope reprocesser (AER) will reduce the contact time (eg, ortho-phthalaldehyde 12 minutes at 20°C but 5 minutes at 25°C in AER). Exposure temperatures for some of the aforementioned high-level disinfectants varies from 20°C to 25°C; check FDA-cleared temperature conditions.[19] Tubing must be completely filled for high-level disinfection and liquid chemical sterilization. Material compatibility should be investigated when appropriate (eg, hydrogen peroxide [HP] and HP with peracetic acid will cause functional damage to endoscopes). Intermediate-level disinfectants destroy vegetative bacteria, mycobacteria, most viruses, and most fungi but not spores and may include chlorine-based products, phenolics, and improved HP. Intermediate-level disinfectants are not included in **Table 1** as there as there is no device or surface for which intermediate-level disinfection is specifically recommended over low-level disinfection.
*Adapted from* Refs.[11–13,20,21]

recommendations requires sterilization technology that achieves a sterility assurance level of $10^{-6}$ of complex medical instruments, such as duodenoscopes. Ideally, this shift would eventually involve not only endoscopes that secondarily enter normally sterile tissue (eg, duodenoscopes, bronchoscopes) but also other semicritical devices (eg, GI endoscopes).[24,25]

### Critical Items

Critical items are so called because of the high risk of infection if such an item is contaminated with any microorganism, including bacterial spores. Thus, it is critical that objects that enter sterile tissue or the vascular system be sterile because any microbial contamination could result in disease transmission. This category includes surgical instruments, cardiac and urinary catheters, and implants used in sterile body cavities. The items in this category should be purchased as sterile or be sterilized by steam sterilization if possible. If heat sensitive, the object may be treated with ethylene oxide (ETO), hydrogen peroxide (HP) gas plasma, vaporized HP, HP vapor (HPV) plus ozone, or by liquid chemical sterilants if other methods are unsuitable. **Table 1** and **Tables 2** and **3** list sterilization processes and liquid chemical sterilants and the advantages and disadvantages of each. With the exception of 0.2% peracetic acid (12 minutes at 50°C–56°C), the indicated exposure times for liquid chemical sterilants range from 3 to 12 hours.[19] Liquid chemical sterilants can be relied on to produce sterility only if cleaning, which eliminates organic and inorganic material, precedes treatment and if proper guidelines as to concentration, contact time, temperature, and pH are met. Another limitation to sterilization of devices with liquid chemical sterilants is that the devices cannot be wrapped during processing in a liquid chemical sterilant; thus, it is impossible to maintain sterility following processing and during storage. Furthermore, devices may require rinsing following exposure to the liquid chemical sterilant with water that, in general, is not sterile. Therefore, because of the inherent limitations of using liquid chemical sterilants in a nonautomated (or automated) reprocessor, their use should be restricted to reprocessing critical devices that are heat sensitive and incompatible with other sterilization methods.

In contrast to semicritical items that have been associated with greater than 100 outbreaks of infection,[6] critical items have rarely,[26] if ever, been associated with disease transmission. For example, any deviation from proper reprocessing (such as crevices associated with the elevator channel) of an endoscope could lead to failure to eliminate contamination with a possibility of subsequent patient-to-patient transmission due to a low or nonexistent margin of safety. This low (or nonexistent) margin of safety associated with endoscope reprocessing compares with the $17\text{-log}_{10}$ margin of safety associated with cleaning and sterilization of surgical instruments (ie, $12\text{-log}_{10}$ reduction via sterilization and at least a net $5\text{-log}_{10}$ reduction based on the microbial load on surgical instruments [2-logs][27] and microbial reduction via a washer disinfector [7-logs]).[18]

### Semicritical Items

Semicritical items are those that come in contact with mucous membranes or nonintact skin. Respiratory therapy and anesthesia equipment, gastrointestinal endoscopes, bronchoscopes, laryngoscopes, endocavitary probes, prostate biopsy probes,[28] cystoscopes,[29] hysteroscopes, infrared coagulation devices,[30] and diaphragm fitting rings are included in this category. These medical devices should be free of all microorganisms (ie, mycobacteria, fungi, viruses, bacteria), although small numbers of bacterial spores may be present. Intact mucous membranes, such as those of the lungs or the gastrointestinal tract, are generally resistant to infection by

**Table 2**
**Summary of advantages and disadvantages of chemical agents used as chemical sterilants[a] or as high-level disinfectants**

| Sterilization Method | Advantages | Disadvantages |
|---|---|---|
| Peracetic acid/HP | • No activation required<br>• Odor or irritation not significant | • Material compatibility concerns (lead, brass, copper, zinc) both cosmetic and functional<br>• Limited clinical experience<br>• Potential for eye and skin damage |
| Glutaraldehyde | • Numerous use studies published<br>• Relatively inexpensive<br>• Excellent material compatibility | • Respiratory irritation from glutaraldehyde vapor<br>• Pungent and irritating odor<br>• Relatively slow mycobactericidal activity (unless other disinfectants added such as phenolic, alcohol)<br>• Coagulates blood and fixes tissue to surfaces<br>• Allergic contact dermatitis |
| HP | • No activation required<br>• May enhance removal of organic matter and organisms<br>• No disposal issues<br>• No odor or irritation issues<br>• Does not coagulate blood or fix tissues to surfaces<br>• Inactivates *Cryptosporidium*<br>• Use studies published | • Material compatibility concerns (brass, zinc, copper, and nickel/silver plating) both cosmetic and functional<br>• Serious eye damage with contact |
| OPA | • Fast-acting high-level disinfectant<br>• No activation required<br>• Odor not significant<br>• Excellent materials compatibility claimed<br>• Does not coagulate blood or fix tissues to surfaces claimed | • Stains protein gray (eg, skin, mucous membranes, clothing, and environmental surfaces)<br>• Limited clinical experience<br>• More expensive than glutaraldehyde<br>• Eye irritation with contact<br>• Slow sporicidal activity<br>• Anaphylactic reactions to OPA in patients with bladder cancer with repeated exposure to OPA through cystoscopy |

| Peracetic acid | • Standardized cycle (eg, Liquid Chemical Sterilant Processing System using Peracetic Acid, rinsed with extensively treated potable water)<br>• Low temperature (50°C–55°C) liquid immersion sterilization<br>• Environmental friendly byproducts (acetic acid, $O_2$, $H_2O$)<br>• Fully automated<br>• Single-use system eliminates need for concentration testing<br>• May enhance removal of organic material and endotoxin<br>• No adverse health effects to operators under normal operating conditions<br>• Compatible with many materials and instruments<br>• Does not coagulate blood or fix tissues to surfaces<br>• Sterilant flows through scope facilitating salt, protein, and microbe removal<br>• Rapidly sporicidal<br>• Provides procedure standardization (constant dilution, perfusion of channel, temperatures, exposure) | • Potential material incompatibility (eg, aluminum anodized coating becomes dull)<br>• Used for immersible instruments only<br>• Biological indicator may not be suitable for routine monitoring<br>• One scope or a small number of instruments can be processed in a cycle<br>• More expensive (endoscope repairs, operating costs, purchase costs) than high-level disinfection<br>• Serious eye and skin damage (concentrated solution) with contact<br>• Point-of-use system, no sterile storage<br>• An AER using 0.2% peracetic acid not FDA cleared as sterilization process but HLD |
| Improved HP (2.0%); HLD | • No activation required<br>• No odor<br>• Nonstaining<br>• No special venting requirements<br>• Manual or automated applications<br>• 12-mo shelf-life, 14-d reuse<br>• 8 min at 20°C HLD claim | • Material compatibility concerns due to limited clinical experience<br>• Antimicrobial claims not independently verified<br>• Organic material resistance concerns due to limited data |

*Abbreviations:* AER, automated endoscope reprocessor; OPA, ortho-phthalaldehyde.

[a] All products effective in presence of organic soil, relatively easy to use, and have a broad spectrum of antimicrobial activity (bacteria, fungi, viruses, bacterial spores, and mycobacteria). The aforementioned characteristics are documented in the literature; contact the manufacturer of the instrument and sterilant for additional information. All products listed are cleared by the FDA as chemical sterilants except ortho-phthalaldehyde, which is an FDA-cleared HLD.

*Adapted from* Refs.[10–13,20]

**Table 3**
**Summary of advantages and disadvantages of commonly used sterilization technologies**

| Sterilization Method | Advantages | Disadvantages |
|---|---|---|
| Steam | • Nontoxic to patients, staff, environment<br>• Cycle easy to control and monitor<br>• Rapidly microbicidal<br>• Least affected by organic/inorganic soils among sterilization processes listed<br>• Rapid cycle time<br>• Penetrates medical packaging, device lumens | • It is deleterious for heat-sensitive instruments.<br>• Microsurgical instruments are damaged by repeated exposure.<br>• It may leave instruments wet, causing them to rust.<br>• There is potential for burns. |
| HP gas plasma | • Safe for the environment and health care personnel<br>• Leaves no toxic residuals<br>• Cycle time ≥28 min, and no aeration necessary<br>• Used for heat- and moisture-sensitive items because process temperature <50°C<br>• Simple to operate, install (208-V outlet), and monitor<br>• Compatible with most medical devices<br>• Only requires electrical outlet | • Cellulose (paper), linens, and liquids cannot be processed.<br>• Endoscope or medical device restrictions are based on lumen internal diameter and length (see manufacturer's recommendations).<br>• It requires synthetic packaging (polypropylene wraps, polyolefin pouches) and a special container tray.<br>• HP may be toxic at levels >1 ppm TWA. |
| 100% ETO | • Penetrates packaging materials, device lumens<br>• Potential for gas leak and ETO exposure minimized by single-dose cartridge and negative-pressure chamber<br>• Simple to operate and monitor<br>• Compatible with most medical materials | • It requires aeration time to remove ETO residue.<br>• ETO is toxic, a carcinogen, and flammable.<br>• ETO emission is regulated by states, but catalytic cell removes 99.9% of ETO and converts it to carbon dioxide and water.<br>• ETO cartridges should be stored in flammable liquid storage cabinet.<br>• It has a lengthy cycle/aeration time. |
| Vaporized HP | • Safe for the environment and health care personnel<br>• Leaves no toxic residue; no aeration necessary<br>• Cycle time 55 min<br>• Used for heat- and moisture-sensitive items (metal and nonmetal devices) | • Medical device restrictions are based on lumen internal diameter and length; see manufacturer's recommendations (eg, stainless steel lumen 1 mm diameter, 125 mm length).<br>• It is not used for liquid, linens, powders, or any cellulose materials.<br>• Requires synthetic packaging (polypropylene).<br>• There are limited materials compatibility data.<br>• There are limited clinical use and comparative microbicidal efficacy data. |

(*continued on next page*)

| Table 3 (continued) | | |
| --- | --- | --- |
| Sterilization Method | Advantages | Disadvantages |
| HP and ozone | • Safe for the environment and health care personnel<br>• Uses dual sterilants, HP, and ozone<br>• Does not need aeration because of no toxic byproducts<br>• Compatible with common medical devices<br>• Cycle time 46 min<br>• FDA cleared for general instruments, single-channel flexible endoscopes, and rigid and semirigid channeled devices | • Endoscope or medical device restrictions are based on lumen internal diameter and length (see manufacturer's recommendations).<br>• There are limited clinical use (no published data on material compatibility/penetrability/organic material resistance) and limited microbicidal efficacy data.<br>• It requires synthetic packaging (polypropylene wraps, polyolefin pouches) and a special container tray. |

*Abbreviations:* ETO, ethylene oxide; HP, hydrogen peroxide; TWA, time-weighted average.
*Adapted from* Refs.[10–13,20]

common bacterial spores but susceptible to other organisms, such as bacteria, mycobacteria, and viruses. Semicritical items minimally require HLD using chemical disinfectants. Glutaraldehyde, HP, ortho-phthalaldehyde (OPA), peracetic acid with HP, and chlorine (via electrochemical activation) are cleared by the FDA[19] and are dependable high-level disinfectants provided the factors influencing germicidal procedures are met (see **Tables 1** and **2**). The exposure time for most high-level disinfectants varies from 8 to 45 minutes at 20°C to 25°C.[19]

Because semicritical equipment has been associated with reprocessing errors that result in patient lookback and patient notifications, it is essential that control measures be instituted to prevent patient exposures.[7] Before new equipment (especially semicritical equipment as the margin of safety is less than that for sterilization)[25] is used for patient care on more than one patient, reprocessing procedures for that equipment should be developed. Staff should receive training on the safe use and reprocessing of the equipment and be competency tested. At the University of North Carolina (UNC) Hospitals, to ensure patient-safe instruments, all staff that reprocess semicritical instruments (eg, instruments which contact a mucous membrane such as vaginal probes, endoscopes, prostate probes) are required to attend a 3-hour class on HLD of semicritical instruments. The class includes the rationale for and importance of high-level disinfection, discussion of high-level disinfectants and exposure times, reprocessing steps, monitoring minimum effective concentration, personal protective equipment, and the reprocessing environment (establish dirty-to-clean flow). Infection control rounds or audits should be conducted annually in all clinical areas that reprocess critical and semicritical devices to ensure adherence to the reprocessing standards and policies. Results of infection control rounds should be provided to the unit managers, and deficiencies in reprocessing should be corrected and the corrective measures documented to infection control within 2 weeks (immediately correct patient safety issues, such as exposure time to high-level disinfectant).

## Noncritical Items

Noncritical items are those that come in contact with intact skin but not mucous membranes. Intact skin acts as an effective barrier to most microorganisms; therefore, the sterility of items coming in contact with intact skin is "not critical." Examples of noncritical items are bedpans, blood pressure cuffs, crutches, bed rails, linens, bedside tables, patient furniture, and floors. In contrast to critical and some semicritical items, most noncritical reusable items may be decontaminated where they are used and do not need to be transported to a central processing area. There is virtually no documented risk of transmitting infectious agents to patients via noncritical items[31] when they are used as noncritical items and do not contact nonintact skin and/or mucous membranes. However, these items (eg, bedside tables, bed rails) could potentially contribute to secondary transmission by contaminating hands of healthcare personnel or by contact with medical equipment that will subsequently come in contact with patients.[32] **Table 1** and **Table 4** list several low-level disinfectants that may be used for noncritical items. **Table 4** lists the advantages and disadvantages of the low-level disinfectants that are used on noncritical patient care items (eg, blood pressure cuffs) and noncritical environmental surfaces. The exposure time for low-level disinfection of noncritical items is at least 1 minute.

## CURRENT ISSUES IN DISINFECTION AND STERILIZATION
### Reprocessing of Endoscopes

Physicians use endoscopes to diagnose and treat numerous medical disorders. Although endoscopes represent a valuable diagnostic and therapeutic tool in modern medicine, more health care–associated outbreaks have been linked to contaminated endoscopes than to any other reusable medical device.[6,8] Additionally, endemic transmission of infections associated with GI endoscopes may go unrecognized for several reasons, including inadequate surveillance of outpatient procedures, long lag time between colonization and infection, low frequency of infection, and because pathogens are the usual enteric flora. In addition, the risk of some procedures might be lower than others (eg, colonoscopy vs ERCP), whereby normally sterile areas are contaminated in the latter. In order to prevent the spread of health care–associated infections (HAIs), all heat-sensitive endoscopes (eg, GI endoscopes, bronchoscopes, nasopharyngoscopes) must be properly cleaned and, at a minimum, subjected to HLD following each use. HLD can be expected to destroy all microorganisms; although when high numbers of bacterial spores are present, a few spores may survive.

Recommendations for the cleaning and disinfection of endoscopic equipment have been published and should be strictly followed.[13,35,36] Unfortunately, audits have shown that personnel often do not adhere to guidelines on reprocessing[5] and outbreaks of infection continue to occur.[3,6,8,37] Additionally, recent studies have suggested that current reprocessing guidelines are not sufficient to ensure successful decontamination.[38] In order to minimize patient risks and ensure that reprocessing personnel are properly trained, there should be initial and annual competency testing for each individual who is involved in reprocessing endoscopic instruments.[13,35,36]

In general, endoscope disinfection or sterilization with a liquid chemical sterilant or high-level disinfectant involves 5 steps after leak testing: (1) clean: mechanically clean internal and external surfaces, including brushing internal channels and flushing each internal channel with water and a enzymatic cleaner or detergent; (2) disinfect: immerse endoscope in high-level disinfectant (or chemical sterilant) and perfuse (eliminates air pockets and ensures contact of the germicide with the internal channels) disinfectant into all accessible channels, such as the suction/biopsy channel and air/water channel, and expose for a time recommended for specific products; (3) rinse: rinse the endoscope and all channels with sterile water, filtered water (commonly used

**Table 4**
**Summary of advantages and disadvantages of disinfectants used as low-level disinfectants**

| Disinfectant Active | Advantages | Disadvantages |
|---|---|---|
| Alcohol | • Bactericidal, tuberculocidal, fungicidal, virucidal<br>• Fast acting<br>• Noncorrosive<br>• Nonstaining<br>• Used to disinfect small surfaces, such as rubber stoppers on medication vials<br>• No toxic residue | • It is not sporicidal.<br>• It is affected by organic matter.<br>• It is slow acting against non-enveloped viruses (eg, norovirus).<br>• It has no detergent or cleaning properties.<br>• It is not EPA registered.<br>• It damages some instruments (eg, harden rubber, deteriorate glue).<br>• It is flammable. (Large amounts require special storage.)<br>• It evaporates rapidly making contact time compliance difficult.<br>• It is not recommended for use on large surfaces.<br>• Outbreaks are ascribed to contaminated alcohol.[33] |
| Sodium hypochlorite | • Bactericidal, tuberculocidal, fungicidal, virucidal<br>• Sporicidal<br>• Fast acting<br>• Inexpensive (in diluted form)<br>• Not flammable<br>• Unaffected by water hardness<br>• Reduces biofilms on surfaces<br>• Relatively stable (eg, 50% reduction in chlorine concentration in 30 d)[34]<br>• Used as the disinfectant in water treatment<br>• EPA registered | • There is a reaction hazard with acids and ammonias.<br>• It leaves a salt residue.<br>• Corrosive to metals (some ready-to-use products may be formulated with corrosion inhibitors)<br>• It is unstable when active. (Some ready-to-use products may be formulated with stabilizers to achieve longer shelf-life.)<br>• It is affected by organic matter.<br>• It discolors/stains fabrics.<br>• A potential hazard is production of trihalomethane.<br>• It has an odor. (Some ready-to-use products may be formulated with odor inhibitors.). It is irritating at high concentrations. |
| Improved HP | • Bactericidal, tuberculocidal, fungicidal, virucidal<br>• Fast efficacy<br>• Easy compliance with wet-contact times<br>• Safe for workers (lowest EPA toxicity category, IV)<br>• Benign for the environment<br>• Surface compatible<br>• Nonstaining<br>• EPA registered<br>• Not flammable | • It is more expensive than most other disinfecting actives.<br>• It is not sporicidal at low concentrations. |

(continued on next page)

**Table 4**
***(continued)***

| Disinfectant Active | Advantages | Disadvantages |
|---|---|---|
| Iodophors | • Bactericidal, mycobactericidal, virucidal<br>• Not flammable<br>• Used for disinfecting blood culture bottles | • It is not sporicidal.<br>• It is shown to degrade silicone catheters.<br>• It requires prolonged contact to kill fungi.<br>• It stains surfaces.<br>• It is used mainly as an antiseptic rather than disinfectant. |
| Phenolics | • Bactericidal, tuberculocidal, fungicidal, virucidal<br>• Inexpensive (in diluted form)<br>• Nonstaining<br>• Not flammable<br>• EPA registered | • It is not sporicidal.<br>• It is absorbed by porous materials and irritates tissue.<br>• Depigmentation of skin is caused by certain phenolics.<br>• It can cause hyperbilirubinemia in infants when phenolic is not prepared as recommended. |
| Quaternary ammonium compounds (eg, didecyl dimethyl ammonium bromide, dioctyl dimethyl ammonium bromide) | • Bactericidal, fungicidal, virucidal against enveloped viruses (eg, HIV)<br>• Good cleaning agents<br>• EPA registered<br>• Surface compatible<br>• Persistent antimicrobial activity when undisturbed<br>• Inexpensive (in diluted form) | • It is not sporicidal.<br>• In general, it is not tuberculocidal and virucidal against nonenveloped viruses.<br>• High water hardness and cotton/gauze can make less microbicidal.<br>• A few reports documented asthma as a result of exposure to benzalkonium chloride.<br>• It is affected by organic matter.<br>• Multiple outbreaks ascribed to contaminated benzalkonium chloride.[33] |
| Peracetic acid/HP | • Bactericidal, fungicidal, virucidal, and sporicidal (eg, *Clostridium difficile*)<br>• Active in the presence of organic material<br>• Environmental friendly by-products (acetic acid, $O_2$, $H_2O$)<br>• EPA registered<br>• Surface compatible | • It lacks stability.<br>• It has potential for material incompatibility (eg, brass, copper).<br>• It is more expensive than most other disinfecting actives.<br>• The odor may be irritating. |

If low-level disinfectant is prepared on-site (not ready to use), document correct concentration at a routine frequency.

*Abbreviations:* EPA, Environmental Protection Agency; HIV, human immunodeficiency virus; HP, hydrogen peroxide.

*Adapted from* Rutala WA, Weber DJ. Selection of the ideal disinfectant. Infect Control Hosp Epidemiol 2014;35:855–65; and Rutala WA, Weber DJ. Disinfection and sterilization in healthcare facilities. In: Han J, editor. SHEA practical healthcare epidemiology. University of Chicago Press.

with automated endoscope reprocessors), or tap water; (4) dry: rinse the insertion tube and inner channels with alcohol and dry with forced air after disinfection and before storage; and (5) store: store the endoscope in a way that prevents recontamination and promotes drying (eg, hung vertically).

*Outbreaks of carbapenem-resistant Enterobacteriaceae infection associated with duodenoscopes: what can we do to prevent infections?*

In the past 3 years, multiple reports of outbreaks have led the FDA, the CDC, and national news to raise awareness among the public and health care professionals that the complex design of duodenoscopes (used primarily for ERCP) may impede effective reprocessing. Several recent publications have associated multidrug-resistant (MDR) bacterial infections, especially due to CRE, in patients who have undergone ERCP with reprocessed duodenoscopes.[3,4,25,37,39] Unlike other endoscope outbreaks,[6] these recent outbreaks occurred even when the manufacturer's instructions and professional guidelines were followed correctly.[3,4]

The key concern raised by these outbreaks is that current reprocessing guidelines are not adequate to ensure a patient-safe GI endoscope (one devoid of potential pathogens), as the margin of safety associated with reprocessing endoscopes is minimal or nonexistent. There are at least 2 (and maybe 3) reasons for this reprocessing failure and why outbreaks continue to occur. First, studies have shown that the internal channel of GI endoscopes, including duodenoscopes, may contain $10^{7-10}$ ($7$–$10$-$\log_{10}$) enteric microorganisms.[40,41] Investigations have demonstrated that the cleaning step in endoscope reprocessing results in a 2- to 6-$\log_{10}$ reduction of microbes and the HLD step results in another 4- to 6-$\log_{10}$ reduction of mycobacteria for a total 6- to 12-$\log_{10}$ reduction of microbes.[40–42] Thus, the margin of safety associated with cleaning and HLD of GI endoscopes is minimal or nonexistent (level of contamination: 4-$\log_{10}$ [maximum contamination, minimal cleaning/HLD] to $-5$-$\log_{10}$ [minimum contamination, maximum cleaning/HLD]). Therefore, any deviation from proper reprocessing (such as crevices associated with the elevator channel) could lead to failure to eliminate contamination with a possibility of subsequent patient-to-patient transmission. This low (or nonexistent) margin of safety associated with endoscope reprocessing compares with the 17-$\log_{10}$ margin of safety associated with cleaning and sterilization of surgical instruments.[23]

Second, GI endoscopes not only have heavy microbial contamination ($10^7$–$10^{10}$ bacteria) but they are also complex with long, narrow channels, right-angle turns, and difficult-to-clean and disinfect components (eg, elevator channel). The elevator channel in duodenoscopes is unique to side-viewing endoscopes. It has a separate channel and provides orientation of catheters, guidewires, and accessories into the endoscopic visual field.[25] This channel is complex in design and has crevices that are difficult to access with a cleaning brush and may impede effective reprocessing.[43] Based on this and other recent studies, it is likely that MDR pathogens are acting as marker or indicator organisms for ineffective reprocessing of the complex design of duodenoscopes, which is an infectious risk to patients.

Third, biofilms could impact endoscope reprocessing failure and continued endoscope-related outbreaks.[44] Biofilms are multilayered bacteria plus exopolysaccharides that cement cells to surfaces. They develop in a wet environment. If reprocessing is performed promptly after use and the endoscope is dry, the opportunity for biofilm formation is minimal.[45,46] However, the formation of endoscopic biofilm during clinical practice may be related to reuse of reprocessing methods, such as reuse of detergent, manual cleaning, and incomplete drying.[47] Ideally, reprocessing should be initiated within an hour of use; however, there are no evidence-based guidelines on delayed endoscope reprocessing.[48] It is unclear if biofilms contribute to failure of endoscope reprocessing.

What should we do now? Unfortunately, there is currently no single, simple, and proven technology or prevention strategy that hospitals can use to guarantee patient safety. Of course, we must continue to emphasize the enforcement of evidenced-based practices, including equipment maintenance, and routine audits with at least yearly competency testing of reprocessing staff.[13,35,36] All reprocessing personnel must be knowledgeable and thoroughly trained on the reprocessing instructions for duodenoscopes. This training includes the new recommendations to use a small bristle cleaning brush and for additional flushing and cleaning steps of the duodenoscope elevator channel (http://medical.olympusamerica.com/sites/default/files/pdf/150326_TJF-Q180V_Customer_letter.pdf). Although these steps were described as validated, no public data are available on the ability of these new cleaning recommendations to yield an ERCP scope devoid of bacteria. But we must do more or additional outbreaks will likely continue. For example, all hospitals that reprocess duodenoscopes should select one of the enhanced methods for reprocessing duodenoscopes. These enhanced methods have been priority ranked with the first providing the greatest margin of safety.[25] They include (1) ETO sterilization after HLD with periodic microbiologic surveillance; (2) double HLD with periodic microbiologic surveillance; (3) HLD with scope quarantine until negative culture results are returned; (4) liquid chemical sterilant processing system using peracetic acid (rinsed with extensively treated potable water) with periodic microbiologic surveillance; (5) other FDA-cleared low-temperature sterilization technology (provided material compatibility and sterilization validation testing performed using the sterilizer and endoscope) after HLD, with periodic microbiologic surveillance; and (6) HLD with periodic microbiologic surveillance. These supplemental measures to enhance duodenoscope reprocessing made in May-June 2015[25] were reinforced by the FDA in August 2015.[43] UNC Hospitals has chosen ETO sterilization after HLD with periodic microbiologic surveillance as its primary reprocessing method for duodenoscopes and if the ETO sterilizer is not available, then double HLD with periodic microbiologic surveillance.[49]

## Role of the Environment in Disease Transmission

There is excellent evidence in the scientific literature that environmental contamination plays an important role in the transmission of several key health care–associated pathogens, including methicillin-resistant *Staphylococcus aureus* (MRSA), vancomycin-resistant *Enterococcus* (VRE), *Acinetobacter sp*, norovirus, and *Clostridium difficile*.[50–53] All these pathogens have been demonstrated to persist in the environment for days (in some cases months), frequently contaminate the environmental surfaces in rooms of colonized or infected patients, transiently colonize the hands of health care personnel, be transmitted by health care personnel, and cause outbreaks in which environmental transmission was deemed to play a role. Importantly, a study by Stiefel and colleagues[54] demonstrated that contact with the environment was just as likely to contaminate the hands of health care personnel as was direct contact with patients. Further, admission to a room in which the previous patient had been colonized or infected with MRSA, VRE, *Acinetobacter* or *C difficile* has been shown to be a risk factor for newly admitted patients to develop colonization or infection.[55–57]

### Improving room cleaning and disinfection and demonstrating the effectiveness of surface decontamination in reducing health care–associated infections

Investigators have reported that intervention programs aimed at improving surface cleaning and disinfection reduced HAIs.[58] Such interventions have generally included multiple activities: disinfectant product substitutions and interventions to improve the effectiveness of cleaning and disinfection (eg, improved housekeeper education, monitoring the thoroughness of cleaning [eg, by use of ATP assays or fluorescent dyes] with feedback of performance to the environmental service workers, and/or use of cleaning checklists).[58–61] Health care facilities must also allow adequate time for room processing to ensure adherence to all steps recommended by institutional policies and professional organization guidelines. The authors have found that collaboration between infection prevention and environmental services staff, nursing, and management is critical to an effective environmental cleaning program. This collaboration includes ensuring that environmental services staff recognize the significance and relationship of adhering to proper work procedures to reduction of microbial contamination. The assignment of cleaning responsibility (eg, medical equipment to be cleaned by nursing; environmental surfaces to be cleaned by environmental service) is also important to ensure all objects and surfaces in a patient room are decontaminated, especially the surfaces of medical equipment (eg, cardiac monitors). Improved environmental cleaning has been demonstrated to reduce the environmental contamination with VRE,[61] MRSA,[62] and *C difficile*.[63] Further, all studies have only focused improvement on a limited number of high-risk objects. Thus, a concern of published studies is that they have only demonstrated improved cleaning of a limited number of high-risk objects (or targeted objects) not an improvement in the overall thoroughness of room decontamination, which is the objective.

To the authors' knowledge only one study has objectively evaluated what constitutes high-touch objects in a patient room and no study has demonstrated epidemiologically what constitutes a high-risk object. Examples of what the literature refers to as high-touch objects includes bed rails, intravenous (IV) poles, call buttons, door knobs, floors, and bathroom facilities[64]; however, a study demonstrated high-touch objects in the intensive care unit were the bed rail, bed surface, and supply cart, whereas the high-touch surfaces in a patient ward were the bed rail, over-bed table, IV pump, and bed surface.[65] Importantly, the level of microbial contamination of room surfaces was not statistically different regardless of how often they were touched before and after cleaning. Until research identifies which objects and surfaces pose the greatest risk of pathogen transmission, all noncritical surfaces that are touched must be cleaned/disinfected.[66]

### No-touch (or mechanical) methods for room decontamination

As noted earlier, multiple studies have demonstrated that environmental surfaces and objects in rooms are frequently not properly cleaned and these surfaces may be important in transmission of health care–associated pathogens. Further, although interventions aimed at improving cleaning thoroughness have demonstrated effectiveness, many surfaces remain inadequately cleaned and, therefore, potentially contaminated. For this reason, several manufacturers have developed room disinfection units that can decontaminate environmental surfaces and objects. These no-touch systems generally use one of 2 methods: either UV light or HPV/mist.[53] These technologies supplement, but do not replace, standard cleaning and disinfection because surfaces must be physically cleaned of dirt and debris.

**Ultraviolet light for room decontamination** UV radiation has been used for the control of pathogenic microorganisms in a variety of applications, such as control of legionellosis, as well as disinfection of air, surfaces, and instruments.[53,67] At certain wavelengths, UV light will break the molecular bonds in DNA, thereby destroying the organism. UV radiation has peak germicidal effectiveness in the wavelength range of 240 to 280 nm. Mercury gas bulbs emit UV-C at 254 nm, whereas xenon gas bulbs produce a broad spectrum of radiation that encompasses the UV (100–280 nm) and the visible (380–700 nm) electromagnetic spectra.[68] The efficacy of UV radiation is a function of many different parameters such as dose, distance, direct or shaded exposure, exposure time, lamp placement, pathogen, carrier or surface tested, inoculum method, organic load and orientation of carriers (eg, parallel vs perpendicular). Data demonstrate that several UV systems have effectiveness (eg, eliminate >3-log$_{10}$ vegetative bacteria [MRSA, VRE, *Acinetobacter baumannii*] and >2.4-log$_{10}$ *C difficile*) at relatively short exposure times (eg, 5–25 minutes for bacteria, 10–60 minutes for *C difficile* spores).[68–70] The studies also demonstrated reduced effectiveness when surfaces were not in direct line-of-sight.[68–72]

**Hydrogen peroxide systems for room decontamination**  Several systems that produce HP (eg, HPV, aerosolized dry mist HP) have been studied for their ability to decontaminate environmental surfaces and objects in hospital rooms. HPV has been used for the decontamination of rooms in health care.[73–83] Studies have demonstrated that HP systems are a highly effective method for eradicating various pathogens (eg, MRSA, *Mycobacterium tuberculosis*, *Serratia*, *C difficile* spores, *Clostridium botulinum* spores) from rooms, furniture, and equipment.

**Comparison of ultraviolet irradiation versus hydrogen peroxide for room decontamination**  UV devices and HP systems have their own advantages and disadvantages (**Table 5**),[53] and there is now ample evidence that these no-touch systems can reduce environmental contamination with health care–associated pathogens and reduce HAIs.[84] However, each specific marketed system should be studied and its efficacy demonstrated before being introduced into health care facilities. The main advantage of both types of units is their ability to achieve substantial reductions in vegetative bacteria. Another advantage is their ability to substantially reduce *C difficile* spores, as low-level disinfectants (such as quaternary ammonium compounds) have only limited or no measurable activity against spore-forming bacteria.[85] Both systems are residual free, and they decontaminate all exposed surfaces and equipment in the room.

Based on data that demonstrated a reduction of colonizations and/or infections associated with these technologies, the authors recommend they should be used for terminal room decontamination after discharge of patients on contact precautions. Because different UV and HP systems vary substantially, infection preventionists should review the peer-reviewed literature and the advantages/disadvantages of each technology (**Box 1**) and choose only devices with demonstrated bactericidal capability as assessed by carrier tests and/or the ability to disinfect actual patient rooms. Ultimately, one would select a device that also has demonstrated the ability to reduce HAIs.[84]

### Assessing Risk to Patients from Disinfection and Sterilization Failures

Disinfection and sterilization are critical components of infection control. Unfortunately, breaches of disinfection and sterilization guidelines are not uncommon. Patient notifications due to improper reprocessing of semicritical (eg, endoscopes) and critical medical instruments have occurred regularly.[7] This referenced article also provides a method for assessing patient risk for adverse events, especially infection. Use of a 14-step algorithm (**Box 2**) can guide an institution in managing potential disinfection and sterilization failures.[7,86]

### Human Papilloma Virus

Human papilloma virus is an extremely common sexually acquired infection and is the most important cause of cervical cancer. A 2014 article reported that the FDA-cleared high-level disinfectants (ie, glutaraldehyde, OPA) tested did not inactivate human papilloma virus, a nonenveloped virus.[87] These findings are inconsistent with many

**Table 5**
Clinical trials using ultraviolet or hydrogen peroxide devices for terminal room disinfection to reduce health care–associated infections

| Author, Year | Design | Setting | Modality Tested | Pathogens | Outcome (HAI) | Assessment of HH Compliance | Assessment of EVS Cleaning | Other HAI Prevention Initiatives |
|---|---|---|---|---|---|---|---|---|
| Boyce, 2008 | Before-after (CDI high incidence wards) | Community hospital | HPV (Bioquell) | CDI | 2.28–1.28 per 1000 Pt-days ($P = .047$) | No | No | NA |
| Cooper, 2011 | Before-after (2 cycles) | Hospitals | HPV (NS) | CDI | Decreased cases (incidence NS) | No | No | Yes |
| Levin, 2013 | Before-after | Community hospital | UV-PX, Xenex | CDI | 9.46–4.45 per 10,000 Pt-days ($P = .01$) | No | No | Yes |
| Passaretti, 2013 | Prospective cohort (comparison of MDRO acquisition; admitted to rooms with or without HPV decontamination) | Academic center | HPV (Bioquell) | MRSA VRE CDI MDRO-all | 2.3–1.2 ($P = .30$) 7.2–2.4 ($P<.01$) 2.4–1.0 ($P=.19$) 12.6–6.2 per 1000 Pt-days ($P<.01$) | No | No | No |
| Manian, 2013 | Before-after | Community hospital | HPV (Bioquell) | CDI | 0.88–0.55 cases per 1000 Pt-days ($P<.0001$) | Yes | No | No |

(continued on next page)

**Table 5**
*(continued)*

| Author, Year | Design | Setting | Modality Tested | Pathogens | Outcome (HAI) | Assessment of HH Compliance | Assessment of EVS Cleaning | Other HAI Prevention Initiatives |
|---|---|---|---|---|---|---|---|---|
| Hass, 2014 | Before-after | Academic center | UV-PX, Xenex | CDI<br>MRSA<br>VRE<br>MDRO-GNB<br>Total | 0.79–0.65 per 1000 Pt-days (P = .02)<br>0.45–0.33 per 1000 Pt-days (P=.007)<br>0.90–0.73 per 1000 Pt-days (P = .002)<br>0.52–0.42 per 1000 Pt-days (P = .04)<br>2.67–2.14 per 1000 Pt-days (P<.001) | No | Yes | Yes |
| Mitchell, 2014 | Before-after | Acute care hospital | Dry hydrogen peroxide vapor (Nocospray, New Work City, NY) | MRSA (colonization and infection) | 9.0–5.3 per 10,000 Pt-days (P<.001) | Yes | No | Yes |
| Miller, 2015 | Before-after | Urban hospital | UV-PX, Xenex | CDI | 23.3–8.3 per 10,000 Pt-days (P = .02) | No | No | Yes |
| Nagaraja, 2015 | Before-after | Academic center | UV-PX, Xenex | CDI | 1.06–0.83 per 1000 Pt-days (P = .06) | No | No | No |
| Pegues, 2015 | Before-after | Academic center | UV-C (Optimum) | CDI | 30.34–22.85 per 10,000 Pt-days (IRR = 0.49, 95% CI 0.26–0.94, P = .03) | Yes | Yes | No |
| Anderson, 2015 | RCT | 9 Hospitals | UV-C (Tru-D) | MRSA, VRE, CDI | 51.3–33.9 per 10,000 Pt-days (P = .036) | Yes | Yes | No |

*Abbreviations:* CDI, *Clostridium difficile* infections; CI, confidence interval; EVS, environmental service; GNB, gram-negative bacteria; HH, hand hygiene; IRR, incidence rate ratio; MDRO, multidrug-resistant organism; NA, not applicable; NS, not stated; Pt, patient; RCT, randomized controlled trial; UV-PX, ultraviolet light, pulsed xenon device.

*Adapted from* Weber DJ, Rutala WA, Anderson DJ, et al. Effectiveness of UV devices and hydrogen peroxide systems for terminal room decontamination: focus on clinical trials. Am J Infect Control 2016;44(5 Suppl):e77–84.

**Box 1**
**Advantages and disadvantages of room decontamination by ultraviolet irradiation units and hydrogen peroxide[1] systems**

*Ultraviolet irradiation*

Advantages
- There is reliable biocidal activity against a wide range of health care–associated pathogens.
- Room surfaces and equipment are decontaminated.
- There is rapid room decontamination ($\sim$5–25 minutes) for vegetative bacteria, which reduces the downtime of the room before another patient can be admitted.
- It is demonstrated to reduce HAIs (eg, *C difficile*, MRSA).
- It is effective against *C difficile*, although requires longer exposure ($\sim$10–50 minutes).
- HVAC system does not need to be disabled and the room does not need to be sealed.
- UV is residual free and does not give rise to health or safety concerns.
- There are no consumable products, so costs include only capital equipment and staff time.
- There is good distribution in the room of UV energy via an automated monitoring system.

Disadvantages
- All patients and staff must be removed from the room before decontamination, thus, limiting use to terminal room decontamination.
- Decontamination can only be accomplished at terminal disinfection (ie, cannot be used for daily disinfection) as room must be emptied of people.
- Capital equipment costs are substantial.
- It does not remove dust and stains, which are important to patients and visitors; hence, cleaning must precede UV decontamination.
- It is sensitive to use parameters (eg, dose, distance, carrier or surface tested, exposure time, pathogen).
- It requires that equipment and furniture be moved away from the walls.

*HP systems*

Advantages
- It has reliable biocidal activity against a wide range of health care–associated pathogens.
- Room surfaces and equipment are decontaminated.
- It has been demonstrated to reduce HAIs (eg, *C difficile*, MRSA, VRE).
- It is useful for disinfecting complex equipment and furniture.
- It does not require that furniture and equipment be moved away from the walls.
- HP is residual free and does not give rise to health or safety concerns (aeration unit converts HP into oxygen and water).
- There is uniform distribution in the room via an automated dispersal system.

Disadvantages
- All patients and staff must be removed from the room before decontamination, thus, limiting use to terminal room decontamination.
- HVAC system must be disabled to prevent unwanted dilution of HP during use, and the doors must be closed with gaps sealed by tape.
- Decontamination can only be accomplished as terminal disinfection (ie, cannot be used for daily disinfection) as room must be emptied of people.
- Capital equipment costs are substantial.
- Decontamination requires approximately 2.0 to 5.0 hours.
- It does not remove dust and stains, which are important to patients and visitors; hence, cleaning must precede UV decontamination.
- It is sensitive to use parameters (eg, HP concentration, pathogen, exposure time).

*Abbreviation:* HVAC, heating, ventilation, and air conditioning.
*Adapted from* Rutala WA, Weber DJ. Disinfectants used for environmental disinfection and new room decontamination technology. Am J Infect Control 2013;41:S36–41.

---

**Box 2**
**Protocol for exposure investigation after the failure to follow disinfection and sterilization principles**

1. Confirm disinfection or sterilization reprocessing failure

2. Embargo any improperly disinfected or sterilized items

3. Do not use the questionable disinfection or sterilization unit (eg, sterilizer, automated endoscope reprocessor)

4. Inform key stakeholders

5. Conduct a complete and thorough evaluation of the cause of the disinfection/sterilization failure

6. Prepare a line listing of potentially exposed patients

7. Assess whether disinfection or sterilization failure increases patient risk for infection

8. Inform expanded list of stakeholders of the reprocessing issue

9. Develop a hypothesis for the disinfection or sterilization failure and initiate corrective action

10. Develop a method to assess potential adverse patient events

11. Consider notification of state and federal authorities

12. Consider patient notification

13. Develop long-term follow-up plan

14. Perform after-action report

*Adapted from* Rutala WA, Weber DJ. How to assess risk of disease transmission to patients when there is a failure to follow recommended disinfection and sterilization guidelines. Infect Control Hosp Epidemiol 2007;28:146–55.

---

articles in the peer-reviewed literature, which demonstrates that high-level disinfectants, such as OPA and glutaraldehyde, inactivate nonenveloped viruses, such as hepatitis A virus, polio, adenovirus, norovirus, and so forth. Because the high-level disinfectants are commonly used to disinfect endocavitary probes (eg, vaginal probes, rectal probes), there is an urgency to corroborating these data. In a conversation with CDC staff regarding this issue, it was determined hospitals should continue to use the FDA-cleared high-level disinfectants consistent with the manufacturers' instructions until the data can be corroborated. Data have demonstrated the activity of a HP mist device to inactivate human papilloma virus.[88]

### Hydrogen Peroxide Mist System for Probes

Although the most common way of performing HLD of contaminated endocavitary probes is by immersion in an FDA-cleared high-level disinfectant (eg, glutaraldehyde), an alternative procedure for disinfecting the endocavitary and surface probes is a HP mist system, which uses 35% HP at 56°C with the probe reaching no more than 40°C (ie, Trophon EPR, Nanosonics, Alexandria, Australia). In one study, the results demonstrated complete inactivation ($>6$-$\log_{10}$ reduction) of VRE and a CRE-*Klebsiella pneumoniae* strain both in the presence and absence of 5% fetal calf serum (FCS). The Trophon EPR system showed good, but not complete, inactivation of *Mycobacterium terrae* (5.2-$\log_{10}$ reduction for *M terrae* with FCS, a 4.6-$\log_{10}$ reduction for *M terrae* without FCS) and *C difficile* spores (5.1-$\log_{10}$ reduction for *C difficile* spores with FCS, 6.2-$\log_{10}$ reduction for *C difficile* spores without FCS).[89] To simulate a worse-case condition, cleaning was not done before disinfection in these experiments; but proper cleaning of probes is necessary to ensure the success of high-level disinfection. Other data have demonstrated the activity of Trophon to inactivate human papilloma virus[88] and other pathogens (eg, bacteria, mycobacteria, viruses) including a greater than 6-$\log_{10}$ reduction of *M terrae* and *C difficile* spores in carrier tests and a greater than 6-$\log_{10}$ reduction in *M terrae* on inoculated ultrasound probes.[90] These results differ slightly from those presented earlier, presumably because of the differences in testing methodology. In the authors' study only the probe devices were inoculated (carriers of different materials were not tested); for recovery of bacteria on the probe, the probes were immersed in media (not swabbed, which would likely result in lower recovery).[89] The Trophon system processes the portion of the probe that has mucous membrane contact but also the handle of endocavitary probes, which may be contaminated; it is an alternative to high-level chemical disinfection for ultrasound probes.

### Do Not Reuse Single-Use Devices

The Department of Justice and the FDA have joined forces in prosecuting health care providers that reuse single-use devices. For example, one physician was criminally prosecuted for reusing needle guides meant for single use during prostate procedures. These prosecutions are based on conspiracy to commit adulteration and Medicare fraud. Third-party reprocessing is allowed by the FDA as the reprocessor is considered the device manufacturer as defined under the Code of Federal Regulations Title 21 Part 820.

### Storage of Semicritical Items

In 2011, The Joint Commission (TJC) recommended that laryngoscope blades be packaged in a way that prevents recontamination. Examples of compliant storage include, but are not limited to, a peel pouch or a closed plastic bag. Examples of noncompliant storage would include unwrapped blades in an anesthesia drawer as well as an unwrapped blade on top of or within a code cart. The packaging not only prevents recontamination but also distinguishes a processed from a nonprocessed semicritical item, such as a specula, laryngoscope blade, or endoscope. The use of a tagging system, in both inpatient and outpatient facilities,[91] that separates processed from nonprocessed items minimizes the risk that a nondisinfected, semicritical device would be used and potentially lead to cross-transmission of a pathogen.[7] This tagging system could involve a tag (eg, green tag, patient ready; red tag, requires reprocessing) for GI endoscopes or a plastic sheath or plastic-paper peel pouch (eg, endocavitary probes). Ideally, hospitals and ambulatory care facilities[91] (as appropriate) should develop a strategy (eg, tagging, storage covers for patient-ready devices) that prevents patient exposures to contaminated devices.

### Immersion Versus Perfusion of Channel Scopes Such as Cystoscopes

In the United States, it is estimated that more than 4 million cystoscopies are performed each year.[29,92] Cystoscopy is a diagnostic procedure that uses an endoscope especially designed to examine the bladder, lower urinary tract, and prostate gland or is used to collect urine samples, perform biopsies, and remove small stones. A flexible or rigid scope can be used to carry out the procedure. Because the procedure, and other channeled scopes (eg, hysteroscopes, some nasopharyngoscopes), involves a medical device in contact with the patients' mucous membranes, it is considered a semicritical device that must minimally be high-level disinfected.

The authors recently evaluated the disinfection of cystoscopes, and their results demonstrated that disinfection (ie, a reduction in bacterial load of greater than

7-$\log_{10}$ colony-forming unit [CFU]) did not occur unless the channel was actively perfused with the glutaraldehyde. In fact, failure to perfuse the channel led to only minimal, if any, reduction in bacterial contamination. However, complete inactivation of $10^8$ CFU of both VRE and CRE was achieved when the channel was actively perfused. It seems that no high-level disinfectant entered the channel unless it was actively perfused, as the level of microbial contamination was not reduced by immersion.[29] This failure to perfuse the channel occurs because the air pressure in the channel is stronger than the fluid pressure at the fluid-air interface. Recommendations are provided for cystoscope HLD and include actively perfusing the device while immersed in the high-level disinfectant.[93] Unfortunately, some cystoscope reprocessing recommendations published in the literature are incorrect. For example, investigators have recommended complete immersion of the cystoscope into the high-level disinfectant but did not mention perfusion of the high-level disinfectant into the channel.[94]

### Laryngoscopes

Laryngoscopes are routinely used to view the vocal cords and larynx and facilitate airway management. It typically consists of a blade that connects to a handle, which usually contains 2 batteries that power the light source. Limited guidelines are available for reprocessing laryngoscope blades and handles, and hospital practices vary.[95–97] For example, some guidelines recommend and hospitals use low-level disinfection of the handle as it does not have direct contact with a mucous membrane, whereas others recommend the handle be high-level disinfected to prevent disease transmission. Although blades have been linked to HAIs, handles have not been directly linked to HAIs. However, reports of contamination with blood (40% of the handles positive for occult blood) and potentially pathogenic microorganisms (86% of the handles deemed ready for patient use were contaminated with pathogens, such as S aureus, Acinetobacter) suggest its potential,[97–100] and the blade and handle function together. For this reason, it is ideal that the blades and handles be high-level disinfected or sterilized even if a protective barrier or sheath is used during the procedure. In 2007, the state of California required that both blades and handles be HLD or sterilized. UNC Hospitals is sterilizing the blades and handles (ie, blades via HP gas plasma, handle [without batteries] by steam). Other methods for HLD or sterilization are acceptable, but one must ensure the blade and handle are compatible with the HLD or sterilization process chosen. After sterilization the blades and handles are checked for function before packaging and then packaged in a Ziploc bag. Per TJC, the laryngoscope blade and handle must be packaged in a way that prevents recontamination after processing (Frequently Asked Questions, The Joint Commission, October 24, 2011). Examples of compliant storage include, but are not limited to, a peel pack after sterilization (long-term storage) or wrapping in a sterile towel (short-term storage).

Recent advances in video technology have led to the development of video laryngoscopes, such as the GlideScope (Verathon Medical, Bothell, WA) and McGrath (Medtronic, Minneapolis, MN) video laryngoscopes.[92] These new intubation devices assist in difficult airway management. For the McGrath an image is displayed on a liquid-crystal display screen that is contained within a monitor mounted to the handle of the device. A sterile, single-use disposable laryngoscope blade covers the camera and light-emitting diode assembly to prevent direct patient contact. Even though a cover is used, HLD or sterilization via ETO or HP gas plasma (battery removed) is recommended for the McGrath MAC video laryngoscope.[93] The manufacturer states, whenever practical, a HLD or sterilization is preferred to a wipe-based process.

The portable GlideScope video laryngoscope system is available in a single-use and a reusable configuration. They should be cleaned and disinfected per the manufacturer's recommendations. The single-use system features a reusable video baton and sterile stats that must be disposed of immediately after use. Low-level disinfection is recommended for the video baton after each use using an Environmental Protection Agency–registered disinfectant (eg, antimicrobial disposable wipe per manufacturer's instructions) after each use. The manufacturer recommends HLD for the video baton when it is visibly soiled.

The manufacturer recommends that the advanced video laryngoscope reusable blade be high-level disinfected and the GlideRite rigid stylets be sterilized.[101]

### Emerging Pathogens, Antibiotic-Resistant Bacteria, and Bioterrorism Agents

Emerging pathogens are of growing concern to the general public and infection control professionals. Relevant pathogens include Ebola,[102] MDR organisms such as CRE, Enterovirus D68, MDR pathogens, Middle East respiratory syndrome-Coronavirus, MDR *M tuberculosis*, human papilloma virus, norovirus, and nontuberculous mycobacteria (eg, *M chelonae*). The susceptibility of each of these pathogens to chemical disinfectants/sterilants has been studied; all of these pathogens (or surrogate microbes such as feline-calicivirus for Norwalk virus, vaccinia for variola,[103] and *Bacillus atrophaeus* [formerly *B subtilis*] for *B anthracis*) are susceptible to currently available chemical disinfectants/sterilants.[19,104] Standard sterilization and disinfection procedures for patient-care equipment (as recommended in this article) are adequate to sterilize or disinfect instruments or devices contaminated with blood or other body fluids from persons infected with blood-borne pathogens, emerging pathogens, and bioterrorism agents, with the exception of prions, HPV, and *C difficile* spores (see earlier discussion). No changes in current procedures for cleaning, disinfecting, or sterilizing need to be made.[13]

In addition, there are no data to show that antibiotic-resistant bacteria (MRSA, VRE, MDR *M tuberculosis*) are less sensitive to the liquid chemical germicides than antibiotic-sensitive bacteria at currently used germicide contact conditions and concentrations.[105–107]

### SUMMARY

When properly used, disinfection and sterilization can ensure the safe use of invasive and noninvasive medical devices. The method of disinfection and sterilization depends on the intended use of the medical device: critical items (contact sterile tissue) must be sterilized before use; semicritical items (contact mucous membranes or nonintact skin) must be high-level disinfected; and noncritical items (contact intact skin) should receive low-level disinfection. Cleaning should always precede HLD and sterilization. Current disinfection and sterilization guidelines must be strictly followed.

### REFERENCES

1. Centers for Disease Control and Prevention. National hospital discharge survey: 2010 table, procedures by selected patient characteristics-number by procedure category and age. 2010.
2. Peery AF, Dellon ES, Lund J, et al. Burden of gastrointestinal disease in the United States: 2012 update. Gastroenterology 2012;143:1179–87.
3. Epstein L, Hunter JC, Arwady MA, et al. New Delhi metallo-beta-lactamase-producing carbapenem-resistant Escherichia coli associated with exposure to duodenoscopes. JAMA 2014;312:1447–55.

4. Wendorf KA, Kay M, Baliga C, et al. Endoscopic retrograde cholangiopancreatography-associated AmpC *Escherichia coli* outbreak. Infect Control Hosp Epidemiol 2015;36:634–42.
5. Ofstead CL, Wetzler HP, Snyder AK, et al. Endoscope reprocessing methods: a prospective study on the impact of human factors and automation. Gastroenterol Nurs 2010;33:304–11.
6. Kovaleva J, Peters FT, van der Mei HC, et al. Transmission of infection by flexible gastrointestinal endoscopy and bronchoscopy. Clin Microbiol Rev 2013;26:231–54.
7. Rutala WA, Weber DJ. How to assess risk of disease transmission to patients when there is a failure to follow recommended disinfection and sterilization guidelines. Infect Control Hosp Epidemiol 2007;28:146–55.
8. Weber DJ, Rutala WA. Lessons learned from outbreaks and pseudo-outbreaks associated with bronchoscopy. Infect Control Hosp Epidemiol 2012;33:230–4.
9. Centers for Disease Control and Prevention. Immediate need for healthcare facilities to review procedures for cleaning, disinfecting, and sterilizing reusable medical devices. 2015. Available at: http://emergency.cdc.gov/han/han00382.asp. Accessed 18 May, 2016.
10. Rutala WA, Weber DJ. Disinfection, sterilization and control of hospital waste. In: Bennett JE, Dolan R, Blaser MJ, editors. Principles and practice of infectious diseases. Philadelphia: Elsevier Saunders; 2015. p. 3294–309.
11. Rutala WA, Weber DJ. Disinfection, Sterilization and Antisepsis: An Overview. Am J Infect Control 2016;44:e1–66.
12. Rutala WA, Weber DJ. Cleaning, disinfection and sterilization. In: Grota P, editor. APIC text of infection control and epidemiology. 4th edition. Washington, DC: Association for Professionals in Infection Control and Epidemiology, Inc.; 2014. p. 31.1–31.15.
13. Rutala WA, Weber DJ, HICPAC. Guideline for disinfection and sterilization in healthcare facilities, 2008. Atlanta (GA): Centers for Disease Control and Prevention; 2008. Available at: http://www.cdc.gov/hicpac/pdf/guidelines/Disinfection_Nov_2008.pdf.
14. Rutala WA, Weber DJ. Disinfection and sterilization in healthcare facilities. In: Han J, editor Practical healthcare epidemiology. 4th edition: University of Chicago Press, in press.
15. Spaulding EH. Chemical disinfection of medical and surgical materials. In: Lawrence C, Block SS, editors. Disinfection, sterilization, and preservation. Philadelphia: Lea & Febiger; 1968. p. 517–31.
16. Sehulster L, Chinn RYW, Healthcare Infection Control Practices Advisory Committee. Guidelines for environmental infection control in health-care facilities. MMWR Morb Mortal Wkly Rep 2003;52:1–44.
17. Rutala WA, Weber DJ. Disinfection and sterilization of prion-contaminated medical instruments, reply to Belay. Infect Control Hosp Epidemiol 2010;31:1306–7.
18. Rutala WA, Gergen MF, Weber DJ. Efficacy of a washer-disinfector in eliminating healthcare-associated pathogens from surgical instruments. Infect Control Hosp Epidemiol 2014;35:883–5.
19. Food and Drug Administration. FDA-cleared sterilants and high level disinfectants with general claims for processing reusable medical and dental devices, March 2015. Available at: http://www.fda.gov/MedicalDevices/DeviceRegulationandGuidance/ReprocessingofReusableMedicalDevices/ucm437347.htm. Accessed 19 May, 2016.

20. Rutala WA, Weber DJ. Disinfection and sterilization in healthcare facilities. In: Han J, ed. SHEA practical healthcare epidemiology University of Chicago Press.
21. Kohn WG, Collins AS, Cleveland JL, et al. Guidelines for infection control in dental health-care settings–2003. MMWR Recomm Rep 2003;52:1–61.
22. McDonnell G, Burke P. Disinfection: is it time to reconsider Spaulding? J Hosp Infect 2011;78:163–70.
23. Food and Drug Administration. Brief summary of the gastroenterology and urology devices panel meeting. 2015.
24. Rutala WA, Weber DJ. Gastrointestinal endoscopes: a need to shift from disinfection to sterilization? JAMA 2014;312:1405–6.
25. Rutala WA, Weber DJ. ERCP scopes: what can we do to prevent infections? Infect Control Hosp Epidemiol 2015;36:643–8.
26. Tosh PK, Disbot M, Duffy JM, et al. Outbreak of *Pseudomonas aeruginosa* surgical site infections after arthroscopic procedures: Texas, 2009. Infect Control Hosp Epidemiol 2011;32:1179–86.
27. Rutala WA, Gergen MF, Weber DJ. Microbial contamination on used surgical instruments. Infect Control Hosp Epidemiol 2014;35:1068–70.
28. Rutala WA, Gergen MF, Weber DJ. Disinfection of a probe used in ultrasound-guided prostate biopsy. Infect Control Hosp Epidemiol 2007;28:916–9.
29. Rutala WA, Gergen MF, Bringhurst J, et al. Effective high-level disinfection of cystoscopes: is perfusion of channels required? Infect Control Hosp Epidemiol 2016;37(2):228–31.
30. Rutala WA, Gergen MF, Weber DJ. Disinfection of an infrared coagulation device used to treat hemorrhoids. Am J Infect Control 2012;40:78–9.
31. Weber DJ, Rutala WA. Role of environmental contamination in the transmission of vancomycin-resistant enterococci. Infect Control Hosp Epidemiol 1997;18:306–9.
32. Weber DJ, Rutala WA, Miller MB, et al. Role of hospital surfaces in the transmission of emerging health care-associated pathogens: norovirus, Clostridium difficile, and Acinetobacter species. Am J Infect Control 2010;38:S25–33.
33. Weber DJ, Rutala WA, Sickbert-Bennett EE. Outbreaks associated with contaminated antiseptics and disinfectants. Antimicrob Agents Chemother 2007;51:4217–24.
34. Rutala WA, Cole EC, Thomann CA, et al. Stability and bactericidal activity of chlorine solutions. Infect Control Hosp Epidemiol 1998;19:323–7.
35. Petersen BT, Chennat J, Cohen J, et al. Multisociety guideline on reprocessing flexible GI endoscopes: 2011. Infect Control Hosp Epidemiol 2011;32:527–37.
36. Society of Gastroenterology Nurses and Associates I. Standards of infection control and reprocessing of flexible gastrointestinal endoscopes. Gastroenterol Nurs 2013;36:293–303.
37. Muscarella LF. Risk of transmission of carbapenem-resistant Enterobacteriaceae and related "superbugs" during gastrointestinal endoscopy. World J Gastrointest Endosc 2014;6:457–74.
38. Ofstead CL, Wetzler HP, Doyle EM, et al. Persistent contamination on colonoscopes and gastroscopes detected by biologic cultures and rapid indicators despite reprocessing performed in accordance with guidelines. Am J Infect Control 2015;43:794–801.
39. Carbonne A, Thiolet JM, Fournier S, et al. Control of a multi-hospital outbreak of KPC-producing Klebsiella pneumoniae type 2 in France, September to October 2009. Euro Surveill 2010;15 [pii:19734].

40. Roberts CG. Studies on the bioburden on medical devices and the importance of cleaning. In: Rutala WA, editor. Disinfection, sterilization and antisepsis: principles and practices in healthcare facilities. Washington, DC: Association for Provessionals in Infection Control and Epidemiology; 2000. p. 63–9.

41. Alfa MJ, Degagne P, Olson N. Worst-case soiling levels for patient-used flexible endoscopes before and after cleaning. Am J Infect Control 1999;27:392–401.

42. Rutala WA, Weber DJ. FDA labeling requirements for disinfection of endoscopes: a counterpoint. Infect Control Hosp Epidemiol 1995;16:231–5.

43. Food and Drug Administration. Brief summary of the gastroeneterology and urology devices panel meeting, May 14-15, 2015. Available at: http://www.fda.gov/AdvisoryCommittees/CommitteesMeetingMaterials/MedicalDevices/MedicalDevicesAdvisoryCommittee/ucm445590.htm. Accessed 18 May, 2016.

44. Pajkos AVK, Cossart Y. Is biofilm accumulation on endoscope tubing a contributor to the failure of cleaning and decontamination. J Hosp Infect 2004;58:224.

45. Roberts CG. The role of biofilms in reprocessing medical devices. In: WA R, editor. Disinfection, sterilization and antisepsis: principles, practices, current issues, new research, and new technologies. Washington, DC: Association for Professionals in Infection Control and Epidemiology; 2010. p. 223–9.

46. Neves MS, daSilva MG, Ventura GM, et al. Effectiveness of current disinfection procedures against biofilm on contaminated GI endoscopes. Gastrointest Endosc 2016;83(5):944–53.

47. Ren-Pei W, Hui-Jun X, Ke Q, et al. Correlation between the growth of bacterial biofilm in flexible endoscopes and endoscope reprocessing methods. Am J Infect Control 2014;42:1203–6.

48. Agrawal D, Muscarella LF. Delayed reprocessing of endoscopes. Gastrointest Endosc 2011;73:853–4.

49. Rutala WA, Weber DJ. Outbreaks of carbapenem-resistant *Enteriobacteriaceae* infections associated with duodenoscopes: what can we do to prevent infections? Am J Infect Control 2016;44(5 Suppl):e47–51.

50. Otter JA, Yezli S, French GL. The role played by contaminated surfaces in the transmission of nosocomial pathogens. Infect Control Hosp Epidemiol 2011;32:687–99.

51. Boyce JM. Environmental contamination makes an important contribution to hospital infection. J Hosp Infect 2007;65(Suppl 2):50–4.

52. Weber DJ, Anderson DJ, Sexton DJ, et al. Role of the environment in the transmission of Clostridium difficile in health care facilities. Am J Infect Control 2013;41:S105–10.

53. Rutala WA, Weber DJ. Disinfectants used for environmental disinfection and new room decontamination technology. Am J Infect Control 2013;41:S36–41.

54. Stiefel U, Cadnum JL, Eckstein BC, et al. Contamination of hands with methicillin-resistant Staphylococcus aureus after contact with environmental surfaces and after contact with the skin of colonized patients. Infect Control Hosp Epidemiol 2011;32:185–7.

55. Carling P. Methods for assessing the adequacy of practice and improving room disinfection. Am J Infect Control 2013;41:S20–5.

56. Huang SS, Datta R, Platt R. Risk of acquiring antibiotic-resistant bacteria from prior room occupants. Arch Intern Med 2006;166:1945–51.

57. Shaughnessy MK, Micielli RL, DePestel DD, et al. Evaluation of hospital room assignment and acquisition of Clostridium difficile infection. Infect Control Hosp Epidemiol 2011;32:201–6.

58. Donskey CJ. Does improving surface cleaning and disinfection reduce health care-associated infections? Am J Infect Control 2013;41:S12–9.
59. Carling PC, Bartley JM. Evaluating hygienic cleaning in health care settings: what you do not know can harm your patients. Am J Infect Control 2010;38: S41–50.
60. Boyce JM, Havill NL, Dumigan DG, et al. Monitoring the effectiveness of hospital cleaning practices by use of an adenosine triphosphate bioluminescence assay. Infect Control Hosp Epidemiol 2009;30:678–84.
61. Hota B, Blom DW, Lyle EA, et al. Interventional evaluation of environmental contamination by vancomycin-resistant enterococci: failure of personnel, product or procedure? J Hosp Infect 2009;71:123–31.
62. Goodman ER, Platt R, Bass R, et al. Impact of an environmental cleaning intervention on the presence of methicillin-resistant Staphylococcus aureus and vancomycin-resistant enterococci on surfaces in intensive care unit rooms. Infect Control Hosp Epidemiol 2008;29:593–9.
63. Eckstein BC, Adams DA, Eckstein EC, et al. Reduction of Clostridium difficile and vancomycin-resistant Enterococcus contamination of environmental surfaces after an intervention to improve cleaning methods. BMC Infect Dis 2007;7:61.
64. Leas BF, SN, Han JH, et al. Environmental cleaning for the prevention of healthcare-associated infection. Technical brief No. 22 (prepared by the ECRI Institute – Penn Agency for Healthcare Research and Quality. Available at: http://effectivehealthcare.ahrq.gov/index.cfm/search-for-guides-reviews-and-reports/?pageaction=displayproduct&productid=1951. Accessed 18 May, 2016.
65. Huslage K, Rutala WA, Sickbert-Bennett E, et al. A quantitative approach to defining "high-touch" surfaces in hospitals. Infect Control Hosp Epidemiol 2010;31:850–3.
66. Huslage K, Rutala WA, Gergen MF, et al. Microbial assessment of high-, medium-, and low-touch hospital room surfaces. Infect Control Hosp Epidemiol 2013;34:211–2.
67. Memarzadeh F, Olmsted RN, Bartley JM. Applications of ultraviolet germicidal irradiation disinfection in health care facilities: effective adjunct, but not stand-alone technology. Am J Infect Control 2010;38:S13–24.
68. Nerandzic MM, Thota P, Sankar CT, et al. Evaluation of a pulsed xenon ultraviolet disinfection system for reduction of healthcare-associated pathogens in hospital rooms. Infect Control Hosp Epidemiol 2015;36:192–7.
69. Rutala WA, Gergen MF, Weber DJ. Room decontamination with UV radiation. Infect Control Hosp Epidemiol 2010;31:1025–9.
70. Rutala WA, Gergen MF, Tande BM, et al. Room decontamination using an ultraviolet-C device with short ultraviolet exposure time. Infect Control Hosp Epidemiol 2014;35:1070–2.
71. Nerandzic MM, Cadnum JL, Pultz MJ, et al. Evaluation of an automated ultraviolet radiation device for decontamination of Clostridium difficile and other healthcare-associated pathogens in hospital rooms. BMC Infect Dis 2010;10:197.
72. Boyce JM, Havill NL, Moore BA. Terminal decontamination of patient rooms using an automated mobile UV light unit. Infect Control Hosp Epidemiol 2011;32:737–42.
73. Boyce JM, Havill NL, Otter JA, et al. Impact of hydrogen peroxide vapor room decontamination on Clostridium difficile environmental contamination and transmission in a healthcare setting. Infect Control Hosp Epidemiol 2008;29:723–9.

74. French GL, Otter JA, Shannon KP, et al. Tackling contamination of the hospital environment by methicillin-resistant Staphylococcus aureus (MRSA): a comparison between conventional terminal cleaning and hydrogen peroxide vapour decontamination. J Hosp Infect 2004;57:31–7.
75. Bartels MD, Kristoffersen K, Slotsbjerg T, et al. Environmental methicillin-resistant Staphylococcus aureus (MRSA) disinfection using dry-mist-generated hydrogen peroxide. J Hosp Infect 2008;70:35–41.
76. Hall L, Otter JA, Chewins J, et al. Use of hydrogen peroxide vapor for deactivation of Mycobacterium tuberculosis in a biological safety cabinet and a room. J Clin Microbiol 2007;45:810–5.
77. Hardy KJ, Gossain S, Henderson N, et al. Rapid recontamination with MRSA of the environment of an intensive care unit after decontamination with hydrogen peroxide vapour. J Hosp Infect 2007;66:360–8.
78. Johnston MD, Lawson S, Otter JA. Evaluation of hydrogen peroxide vapour as a method for the decontamination of surfaces contaminated with Clostridium botulinum spores. J Microbiol Methods 2005;60:403–11.
79. Heckert RA, Best M, Jordan LT, et al. Efficacy of vaporized hydrogen peroxide against exotic animal viruses. Appl Environ Microbiol 1997;63:3916–8.
80. Klapes NA, Vesley D. Vapor-phase hydrogen peroxide as a surface decontaminant and sterilant. Appl Environ Microbiol 1990;56:503–6.
81. Bates CJ, Pearse R. Use of hydrogen peroxide vapour for environmental control during a Serratia outbreak in a neonatal intensive care unit. J Hosp Infect 2005; 61:364–6.
82. Shapey S, Machin K, Levi K, et al. Activity of a dry mist hydrogen peroxide system against environmental Clostridium difficile contamination in elderly care wards. J Hosp Infect 2008;70:136–41.
83. Falagas ME, Thomaidis PC, Kotsantis IK, et al. Airborne hydrogen peroxide for disinfection of the hospital environment and infection control: a systematic review. J Hosp Infect 2011;78:171–7.
84. Weber DJ, Rutala W, Anderson DJ, et al. Effectiveness of UV devices and hydrogen peroxide systems for terminal room decontamination: focus on clinical trials. Am J Infect Control, 2016.;44(5 Suppl):e77-e84.
85. Rutala WA, Weber DJ. Selection of the ideal disinfectant. Infect Control Hosp Epidemiol 2014;35:855–65.
86. Weber DJ, Rutala WA. Assessing the risk of disease transmission to patients when there is a failure to follow recommended disinfection and sterilization guidelines. Am J Infect Control 2013;41:S67–71.
87. Meyers J, Ryndock E, Conway MJ, et al. Susceptibility of high-risk human papillomavirus type 16 to clinical disinfectants. J Antimicrob Chemother 2014;69(6): 1546–50.
88. Ryndock E, Robison R, Meyers C. Susceptibility of HPV 16 and 18 to high-level disinfectants indicated for semi-critical ultrasound probes. J Med Virol 2015; 88(6):1076–80.
89. Rutala WA, Gergen MF, Sickbert-Bennett EE. Effectiveness of a hydrogen peroxide mist (Trophon®) system in inactivating healthcare pathogens on surface and endocavitary probes. Infect Control Hosp Epidemiol 2016;37(5):613–4.
90. Vickery K, Gorgis VZ, Burdach J, et al. Evaluation of an automated high-level disinfection technology for ultrasound transducers. J Infect Public Health 2014;7:153–60.
91. Bringhurst J. Disinfection and sterilization in physician practices and specialty clinics. Am J Infect Control 2016;44:e63–7.

92. Rutala WA, Weber DJ. Reprocessing semicritical items: current issues and new technologies. Am J Infect Control 2016;44(5 Suppl):e53–62.
93. Anonymous. McGrath MAC video laryngoscope operator's manual. Available at: https://www.physio-control.com/uploadedFiles/Physio85/Contents/Emergency_ Medical_Care/Products/PreHospital/MAC%20EMS%20IFU.pdf. Access 18 May, 2016.
94. Wendelboe AM, Bauchman J, Blossom DB, et al. Outbreak of cystoscopy related infections with Pseudomonas aeurginosa: New Mexico, 2007. J Urol 2008;180:588–92.
95. Muscarella LF. Recommendations to resolve inconsistent guidelines for the re-processing of sheathed and unsheathed rigid laryngoscopes. Infect Control Hosp Epidemiol 2007;28:504–7.
96. Muscarella LF. Prevention of disease transmission during flexible laryngoscopy. Am J Infect Control 2007;35:536–44.
97. Muscarella LF. Reassessment of the risk of healthcare-acquired infection during rigid laryngoscopy. J Hosp Infect 2008;68:101–7.
98. Call TR, Auerbach FJ, Riddell SW, et al. Nosocomial contamination of laryngo-scope handles: challenging current guidelines. Anesth Analg 2009;109:479–83.
99. Williams D, Dingley J, Jones C, et al. Contamination of laryngoscope handles. J Hosp Infect 2010;74:123–8.
100. Phillips RA, Monaghan WP. Incidence of visible and occult blood on laryngo-scope blades and handles. AANA J 1997;65:241–6.
101. Anonymous. GlideScope. Available at: http://www.verathon.com/assets/0900-4200-02-60.pdf. Accessed 18 May, 2016.
102. Cook BWM, Cutts TA, Nikiforuk AM, et al. Evaluating environmental persistence and disinfection of the Ebola virus Makona variant. Viruses 2015;7:1975–86.
103. Klein M, DeForest A. The inactivation of viruses by germicides. Chem Special-ists Manuf Assoc Proc 1963;49:116–8.
104. Rutala WA, Gergen MF, Weber DJ. Sporicidal activity of a new low-temperature sterilization technology: the Sterrad 50 sterilizer. Infect Control Hosp Epidemiol 1999;20:514–6.
105. Rutala WA, Stiegel MM, Sarubbi FA, et al. Susceptibility of antibiotic-susceptible and antibiotic-resistant hospital bacteria to disinfectants. Infect Control Hosp Epidemiol 1997;18:417–21.
106. Anderson RL, Carr JH, Bond WW, et al. Susceptibility of vancomycin-resistant enterococci to environmental disinfectants. Infect Control Hosp Epidemiol 1997;18:195–9.
107. Rutala WA, Barbee SL, Aguiar NC, et al. Antimicrobial activity of home disinfec-tants and natural products against potential human pathogens. Infect Control Hosp Epidemiol 2000;21:33–8.

# Optimizing Health Care Environmental Hygiene

Philip C. Carling, MD

## KEYWORDS

- Hygienic practice • Hand hygiene • Environmental hygiene
- Optimizing disinfection cleaning

## KEY POINTS

- During the past decade it has become widely appreciated that patient area environmental surfaces play an important role in the transmission of all health care–associated pathogens (HAPs).
- Clarification of opportunities to have a favorable impact on such transmission has led to new approaches for optimizing the structure and practice of health care environmental hygiene.
- Although both hand hygiene and environmental hygiene represent basic horizontal interventions to prevent transmission of HAPs, there is a need for these 2 interventions to be recognized as interdependent.
- Several technologic interventions to augment environmental hygiene have been recently developed but remain to be objectively evaluated in well-designed clinical studies.

## INTRODUCTION

As recently noted by the Centers for Disease Control and Prevention (CDC), "In the 1970s and 1980s the transmission of pathogens from healthcare surface to susceptible patients was thought to be insignificant."[1] As a result of epidemiologic and microbiologic studies over the past decade, it has become increasingly evident that interventions to mitigate environmental surface pathogen contamination constitute an important component of health care–associated infection (HAI) prevention. During this time it has become widely appreciated that, "Cleaning of hard surfaces in hospital rooms is critical for reducing healthcare-associated infections."[2] Unfortunately, the complexity of the interrelated factors necessary to optimize the safety of surfaces in the patient zone remains an evolving challenge. Precisely defining how the impact of various surface cleaning interventions and optimized hand hygiene practice can

Disclosure Statement: The author reports having served as a consultant to AORN and Ecolab and has licensed patents to Ecolab.
Department of Infectious Diseases, Carney Hospital, 2100 Dorchester Avenue, Boston, MA 02124, USA
E-mail address: pcarling@comcast.net

Infect Dis Clin N Am 30 (2016) 639–660
http://dx.doi.org/10.1016/j.idc.2016.04.010
**id.theclinics.com**

be validated to develop clinically grounded implementation guidance has yet to be substantially realized.[1,3] Despite such ongoing challenges, it is important to recognize that environmental hygiene represents a critical element of what Wenzel and Edmond define as "horizontal interventions" that are central to mitigating a wide range of HAIs.[4,5] These approaches aim to reduce the risk of infections caused by a broad range of pathogens by the implementation of standard practices that are effective regardless of patient-specific conditions.[6] In contrast to the horizontal interventions, "vertical interventions" are pathogen and/or condition specific. They remain important in defined settings and become most cost effective when the indications for their use are most clearly defined. Although vertical and horizontal approaches are not mutually exclusive, there is evolving evidence that horizontal interventions in endemic situations may represent a best use of HAI prevention resources.[6] Recent well-designed studies of chlorhexidine bathing and decolonization as well as expanded use of contact precautions in ICUs seem to have significant potential for HAI reduction, at least in certain settings.[6] Furthermore, the use of vertical interventions has recently been shown of critical value in optimizing safety with emerging pathogens, such as Ebola virus and the Corona virus associated with MeRS.[7,8]

To facilitate discussion of the many elements necessary to optimize health care hygienic cleaning, it is useful to put these interventions into a defined construct of HAI prevention activities. As indicated in **Fig. 1**, hygienic cleaning and hand hygiene as well as interventions related to instrument reprocessing, air quality, water quality, and physical setting design are all horizontal interventions. All these horizontal interventions represent elements of health care hygienic practice. Although these elements have traditionally been discussed independently, their effectiveness in clinical settings is substantially interrelated, in particular environmental hygiene and hand hygiene, as discussed later. The term, *environmental hygiene*, with respect to health care, can be defined as cleaning activities directed at removing and/or killing potentially harmful pathogens capable of being transmitted directly from surfaces or indirectly to susceptible individuals or other surfaces. As such it consists of both the physical cleaning of surfaces as well as surface disinfection cleaning (see **Fig. 1**). Although liquid chemistries are well established as the most clinically useful

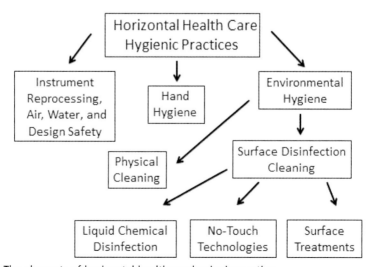

**Fig. 1.** The elements of horizontal healthcare hygienic practice.

approach to surface disinfection, innovative approaches that may have the potential for complementing traditional liquid chemistry have been developed over the past several years. Each of these aspects of environmental hygiene is discussed in detail whereas the other components of health care hygienic practice (see **Fig. 1**) are addressed in other articles of this issue.

## EPIDEMIOLOGY OF CONTAMINATED SURFACES

Although minimizing health care surface pathogens has long been considered a useful aspect of optimizing patient safety, it was not until the landmark study by Huang and colleagues[9] quantified the risk of methicillin-resistant *Staphylococcus aureus* (MRSA) and VRE acquisition posed by occupying a room previously occupied by a patient colonized or infected by these pathogens that the clear risk of suboptimal disinfection cleaning became widely appreciated. Eight similar studies have confirmed an average 120% increased risk of the subsequent occupant becoming colonized or infected with MRSA, vancomycin-resistant enterococci (VRE), *Clostridium difficile*, pseudomonas, and Acinetobacter.[10,11] As a result of a range of investigations, important insights have been gained into the basic epidemiology of health care surface pathogen transmission, as summarized in **Table 1**. Current understanding of these features provides a critical context, both for optimizing current practices and for designing future research to objectively evaluate the importance of intervention strategies aimed at optimizing environmental hygiene.

**Table 1**
**The key epidemiologic features of HAP transmission.**

| Epidemiologic Feature | References |
|---|---|
| Shedding of gastrointestinal tract colonizing pathogens is unpredictable and prolonged; it fluctuates; and it is impacted by colonic flora disbiosis. | Donskey et al,[12] 2000; Chang et al,[13] 2009; Sethi et al,[14] 2009, Sethi et al,[15] 2010; Kundrapu et al,[16] 2015; Faired et al,[17] 2013; Miles et al,[18] 2015; Tschudin-Sutter et al,[19] 2015 |
| Environmental contamination by HAI pathogens is common, greatest on surfaces closest to the patient, quantitatively variable, and often sparse. | Chang et al,[20] 2011; Weber et al,[21] 2010; Donskey,[22] 2013; Sitzlar et al,[23] 2013; Linder et al,[24] 2014; Creamer et al,[25] 2014 |
| Environmental contamination is almost equally associated with colonize or infect a recipient patients. | Guerrero et al,[26] 2013; Linder et al,[24] 2014; Kundrapu et al,[16] 2015; Gavalda et al,[27] 2015 |
| All common HAI pathogens survive for many hours to months on a wide range of patient zone surfaces. | Kramer et al,[28] 2006; Dancer,[11] 2014; Munoz-Price & Weinstein,[29] 2015 |
| Health care personnel have frequent contact with HAP-contaminated surfaces | Guerrero et al,[30] 2012; Kundrapu et al,[31] 2012; Morgan et al,[32] 2012; Dancer,[11] 2014 |
| Contact with the environment is as likely to contaminate health care workers' hands. | Donskey,[22] 2013; Weber et al,[21] 2013; Ferng et al,[33] 2015, Thomas et al,[34] 2015 |
| The dose of pathogen needed to colonization or infect of a recipient with most HAPs is typically very low. | Weber et al,[21] 2013; Dancer,[11] 2014 |
| Surface-contaminating HAPs range widely in their sensitivity to chemical disinfects UV light and antimicrobial surface treatments. | Rutala & Weber,[35] 2014; Nerandzic et al,[36] 2015 |

## CLEANING HEALTH CARE SURFACES

The importance of physically removing visible dirt and soil from surfaces in hospitals has been recognized for more than 150 years.[37] Consequently, acute care hospitals have developed policies and procedures to define the role of environmental services (EVS) personnel for cleaning surfaces in all patient care areas. EVS managers and infection preventionists had implemented joint visual inspection of surfaces in patient care areas well before the CDC recommended that hospitals were to clean and disinfect "high-touch surfaces" in 2003[38] and that hospitals monitor (ie, supervise and inspect) cleaning performance to insure consistent cleaning and disinfection of surfaces in close proximity to patients and likely to be touched by patients and health care professionals in 2006.[39] Such monitoring, referred to as *environmental rounds* in the United States and *visual audits* in Great Britain, is used primarily to identify cleaning deficiencies.[40] Unfortunately, the intrinsically subjective nature of such monitoring along with its episodic and deficiency-oriented features limit its ability to accurately assess the thoroughness of day-to-day cleaning activity. Preliminary studies documenting patient zone surface contamination with HAPs raised concerns that cleaning practice should be improved.[41] It was not until actual cleaning practice was objectively monitored, initially using a covert visual monitoring system[42] and later with covertly applied fluorescent markers, that actual cleaning practice was objectively evaluated.[43,44] This made it possible to contrast conventional visual monitoring to objective monitoring of cleaning practice (**Box1**).[10]

After the identification of opportunities to improve the thoroughness of patient zone surface cleaning as part of discharge cleaning in acute care hospitals,[43,44] cleaning practice was similarly evaluated in multiple venues within hospitals, including the operating room between cases and end-of-day cleaning, emergency departments, outpatient clinics, and chemotherapy administration suites.[45] Identical studies have been extended to long-term care facilities and dialysis units as well as dental clinics and emergency medical services vehicles.[45] The evaluations were done in a standardized manner with an identical fluorescent marking system. The outcome measured was the actual thoroughness of cleaning expressed as a thoroughness of disinfection

---

**Box 1**
**Approaches to evaluating environmental hygiene performance**

*Conventional Program*

- Subjective visual assessment
- Deficiency oriented
- Episodic evaluation
- Problem detection feedback
- Unable to covertly assess cleaning practice
- Open definition of remedial interventions

*Objective Monitoring Program*

- Objective quantitative assessment
- Performance oriented
- Ongoing cyclic monitoring
- Objective performance feedback
- Goal-oriented structured process improvement model

cleaning (TDC) score. TDC is an expression of the proportion of actual cleaning documented in comparison to the cleaning expected to be done according to the relevant cleaning policy.[43,46] As shown in **Fig. 2**, these studies consistently identified substantial opportunities for improving practice in all settings.[45] Although visual monitoring as part of environmental rounds remains important for detecting substantial oversights in cleaning practice, there are many advantages to the objective monitoring of disinfection cleaning practice.[10]

Shortly after confirming the sensitivity and specificity of covert use of fluorescent markers to objectively and reproducibly identify opportunities to improve terminal cleaning thoroughness, process improvement interventions based on structured educational activities and direct performance feedback to EVS staff was shown highly effective in improving cleaning thoroughness.[47] Published reports have now confirmed the effectiveness of such programs in more than 120 hospitals in the United States, Canada, and Australia.[45,47–51] In the study hospitals, not only has the thoroughness of cleaning improved from TDC scores of approximately 40% to 60% to 80% to 90% or higher as a result of similar programmatic intervention but also there has been excellent sustainability of the results over at least 3 years where ongoing programs have been evaluated.[50]

Several reports have now shown that improved environmental cleaning decreases HAP contamination of surfaces. As shown in **Fig. 3**, 4 comparable clinical studies objectively evaluating thoroughness of environmental cleaning over many months found contamination of patient zone surfaces decreased an average of 64% as a result of an average 80% improvement in thoroughness of environmental disinfection cleaning.[10] Although the complexity and cost of studies to evaluate the impact of decreased patient zone HAP contamination on acquisition has limited such

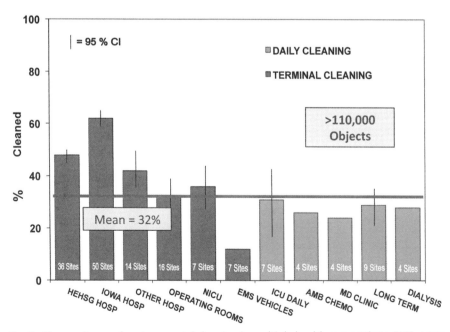

**Fig. 2.** Thoroughness of environmental cleaning in multiple health care settings. EMS, emergency medical service; HE HSG, healthcare environmental hygiene study group; Hosp, hospitals; AMB, ambulatory.

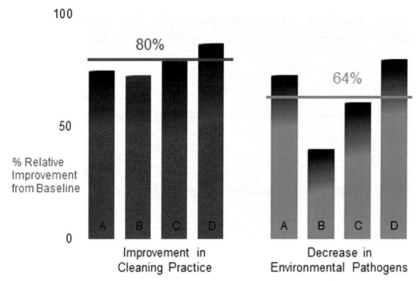

**Fig. 3.** Improving disinfection cleaning to decrease environmental surface contamination.

undertakings, 2 landmark studies found similar statistically significant results. The 2006 study by Hayden and colleagues[42] confirmed a 66% (P<.001) reduction in VRE acquisition as a result of a 75% improvement TDC. A more recent study by Datta and colleagues[52] found a 50% (P<.001) reduction in MRSA acquisition and a 28% (P<.001) reduction in VRE acquisition as a result of an 80% improvement in environmental cleaning. The latter study also confirmed significantly decreased prior room occupant transmission for both pathogens during the intervention period. These studies clearly show that direct patient safety benefits can be realized by improving the thoroughness of patient zone surface cleaning.

Based on published evidence supporting objective monitoring to evaluate surface cleaning processes and improved patient outcomes as a result of improved environmental hygiene, the CDC developed the guidelines, *Options for Evaluating Environmental Cleaning* in 2010.[46] This guidance recommends that all hospitals implement methods to objectively monitor environmental cleaning (**Box 2**).[46]

### Methods for Evaluating Physical Cleaning

Direct overt monitoring of individual EVS workers as they clean with or without some form of testing, such as fluorescent marking or an adenosine triphosphate (ATP)

---

**Box 2**
**Centers for Disease Control and Prevention environmental hygiene monitoring guidance**

Hospitals should implement programs to improve current environmental hygiene practice by adopting a 2-phase stepwise programmatic approach:

Level I program
   Basic interventions to optimize disinfection cleaning policies, procedures, and environmental services staff education and practice. When completed move to level II program.

Level II program
   All elements of level I program + objective monitoring

measurement (discussed later), can be used by EVS managers to teach proper cleaning of patient zone surfaces[53,54] as part of a certification process.[55] Unfortunately, such activity typically leads to a Hawthorne effect, whereby the knowledge of observation affects observed behavior.[56] In addition, substantial resources are needed to broadly implement such activities for large numbers of individuals. For these reasons, the use of direct overt monitoring of EVS workers to quantifiably assess cleaning practice is not feasible. As discussed in the CDC guidelines and the 2015 Agency for Healthcare Research and Quality (AHRQ) Technical Brief 22, *Environmental Cleaning for the Prevention of Healthcare-Associated Infections*,57 5 methods have the potential for being used within a structured process improvement program to objectively monitor cleaning practice, if performed as recommended.[46,47,57]

### Covert direct practice observation

As demonstrated by Hayden and colleagues,[42] this form of monitoring of actual cleaning practice, covert direct practice observation, can provide an objective assessment of individual EVS worker performance and compliance with cleaning protocols. Unfortunately, logistical issues, cost, and challenges with standardization across multiple settings limit the use of this form of monitoring to research settings.

### Basic culture methods

Various culture methods have been used to study microbial contamination of environmental surfaces. Swab cultures or replicate organism direct agar contact (RODAC) contact plates are often used for such assessments. Recently, sterile sponge cultures as well as Petrifilm have shown a potential for increasing the sensitivity of such cultures.[58] No matter which system is used, cultures are most helpful when it is necessary to identify specific pathogens during epidemiologic investigations of outbreaks. Unfortunately all these basic culture methods are difficult to use for programmatically monitoring cleaning practice because of the need to determine precleaning levels of contamination for each object evaluated to accurately assess cleaning practice due to the intrinsically low bioburden of health care environmental surfaces.[10] For this reason, swab system cultures are used primarily to identify specific pathogens to help clarify the epidemiology of possible environmental hygiene–related outbreaks or hyperendemic transmission problems.[46]

### Agar slide cultures

Agar-coated glass slides, initially developed to simplify quantitative cultures of liquids, have been used to evaluate the cleanliness of environmental surfaces in health care settings.[53,59,60] Although the ability of the fixed surface area of the slide to quantify viable bioburden (expressed as aerobic colony counts/cm$^2$), is useful, any culture-based system to evaluate the environmental cleaning practice has the same limitations noted for swab cultures, necessitating the comparison of precleaning cultures with postcleaning, as discussed previously. A recent study confirmed the ability of such a process to evaluate thoroughness of cleaning practice.[61] In the study, 10.5% of precleaning cultures were without measureable bioburden using this system before cleaning. This decreased the sensitivity of this form of monitoring, which necessitated the monitoring of a greater number of objects to develop an accurate analysis of cleaning practice.

### Adenosine triphosphate assays

ATP bioluminescence technology detects the presence of organic material, including viable and nonviable bioburden, on surfaces. Semiautomated ATP measurement systems have been in use in the food processing industry for more than 30 years.

Although their ease of use led to an attempt to use them to quantify health care surface bioburden, the high sensitivity of the system to nonmicrobiologic and nonviable organic matter and its relative insensitivity to some HAPs have now been clarified.[53,62,63] As recently reported by Mulvey and colleagues in a detailed evaluation of the ATP technology, "Sensitivity and specificity of 57% (with the ATP tool) means that the margin for error is too high to justify stringent monitoring of the hospital environment (with ATP technology) at present."[60(p29)] Furthermore, significant intrinsic limitations of the technology, which would have an impact on its use in objectively monitoring cleaning practice, have been recently identified by Whitley and colleagues.[62,64]

Although not yet investigated, it is plausible that the ATP assay could be used for prospective monitoring of cleaning practice over time if the type of pre–post cleaning target evaluation system recommended for culture-based symptoms is used. Although several reports discussed previously have used ATP tools for education, the frequently low bioburden of most clinical surfaces as well as the limitations of the technology have made it difficult to use ATP assays for other than immediate performance feedback.

### Fluorescent markers

As discussed previously, studies in the United States and abroad during the past 10 years have used a specially developed fluorescent gel test soil to covertly evaluate environmental cleaning in a wide range of health care settings.[43,47–51,65–67] These studies have used a standardized transparent gel specifically formulated for the covert evaluation of health care surface cleaning. Although nonstandardized fluorescent powders and lotions have been used in a noncovert manner for education,[68] the fact that these substances are visible in ambient light precludes their use in programs to objectively monitor cleaning practice as a result of their ability to induce a Hawthorne effect.[66,67] Because fluorescent gel cannot be used to detect the presence or absence of specific organisms, its exclusive use in pathogen-specific outbreak evaluations is not feasible.[46] Because the removal of the fluorescent gel represents a physical removal of an applied substance, the possibility has been raised that surfaces may have been effectively disinfected but not necessarily cleaned well and may be flagged as not being effectively cleaned.[57] Because the use of liquid disinfectant chemistries involve a concomitant physical cleaning process, that is, wiping the surface, which has been shown to result in the easy removal of the standardized fluorescent gel, such a hypothetical concern seems unwarranted.[43,66] As noted in the 2015 AHRQ technical brief, "Fluorescent gel is the most commonly used formulation because it dries to a transparent finish on surfaces, it is abrasion-resistant, and unlike powder, is not easily disturbed. For these reasons, the fluorescent gel formulation has been the most well-studied method to assess surface disinfection and to quantify the impact of educational interventions."[57(p14)] The report adds that additional advantages of fluorescent surface markers include their "relatively low cost, ease of implementation and their use for direct feedback to the EVS staff."[57(p14)]

### Programmatic Benefits and Challenges of Environmental Cleaning Monitoring

Although process improvement programs developed in accordance with the CDC 2010 guidelines have been successful in improving patient zone cleaning as well as decreasing HAP surface contamination and transmission (as discussed previously), recent studies have begun to identify both the collateral benefits and the challenges of these programs.

As part of an HAI prevention initiative in Iowa, a diverse group of 56 hospitals implemented objective monitoring and process improvement activities for discharge cleaning practice using the fluorescent marking system and programmatic interventions as previously modeled.[47,50] Preintervention cleaning thoroughness averaged 60% and was similar in most hospitals (95% CI, 56.7–64.4). As indicated in **Fig. 4**, after education and ongoing feedback of performance to the EVS staff, cleaning ultimately improved to 89% for the group (*P*<.001).[50] A structured questionnaire by the hospitals completing the project found that the EVS staff at all hospitals appreciated and were enthusiastic about being evaluated, particularly because the program provided them with a new and unique opportunity to show other health care workers how well they were performing disinfection cleaning activities. Approximately half the sites reported that the program led to new senior management recognition of the value of the patient safety oriented work performed by EVS personnel, that the program redefined the EVS role in patient safety, and that the targeting system was valuable for one-on-one training. Twenty percent of the hospitals reported that the study led to identification of opportunities for improving EVS program issues related to manpower resources and communication. A similar number of sites commented on the very favorable response the program received from the board of trustees. Three of 20 sites (15%) noted that the program initially met resistance from EVS management. Three other sites noted that the program resulted in some transient anxiety among the EVS personnel, which resolved once the value of the program and its nonpunitive orientation was understood.

Although the study confirmed the value of an objective structured programmatic process to broadly improve cleaning practice, it also documented the challenges of implementing such activities. Due primarily to resource limitations (infection preventionists' time constraints) and personnel turnover, more than one-third (23/56 [41%]) of the sites, which likely could have benefitted significantly from the program, withdrew from the study prior to achieving cleaning scores of greater than 80% (see **Fig. 4**). Although it is not possible to exclude the impact of motivational issues on the decision by some of these sites to withdraw from the program, recent reports

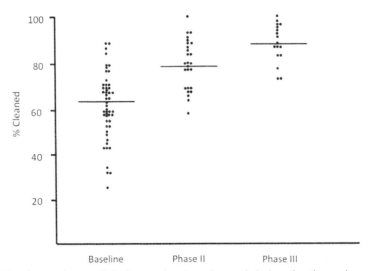

**Fig. 4.** The thoroughness of discharge cleaning observed during the three phases of the Iowa disinfection cleaning project.[50]

have confirmed high levels of administrative pressures on infection preventionists working in acute care hospitals.[69] Conversely, 71% of the sites in which the initial assessment disclosed opportunities to improve disinfection cleaning were motivated enough to pursue the study and to achieve cleaning scores of greater than 80%. Furthermore, 27% of the hospitals completing the study independently maintained cleaning thoroughness at greater than 90% for more than 3 years.[50] Similar sustainability of cleaning thoroughness (92%) was also found in a group of 14 hospitals in California using the same program for more than a year.[70]

As stated in the 2010 CDC guidelines, "It is important that the monitoring be performed by hospital epidemiologists, infection preventionists or their designees who are not part of the actual EVS cleaning program. Such an approach assures the validity of the information collected."[46(Appendix B, p1)] A recent study in 2 hospitals found that when EVS managers monitored the discharge room TDC, they documented an average score of 82.5% whereas a research team covertly evaluating the same hospitals documented an average score of 52.4%.[71] Given that neither the Joint Commission nor the World Health Organization considers self-monitoring of hand hygiene practice acceptable, it seems reasonable that a similar expectation should be applied to monitoring disinfection cleaning activities.

## DISINFECTING ENVIRONMENTAL SURFACES
### Chemical Disinfectants

The use of EPA-registered hospital-grade disinfectants to clean patient zone hard surfaces has been considered an important element of health care environmental cleaning for many years.[35] As recommended by the CDC, disinfectants are used on all such surfaces in US hospitals.[38] Their use in some other countries has been limited to special areas, such as intensive treatment units and operating theaters.[11] Given the recent detailed review related to disinfectant choice and utilization,[35] the following discussion focuses only on several important generalizations.

During the past 2 years, the traditional use of EPA-registered hospital-grade disinfectants on noncritical patient zone surfaces has been profoundly impacted by the development of sporicidal chemistries that are at least as effective as bleach, are not associated with significant damage to surfaces, and are not associated with potentially toxic residuals during either their use or disposal.[72]

Recent published reports have confirmed both equal sporicidal potency to bleach as well as an absence of any discernable damage to a range of surfaces after repeated exposure for 1 hydrogen proxide/peroxy acetic acid disinfectant.[72,73] In a clinical study, the peroxide/peroxy acetic acid formulation was found approximately twice as potent as a quartenary ammonium compound in surface bioburden reduction and as effective as bleach in clinical use.[61,74] Although studies to further quantify the relative clinical value of both peroxide/paracedic acid formulations as well as chlorinated hydrogen peroxide are warranted, these new chemistries have the potential for substantially improving the effectiveness of patient zone surface disinfection cleaning. Given the numerous traditional hospital-grade disinfectants currently marketed and the ongoing development of new chemistries, it is critically important that all disinfectant systems undergo rigorously designed comparative studies in actual clinical settings to quantify their efficacy, similarities, differences, and potential limitations.[35,57,61] Although the development of new disinfectants and delivery systems may hold the promise of more effective and less difficult to use disinfection of patient zone surfaces, in 2014 Rutala stated, "Nothing is more important than the thoroughness of cleaning/disinfecting all hand contact (eg, environmental surfaces or patient care equipment) as current studies demonstrate that less than 50% of high risk objects are cleaned/disinfected at terminal cleaning."[35(p859)]

Although premoistened disposable wipes have been widely used to clean surfaces in health care settings, their clinical effectiveness has yet to be evaluated in comparative studies. Over the past 5 years, reports have documented the spread of HAPs from contaminated to noncontaminated surfaces by wipes.[75,76] In a review of health care cleaning practices, Sattar and Millard[76] in 2013 recommended that a moist wipe using a single-direction application be used on only 1 surface before being discarded. The validity of this approach was confirmed by the recently approved American Society for Testing and Materials standard E2967-15 test. All the 5 wipes tested by 3 independent testing sites confirmed a greater than 4 $\log_{10}$ reduction in *Staphylococcus aureus* and *Acinetobacter baumanii* on seeded surfaces but only a wipe using 0.5% accelerated $H_2O_2$ prevented transfer of the test bacteria to another surface.[77]

## Technologies to Augment Disinfection Cleaning

Although the use of EPA-registered hospital-grade disinfectants is intrinsic to surface disinfection cleaning, the concomitant recognition of suboptimal cleaning practice in many health care settings along with the evolving recognition of the role of the HAP-contaminated surfaces in pathogen acquisition has led to the development of technological interventions designed to augment physical cleaning of patient zone surfaces. Over the past decade, many innovative approaches have been developed and can be categorized broadly as no-touch technologies and self-disinfecting surfaces.

### No-touch technologies

Over the past several years, innovative technologies using hydrogen peroxide vapor or UV light systems have been developed and used to augment traditional chemical-based disinfection cleaning at the time of discharge. As stated by Otter[78] in a recent review, "The key question for some time has been whether automated room disinfection systems are able to reduce the rate of transmission compared with conventional cleaning and disinfection. HPV technologies are more potent systems but have logistical disadvantages. Recommendations would be premature for the routine use of such novel technology, primarily because research on microbial effectiveness, cost effectiveness and pragmatic application is still underway."[78(p234)] Ultimately, well-designed, independent, controlled, comparative studies will be needed to objectively quantify the cost and possible added value of such technologies when routine cleaning and disinfection has been sustainably optimized.[3]

### Self-disinfecting surfaces

Although the antibacterial properties of heavy metals, in particular silver, have led to its use in central venous and Foley catheters to decrease colonization and possibly infection, only recently have such materials been proposed as health care surface treatments to augment traditional chemical disinfection. Although in vitro studies of copper, silver, and other treated surfaces have confirmed modest but slow killing of most HAPs other than *C difficile* spores, substantial concerns have been raised regarding factors that could limit the clinical effectiveness of such surface treatments over time.[79] Although the concept of patient zone surfaces that are intrinsically inhospitable to HAPs is an attractive one, as noted by Humphries[79] in a recent review of disinfecting and microbocide impregnated surfaces and fabrics, "Larger and better designed studies are required to determine if these approaches augment current hygiene regimens, especially when these (current hygienic regimens) are optimally implemented."[79]

## Challenges of Measuring Cleanliness Versus Cleaning

According to the summary of the AHRQ technical brief developed by Han and colleagues,[2] "Environmental cleaning is a complex, multi-faceted process and involves the physical action of cleaning surfaces to remove organic and inorganic material followed by the application of a disinfectant as well as monitoring strategies to insure the appropriateness of these practices."[2(p1)] Before discussing the challenges of such monitoring by evaluating the process of cleaning or its outcome, cleanliness, it is important to clarify the critical difference between these 2 similar terms. As indicated in **Table 2**, monitoring cleaning represents a process measure of practice. It is expressed as a TDC score and may be applicable to an object, a defined set of surfaces, a defined geographic entity such as an ICU, or monitoring a hospital or even a group of hospitals.[46] When used generally, the term, *cleanliness*, may be used to describe a surface free from visible soil. In contrast, when discussing patient zone hygiene, cleanliness represents a quantitative measure of viable bacteria on a surface after the surface has been cleaned.

### Cleanliness

Given that truly sterile patient zone surfaces are not feasible in the context of the epidemiology of HAPs (discussed previously), it has been suggested that a microbiologically definable threshold, or cleanliness standard, may exist below which transmission of HAPs would not occur.[11] Although, as Rutala and Weber have noted, the value of having patient zone surfaces "hygienically clean, that is, free of pathogens in significant numbers to cause human disease"[35(p863)] is widely appreciated, it has not yet been possible to define or quantify such a condition.[57] Because the realistic goal of environmental cleaning and disinfection of patient care areas is not to produce a continuously sterile surface environment but rather to effectively decrease pathogen transmission, the identification of a threshold of environmental contamination below which transmission would not be expected to occur could be valuable.[3] Furthermore, the challenges of evaluating cleanliness over time as a process measure include the typically low bioburden of HAPs on contaminated surfaces, the need to measure cleanliness immediately after cleaning to eliminate the variable of recontamination

**Table 2**
**The difference between cleaning and cleanliness**

|  | Cleaning | Cleanliness |
|---|---|---|
| Definition | A measure of the physical cleaning process | A measure of viable bacteria on a surface |
| Defined criteria | Compliance with existing cleaning policy | No cleanliness standard |
| Improvement shown to decrease bacterial transmission (published) | Multiple studies | No direct studies |
| Impacted by | Thoroughness of cleaning practice, potential observer bias | Type and magnitude of bioburden, thoroughness of cleaning contamination since cleaning, culture system used |

before measurement, the relative clinical efficacy of different hospital-grade disinfectants and the biostability of various surface materials to support or inhibit microbial growth. If a basic cleanliness standard were defined, it would then need to be validated across diverse clinical venues within the hospital as well as in nonhospital health care settings.

### Cleaning
Objectively monitoring the process of cleaning as recommended by the CDC guidelines has been shown to decrease both HAP environmental contamination and HAP transmission to patients. As discussed previously, many studies over the past decade have documented its value in mitigating environmental HAP contamination while improving patient safety with respect to these pathogens.

## ENVIRONMENTAL HYGIENE AND HAND HYGIENE—AN INTEGRATED APPROACH

Over the past several years, it has become increasingly evident that infection prevention initiatives focused on optimizing hand hygiene have not realized their hoped-for impact on HAP transmission in well-resourced health care settings.[80–84] Accepting an inability to quantify the absolute risk of pathogen acquisition directly from health care workers' hands, there is good circumstantial evidence that such transmission accounts for a substantial proportion of HAP transmission. It has become widely accepted that hand hygiene, as noted by Palamore and Henderson, is "critically important for the prevention of HAIs."[85(p8)] In response, many health care organizations have undertaken extensive, resource-intensive efforts to improve hand hygiene compliance.[86] Despite extensive translational research and strong support from accrediting institutions over the past 10 years, the enthusiasm for quickly reaping substantial benefits from optimizing hand hygiene practice has been tempered by the realization that acceptance inertia, psychological barriers, suboptimal application of technique, and, most particularly, the pressures of providing direct patient care have had an adverse impact on the effectiveness of this intervention.[87] These issues, along with the challenges of performing hand hygiene as recommended by the World Health Organization "five moments" construct while caring for acutely ill patients and the fact that 10% to 60% of patient zone surfaces contain HAPs, make it likely that pathogen-contaminated environmental surfaces will negate some of the benefits of optimized hand hygiene practice.[11,43,88]

   Given that patient zone surfaces not contaminated by HAPs cannot be a source of pathogen transmission even in the absence of hand hygiene, further consideration must be given to viewing both environmental hygiene and hand hygiene as interdependent interventions. When viewed in this manner, it becomes evident that the mandates and challenges of these 2 interventions represent an inverse continuum (**Fig. 5**). For example, in the ICU setting, where hand hygiene often becomes logistically challenging and glove use without hand hygiene is frequent, there would be a particularly strong mandate to optimize hygienic cleaning. In contrast, in ambulatory settings, where there are few intrinsic barriers to hand hygiene, enhanced hygienic cleaning practices would not be strongly mandated. In this context, the specific elements of hygienic practice can be characterized along a complexity gradient (**Fig. 6**). By relating these constructs to the various settings (**Fig. 7**), interventions can be defined along the continuum outlined to provide a framework for analyzing and prioritizing the relative cost/benefit of different levels of complementary hygienic practices (see **Fig. 7**). By characterizing intrinsic patient/personnel risk and setting modifiers, a particular site can be moved up or down diagonally along the range of settings. For example, if an immunologically compromised person was in an ambulatory care setting, it would

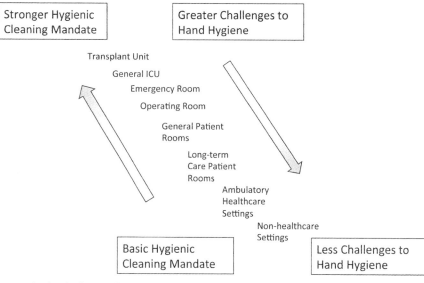

Transplant Unit
General ICU
Emergency Room
Operating Room
General Patient Rooms
Long-term Care Patient Rooms
Ambulatory Healthcare Settings
Non-healthcare Settings

Stronger Hygienic Cleaning Mandate

Greater Challenges to Hand Hygiene

Basic Hygienic Cleaning Mandate

Less Challenges to Hand Hygiene

**Fig. 5.** The hygienic practice continuum.

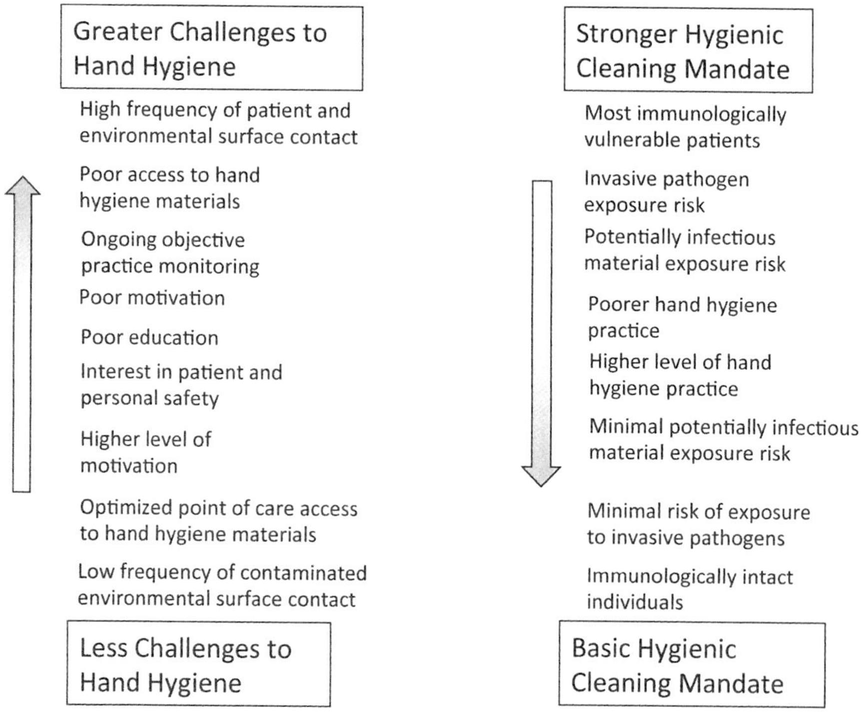

Greater Challenges to Hand Hygiene

High frequency of patient and environmental surface contact

Poor access to hand hygiene materials

Ongoing objective practice monitoring

Poor motivation

Poor education

Interest in patient and personal safety

Higher level of motivation

Optimized point of care access to hand hygiene materials

Low frequency of contaminated environmental surface contact

Less Challenges to Hand Hygiene

Stronger Hygienic Cleaning Mandate

Most immunologically vulnerable patients

Invasive pathogen exposure risk

Potentially infectious material exposure risk

Poorer hand hygiene practice

Higher level of hand hygiene practice

Minimal potentially infectious material exposure risk

Minimal risk of exposure to invasive pathogens

Immunologically intact individuals

Basic Hygienic Cleaning Mandate

**Fig. 6.** Elements of hygienic practice.

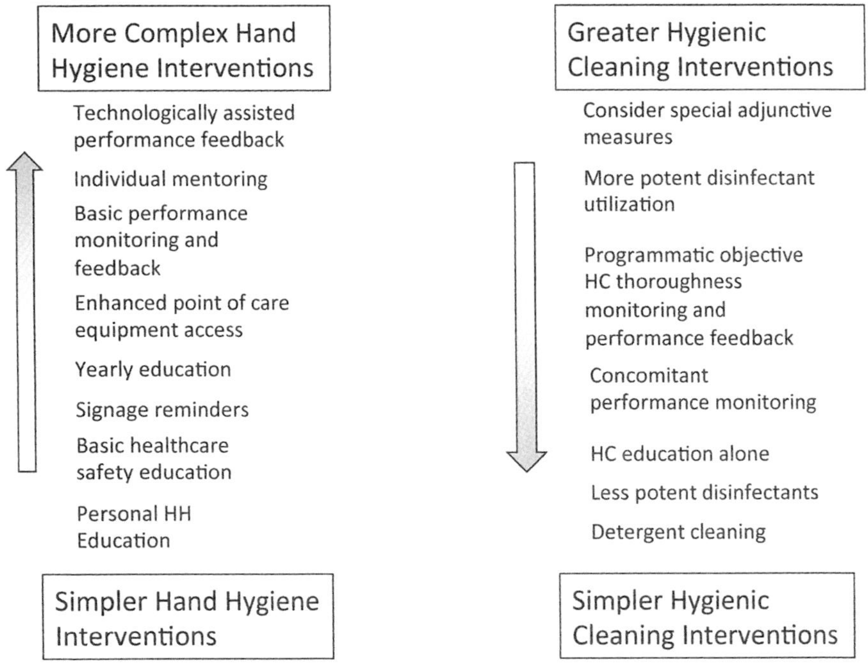

| More Complex Hand Hygiene Interventions | Greater Hygienic Cleaning Interventions |
|---|---|
| Technologically assisted performance feedback | Consider special adjunctive measures |
| Individual mentoring | More potent disinfectant utilization |
| Basic performance monitoring and feedback | |
| | Programmatic objective HC thoroughness monitoring and performance feedback |
| Enhanced point of care equipment access | |
| Yearly education | Concomitant performance monitoring |
| Signage reminders | |
| Basic healthcare safety education | HC education alone |
| | Less potent disinfectants |
| Personal HH Education | Detergent cleaning |
| Simpler Hand Hygiene Interventions | Simpler Hygienic Cleaning Interventions |

**Fig. 7.** Hygienic practice interventions.

be reasonable to consider moving to a higher level of hygienic cleaning intervention than otherwise is warranted. Similarly if the patient population in a long-term care setting required only minimal assistance, it would be reasonable to move down the intervention continuum toward noninpatient health care settings. Once the particular features of a setting are defined in this manner, the constructs can be used to develop programmatic interventions that maximize the components of health care hygienic practice for the best cost/benefit to improving patient/personnel safety.

## RESEARCH OPPORTUNITIES AND CHALLENGES

Along with an evolving awareness of the need to optimize both the process and structural elements of hygienic cleaning (see **Box 1**), it has become increasingly evident that there is limited objectively developed evidence to guide best practices.[1,3,11,57]

### Improving Study Design

During the past 20 years, many published reports have described improved outcomes as the result of modifications in basic hygienic cleaning. Unfortunately, causal analysis of almost all these studies has been greatly hampered by the simultaneous implementation of multiple interventions in addition to improved cleaning. This issue is particularly well illustrated by the reports of interventions to minimize health care–onset C difficile infection beginning in the mid-1980s. Although more than 20 quasiexperimental, often outbreak-associated, studies have supported the likely role of improved environmental hygiene on C difficile transmission, all these studies consist of several interventions implemented simultaneously. Because of confounding variables (some known and some unknown) in each study, it has been impossible to specifically quantify the impact of disinfection cleaning on C difficile transmission.[89] Even when a single environmental intervention, such as cleaning agent change, is pursued, published studies have not separated the thoroughness of cleaning from the specific cleaning agent being tested.[90,91] For example, it is possible that the novelty of a new cleaning agent resulted in better attention to the process of cleaning. As a result, the improved outcome may have actually been due to the heightened attention to cleaning surrounding the change in disinfectant. To date, only 2 clinical studies have compared the relative effectiveness of 2 disinfectant chemistries while controlling for this phenomenon by objectively monitoring the thoroughness of the hygienic cleaning processes in addition to microbiologic[61,74] and outcomes.[74]

There is also a need to substantially move environmental hygiene research from evaluation of practice to evaluation of objectively defined and reproducible clinically meaningful outcomes.[11,61,92] Several studies have successfully used objective cleaning process monitoring and documented significantly decreased environmental contamination by clinically important bacterial pathogens, such as methicillin-sensitive *Staphylococcus aureus*, VRE, *C difficile*, and mixed bowel flora.[23,42,87,93] There remains a need, however, for large well-conducted studies that use pathogen acquisition and, if feasible, clinical infection as outcomes to quantify the clinical impact of disinfection cleaning agents and thoroughness of practice.[3,92,94] Such outcome studies, although logistically complex and costly, will provide critical validation of the benefit of improving routine disinfection cleaning practice. Similar studies could also be used to clarify the potential benefits of no-touch technologies and self-cleaning surfaces.[3,11,92]

### A Proposed Hygienic Practice Research Agenda

The critical importance of developing a consensus-based research agenda focused on broad as well as specific needs led the CDC to convene a round table meeting, *Environmental Hygiene in Healthcare,* in September 2015.[1] The meeting brought together more than 30 clinical and academic experts, members of industry, patient advocates, federal agencies (Food and Drug Administration) and union representatives to "discuss the current state of knowledge regarding how patient care surfaces become contaminated, how transmission of infections occurs from the surfaces, and importantly, what facilities can do to improve the cleanliness of these surfaces."[1] There were 5 presentations given related to specific topics, including the presentation of a proposed environmental hygiene agenda.[95] Subsequently, a roundtable discussion led to the development of a consensus related to 4 key areas of interest for further research.

### Understanding transmission events related to patient room surfaces
As discussed previously, hand hygiene and hygienic cleaning are critical and interdependent elements of hygienic practice, although the quantitative impact of these 2 interventions has yet to be well defined.[11] In this regard it is hoped that the rapidly evolving technology, including the use of genomic epidemiology tools, highly sensitive and standardized surface culture methods, and sensitive approaches to pathogen acquisition monitoring will begin to clarify ways to optimize these interventions.

### Measuring cleanliness
Although the value as well as significant challenges of defining a so-called cleanliness standard are discussed previously, it is hoped that standardized surface culturing methods and sensitive systems to quantify transmission events will lead to defining when in-use patient zone surfaces are a transmission risk to patients.

*Improving cleanliness by focusing on process*
The opportunities and challenges of the important EVS activities were discussed extensively during the meeting. It was observed that some subject areas need further study and guidance, including methods of education and training of EVS personnel, methods for monitoring cleaning and disinfection, and ways to overcome organizational challenges of the work that EVS personnel perform.

*Improving cleanliness by evaluating emerging interventions*
The role of no-touch technologies and self-disinfecting surfaces was acknowledged as was the fact that the body of evidence to define the appropriate role for these interventions is limited. There was unanimous agreement that comparative studies of these technologies are urgently needed.[1]

The importance of developing such a consensus research agenda has become a critical guide to the 6 previous and 5 new CDC Epicenter programs, recently the recipients of almost $11 million in federal funding specifically to further research in these areas.[96]

## ACKNOWLEDGMENTS

This review is dedicated to the memory of Judeen Bartley, MS, MPH, CIC, whose insight and leadership related to health care environmental hygiene science greatly influenced the development of the field. The author acknowledges editorial guidance and assistance from Hilary Humphreys, MD, and Linda Homan, RN, CIC.

## REFERENCES

1. Centers for Disease Control and Prevention. Environmental Hygiene in Healthcare. 2015. Available at: http://www.cdc.gov/hai/research/eic-meeting.html. Accessed December 10, 2015.
2. Han JH, Sullivan N, Leas BF, et al. Cleaning hospital room surfaces to prevent healthcare-assocaited infections. Ann Intern Med 2015;163(8):598–607.
3. Carling PC, Huang SS. Improving healthcare environmental cleaning and disinfection: current and evolving issues. Infect Control Hosp Epidemiol 2013;34(5): 507–13.
4. Wenzel RP, Edmond MB. Infection Control: The case for horizontal rather than vertical interventional programs. Int J Infect Dis 2010;14:S3–5.
5. Edmond MB, Wenzel RP. Screening inpatients for MRSA - Case Closed. N Engl J Med 2013;368(24):2314.
6. Septimus E, Weinstein A, Perl T, et al. Approaches for preventing healthcare-associated infections: Go long or go wide? Infect Control Hosp Epidemiol 2014;35(7):797–801.
7. Jeong H, Heo J, Kim H, et al. Persistent environmental contamination and prolonged viral shedding in MERS patients during MERS-CoV outbreak in South Korea. Abstract 1978a. ID Week. San Diego (CA), October 6, 2015.
8. Donskey C, Hayden M, Huang S, et al. for the Department of Health & Human Services. Environmental hygiene: Ebola and other emerging pathogens in healthcare. Available at: http://www.cdc.gov/hai/researcj/eic-meeting.html. Accessed December 10, 2015.
9. Huang S, Datta R, Platt R. Risk of acquiring antibiotic-resistant bacteria from prior room occupants. Arch Intern Med 2006;166:1945–51.
10. Carling P. Methods for assessing the adequacy of practice and improving room disinfection. Am J Infect Control 2013;14(5 Suppl):S20–5.

11. Dancer S. Controlling hospital-acquired infection: focus on the role of the environment and new technologies for decontamination. Clin Microbiol Rev 2014;27(4): 665–90.

12. Donskey C, Chowdhry T, Hecker M, et al. Effect of antibiotic therapy on the density of vancomycin-resistant enterococci in the stool of colonized patients. N Engl J Med 2000;343(26):1925–32.

13. Chang S, Sethi AK, Eckstein BC, et al. Skin and environmental contamination with methicillin-resistant Staphylococcus aureus among carriers identified clinically versus through active surveillance. Clin Infect Dis 2009;48(10):1423–8.

14. Sethi AK, Al-Nassir WN, Nerandzic MM, et al. Skin and environmental contamination with vancomycin-resistant Enterocci in patients receiving oral metronidazole or oral vancomycin treatment for Clostridium difficile-associated disease. Infect Control Hosp Epidemiol 2009;30(1):13–7.

15. Sethi AK, Al-Nassir WN, Nerandzic MM, et al. Persistence of skin contamination and environmental shedding of Clostridium difficile during and after treatment of C. difficile infection. Infect Control Hosp Epidemiol 2010;31(1):21–7.

16. Kundrapu S, Sunkesula V, Tomas M, et al. Skin and environmental contamination in patients diagnosed with Clostridium difficile infection but not meeting clinical criteria for testing. Infect Control Hosp Epidemiol 2015;36(11):1348–50.

17. Faired MC, Pearl DL, Berke O, et al. The identification and epidemiology of meticillin-resistant Staphylococus aureus and Clostridium difficile in patient rooms and the ward environment. BMC Infect Dis 2013;13:342.

18. Miles J, Holt J, Handelsman J. Allies and adversaries: roles of the microbiome in infectious disease. Microbe 2015;10(9):368–74.

19. Tschudin-Sutter S, Carroll K, Tamma P, et al. Impact of toxigenic Clostridium difficile colonization on the risk of subsequent C. difficile infection in Intensive Care Unit patients. Infect Control Hosp Epidemiol 2015;36(11):1324–9.

20. Chang S, Sethi A, Stiefel U, et al. Occurrence of skin and environmental contamination with methicillin-resistant Staphylococcus aureus before results of polymerase chain reaction at hospital admission become available. Infect Control Hosp Epidemiol 2011;31(6):607–12.

21. Weber D, Rutala W, Miller M, et al. Role of hospital surfaces in the transmission of emerging health care-associated pathogens: Norovirus, Clostridium difficile, and Acinetobacter species. Am J Infect Control 2010;38:S25–33.

22. Donskey C. Does improving surface cleaning and disinfection reduce health care-associated infections? Am J Infect Control 2013;41:S12–9.

23. Sitzlar B, Deshparade A, Fentelli D, et al. An environmental disinfection oddssey: evaluation of dequential interventions to improve disinfection of Clostridium difficile patient rooms. Infect Control Hosp Epidemiol 2013;34:459–65.

24. Linder K, Hecker M, Kundrapu S, et al. Evaluation of patients' skin, environmental surfaces, and urinary catheters as sources for transmission of urinary pathogens. Am J Infect Control 2014;42(7):810–2.

25. Creamer E, Shore AC, Deasy EC, et al. Air and surface contamination patterns of meticillin-resistant Staphylococcus aureus on eight acute hospital wards. J Hosp Infect 2014;86:201–8.

26. Guerrero D, Becker J, Eckstein E, et al. Asymptomatic carriage of toxigenic Clostridium difficile by hospitalized patients. J Hosp Infect 2013;85(2):155–8.

27. Gavalda L, Pequeno S, Soriano A, et al. Environmental contamination by multidrug-resistant microorganisms after daily cleaning. Am J Infect Control 2015;43:776–8.

28. Kramer A, Schwebke I, Kamp FG. How long do nosocomial pathogens survive on an inanimate surface? BMC Infect Dis 2006;6:130.

29. Munoz-Price L, Weinstein A. Fecal patina in the anesthesia work area. Anesth Analg 2015;120(4):703–5.

30. Guerrero D, Nerandzic M, Jury L, et al. Acquisition of spores on gloved hands after contact with the skin of patients with Clostridium difficile infection and with environmental surfaces in their rooms. Am J Infect Control 2012;40(6):556–8.

31. Kundrapu S, Sunkesula V, Jury L, et al. Daily disinfection of high-touch surfaces in isolation rooms to reduce contamination of healthcare worker's hands. Infect Control Hosp Epidemiol 2012;33(10):1039–42.

32. Morgan DJ, Liang SY, Smith CL. Frequent multidrug-resistant Acinetobacter baumannii contamination of gloves, gowns, and hands of healthcare workers. Infect Control Hosp Epidemiol 2012;31(7):716–21.

33. Ferng YH, Clock SA, Wong-Mcloughlin J, et al. Multicenter study of hand carriage of potential pathogens by Neonatal ICU healthcare personnel. J Pediatr Infect Dis Soc 2015;4(3):276–9.

34. Thomas ME, Sunkesula V, Kundrapu S, et al. An intervention to reduce healthcare personnel hand contamination during care of patients with Clostridium difficile infection. Am J Infect Control 2015;43:1366–7.

35. Rutala WA, Weber DJ. Selection of the ideal disinfectant. Infect Control Hosp Epidemiol 2014;35(7):855–65.

36. Nerandzic M, Thota P, Sankar C, et al. Evaluation of a pulsed xenon ultraviolet disinfection system for reduction of healthcare-associated pathogens in hospital rooms. Infect Control Hosp Epidemiol 2015;36(2):192–7.

37. Smith P, Watkins K, Hewlett A. Infection control through the ages. Am J Infect Control 2012;40:35–42.

38. Centers for Disease Control and Prevention/Healthcare Infection Control Advisory Committee (HICPAC). Guidelines for environmental infection control in healthcare facilities. Atlanta (FA): Centers for Disease Control and Prevention; 2003. Available at: http://www.cdc.gov/hicpac/pdf/guidelines/eic_in_HCF_03.pdf. Accessed December 10, 2015.

39. Siegel JD, Rhinehart E, Jackson M, et al. Healthcare infection control practices Advisory Committee. Management of multi-drug-resistant organisms in healthcare settings. 2006. Available at: http://www.cdc.gov/ncidod/dhqp/pdf/ar/mdroGuideline 2006.pdf. Accessed January 15, 2009.

40. Carling PC, Bartley JM. Evaluating hygienic cleaning in healthcare settings: what you do not know can harm your patients. Am J Infect Control 2010;38:S41–50.

41. Dancer SJ. How do we assess hospital cleaning? A proposal for microbiological standards for surface hygiene in hospitals. J Hosp Infect 2004;56:10–5.

42. Hayden MK, Bonten MJ, Blom DW, et al. Reduction in acquisition of vancomycin-resistant enterococcus after enforcement of routine environmental cleaning measures. Clin Infect Dis 2006;42(11):1552–60.

43. Carling PC, Briggs J, Hylander D, et al. Evaluation of patient area cleaning in 3 hospitals using a novel targeting methodology. Am J Infect Control 2006;34:513–9.

44. Carling PC, Parry MF, Von Beheren SM. Identifying Opportunities to Enhance Environmental Cleaning in 23 Acute Care Hospitals. Infect Control Hosp Epidemiol 2008;29(1):1–7.

45. Carling PC, Po JL, Bartley J, et al; Healthcare Environmental Hygiene Group. Identifying opportunities to improve environmental hygiene in multiple healthcare

settings. Abstract 908. Fifth Decennial International Conference on Healthcare-Associated Infections. Atlanta (GA), March 10, 2010.

46. Guh A, Carling P; for the Environmental Evaluation Workgroup. Options for evaluating environmental cleaning. 2010. Available at: http://www.cdc.gov/HAI/toolkits/Evaluating-Environmental-Cleaning.html. Accessed December 10, 2015.

47. Carling PC, Parry MM, Rupp ME, et al. Improving cleaning of the environment surrounding patients in 36 acute care hospitals. Infect Control Hosp Epidemiol 2008; 29(11):1035–41.

48. Carling P, Briggs J, Perkins J, et al. Improving cleaning of patient rooms using a new targeting method. Clin Infect Dis 2006;42:385–8.

49. Carling PC, Eck EK. Achieving sustained improvement in environmental hygiene using coordinated benchmarking in 12 hospitals. Abstracts of the SHEA Fifth Decennial Meeting. Atlanta (GA), March 18-22, 2010.

50. Carling PC, Herwaldt LA, VonBeheren S. The Iowa disinfection cleaning project: opportunities, successes and challenges of a structured intervention project in 56 hospitals. Infect Control Hosp Epidemiol. Abstract 1024. ID Week, San Diego(CA), October 6, 2015.

51. Murphy CL, Macbeth DA, Derrington P, et al. An assessment of high touch object cleaning thoroughness using a fluorescent marker in two Australian hospitals. Healthc Infect 2012;16(4):156–63.

52. Datta R, Platt R, Yokoe DS, et al. Environmental cleaning intervention and risk of acquiring multidrug-resistant organisms from prior room occupants. Arch Intern Med 2011;171(6):491–4.

53. Boyce JM, Havill NL, Havill HL, et al. Comparison of fluorescent marker systems with 2 quantitative methods of assessing terminal cleaning practices. Infect Control Hosp Epidemiol 2011;32:1187–93.

54. Branch-Ellman W, Robilland E, McCarthy G Jr, et al. Direct feedback with the ATP liminometer as a process improvement tool for the terminal cleaning of patient rooms. Am J Infect Control 2014;42:195–7.

55. Association for the Healthcare Environment of the American Hospital Association. Curriculum for the Certified Healthcare Environmental Services Technician (TM). Available at: http://www.ahe.org/ahe/lead/CHEST/curriculum.shtml. Accessed December 10, 2015.

56. Chen L, Vander Weg M, Hofmann D, et al. The Hawthorne Effect in infection prevention and Epidemiology. Infect Control Hosp Epidemiol 2015;36(12):1444–50.

57. Agency for Healthcare Research and Quality Technical brief 22 Environmental Cleaning for the Prevention of Healthcare-Associated Infections (HAI). Available at: http://effectivehealthcare.ahrq.gov/index.cfm/search-for-guides-reviews-and-reports/?pageaction=displayproduct&productid=2103. Accessed December 10, 2015.

58. Claro T, Galvin S, Cahill O, et al. What is the best method? Recovery of methicillin-resistant Stahylococcus aureus and extended-spectrum B-lactamase-producing Escherichia coli from inanimate hospital surfaces. Infect Control Hosp Epidemiol 2014;35(7):869–71.

59. Dancer SJ. The role of environmental cleaning in the control of hospital-acquired infection. J Hosp Infect 2009;73:378–85.

60. Mulvey D, Redding P, Robertson C, et al. Finding a benchmark for monitoring hospital cleanliness. J Hosp Infect 2011;77(1):25–30.

61. Carling PC, Perkins J, Ferguson J, et al. Evaluating a new paradigm for company surface disinfection in clinical practice. Infect Control Hosp Epidemiol 2014; 35(11):1349–55.

62. Whiteley GS, Derry C, Glasbey T. A comparative performance of three brands of portable ATP – bioluminometers intended for use in hospital infection control. Healthc Infect 2012;73:4–9.
63. Malik DJ, Shama G. Estimating surface contamination by means of ATP determinations: 20 pence short of a pound. J Hosp Infect 2012;80(4):354–5.
64. Whiteley GS, Derry C, Glasbey T, et al. The perennial problem of variability in adenosine triphosphate (ATP) tests for hygiene monitoring within healthcare settings. Infect Control Hosp Epidemiol 2015;36(6):658–63.
65. Munoz-Price LS, Bimbach DJ, Lubarsky DA, et al. Decreasing operating room environmental pathogen contamination through improved cleaning practice. Infect Control Hosp Epidemiol 2012;33(9):897–904.
66. Munoz-Price LS, Fajardo-Aquino Y, Arheart KL. Ultraviolet powder versus ultraviolet gel for assessing environmental cleaning. Infect Control Hosp Epidemiol 2012;33(2):192–5.
67. Munoz-Price LS. Controlling multidrug-resistant gram-negative bacilli in your hospital: a transformational journey. J Hosp Infect 2015;89:254–8.
68. Gillespie E, Wright P, Snook K, et al. The role of ultraviolet marker assessments in demonstrating cleaning efficacy. Am J Infect Control 2015;43:1347–9.
69. Conway LJ, Raveis VH, Pogorzelska-Maziarz M, et al. Tensions inherent in the evolving role of the infection preventionist. Am J Infect Control 2013;41(11):959–64.
70. Holmer L, Russell D, Steger P, et al. Sustainability of an environmental cleaning program in California small and critical access hospitals. Abstract presented at the Annual Meeting of the Association for Infection Control Professionals. San Diego (CA), June 16, 2014.
71. Knelson LP, Ramadanovic G, Chen L, et al. Self-monitoring of hospital room cleaning by Environmenal Services (EVS) may not accurately measure cleanliness. Abstract 732. ID week, San Diego (CA), October 6, 2015.
72. Cadnum JL, Jencson A, Thriveen J, et al. Evaluation of Real-World Materials Compatibility of OxyCide Daily Disinfectant Cleaner versus Sodium Hypochlorite. Abstract 7202. Presented at the Society for Healthcare Epidemiology Meeting. Orlando, FL, May 5, 2015.
73. Deshpande A, Mana TSC, Cadnum JL, et al. Evaluation of a sporicidal peracetic acid/Hydrogen Peroxide-based daily disinfectant cleaner. Infect Control Hosp Epidemiol 2014;35(11):1414–6.
74. Haider S, Moshos J, Burger T, et al. Impact of QxyCide™ on environmental contamination and infection rates compared to standard cleaning practice. Abstract 1437, ID Week. San Diego (CA), 2014.
75. Ramm L, Siani S, Westgate R, et al. Pathogen transfer and high variability in pathogen removal by detergent wipes. Am J Infect Control 2015;43:724–8.
76. Sattar SA, Millard J. The enveial role of wiping in decontamination of high-touch environmental surfaces: A review of current status and directions for the future. Am J Infect Control 2013;41:S97–104.
77. Sattar SA, Bradley C, Kibbee R, et al. Disinfectant wipes are appropriate to control microbial bioburden from surfaces: use of a new ASTM standard test protocol to demonstrate efficacy. J Hosp Infect 2015;91:319–25.
78. Otter JA. What's trending in the infection prevention and control literature? From HIS 2012 to HIS 2014, and beyond? J Hosp Infect 2015;89:229–36.
79. Humphreys H. Self-disinfecting and microbiocide-impregnated surfaces and fabrics: What potential in interrupting the spread of healthcare-associated infection? Clin Infect Dis 2014;58(6):848–53.

80. Silvestri L, Petros AJ, Sarginson RE, et al. Hand washing in the intensive care unit: a big measure with modest effects. J Hosp Infect 2005;59:172–9.
81. Rupp M, Fitzgerald T, Puumala S, et al. Prospective, controlled, cross-over trial of alcohol-based hand gel in critical care units. Infect Control Hosp Epidemiol 2008; 29(1):8–15.
82. Sepkowitz KA. Why doesn't hand hygiene work better? Lancet Infect Dis 2012;12: 96–7.
83. Smiddy M, O'Connell R, Creedon S. Systematic qualitative literature review of health care worker's compliance with hand hygiene guidelines. Am J Infect Control 2015;43:269–74.
84. Graves N. It's not all about hand hygiene – other measures are at least that important. Conturunsies Infection Control and Prevention. Presented at the Interscience Conference on Antimicrobial Agents and Chemotherapy 2015. San Diego (CA), September 6, 2015.
85. Palmore T, Henderson D. Big brother is washing...video surveillance for hand hygiene adherence, through the lenses of efficacy and privacy. Clin Infect Dis 2012;54(1):8–9.
86. Page K, Barnett A, Campbell M, et al. Costing the Australian national hand hygiene initiative. J Hosp Infect 2014;88:141–8.
87. Conway L, Riley L, Saiman L, et al. Implementation and impact of an automated group monitoring and feedback system to promote hand hygiene among health care personnel. Jt Comm J Qual Patient Saf 2014;40(9):408–17.
88. Sax H, Allegranzi B, Uckay I, et al. "My five moments of hand hygiene": a user-centered design approach to understand, train, monitor and report hand hygiene. J Hosp Infect 2007;67:9–21.
89. Carling PC. Optimizing environmental hygiene: the Key to C. difficile control. 2012. Available at: http://www.webbertraining.com/files/library/docs/416.pdf. Accessed December 20, 2015.
90. Mayield JL, Lee T, Miller J, et al. Environmental control to reduce transmission of Clostridium difficile. Clin Infect Dis 2000;31(4):995–1000.
91. Wilcox MH, Fawley WN, Wigglesworth N, et al. Comparisonof the effect of detergent versus hypochlorite on environmental contamination and incidence of Clostridium difficile infection. J Hosp Infect 2003;54(2):109–14.
92. McDonald LC, Arduino M. Climbing the evidentiary hierarchy for environmental infection control. Clin Infect Dis 2013;56(1):36–9.
93. Goodman ER, Platt R, Bass R, et al. Impact of an environmental cleaning intervention on the presence of methicillin-resistant Staphylococcus aureus and vancomycin-resistant enterococci on surfaces in intensive care unit rooms. Infect Control Hosp Epidemiol 2008;29(7):593–9.
94. Safdar N, Anderson D, Braun B, et al. The evolving landscape of healthcare-associated infections: Recent advances in prevention and a road map for research. Infect Control Hosp Epidemiol 2014;35(5):480–93.
95. Reddy S. Draft framework for environmental infection control research focused on non-critical surfaces. Centers for Disease Control and Prevention. Environmental Hygiene in Healthcare; 2015. Available at: http://www.cdc.gov/hai/research/eic-meeting.html. Accessed December 10, 2015.
96. Centers for Disease Control and Prevention. CDC Names Six New Medical Research Centers to Accelerate Health Care Innovations. Available at: http://www.cdc.gov/media/releases/2015/p1005-medical-research-centers.html. Accessed December 20, 2015.

# Outbreaks in Health Care Settings

Geeta Sood, MD[a],*, Trish M. Perl, MD, MSc[b]

KEYWORDS

- Outbreaks • Health care settings • Sources of outbreaks • Evaluation • Review

KEY POINTS

- Outbreaks and pseudo-outbreaks that occur in health care settings should be approached systematically using advanced laboratory testing and epidemiologic tools to guide evaluation of events and to determine course of action.
- Multiple sources, such as health care personnel, the health care environment, supplies and equipment, and potable water, have been associated with outbreaks.
- Multiple organisms, such as atypical mycobacteria, *Acinetobacter*, *Pseudomonas*, *Staphylococcus aureus*, and carbapenem-resistant Enterobacteriaceae and fungal species have been associated with outbreaks in health care settings.
- Certain settings, including the neonatal intensive care unit, endoscopy, oncology, and transplant units, have specific issues that impact the approach to investigation and control of outbreaks in these settings.

## OUTBREAKS

Health care settings, while providing a safe environment for patient care, are complex settings and can produce conditions that facilitate the transmission of organisms and outbreaks. First, patients are vulnerable hosts due to immunosuppressive conditions, disruptions of their skin and mucous membranes, medications, and extremes of age. Second, the facility design, the multitude of life-saving invasive procedures using complicated equipment, contamination of the hospital environment with organisms (including multidrug-resistant organisms), the close proximity of patients who harbor transmissible organisms, and frequent contact with health care personnel, who can themselves transmit organisms, can provide an ideal environment for the propagation of an infectious agent.

---

Disclosure Statement: The authors have nothing to disclose.
[a] Division of Infectious Diseases, Johns Hopkins University School of Medicine, Johns Hopkins Bayview Medical Center, Mason F. Lord Building Center Tower, 3rd Floor, 5200 Eastern Avenue, Baltimore, MD 21224, USA; [b] Bloomberg School of Public Health, Johns Hopkins School of Medicine, 725 North Wolfe Street, Suite 228 PCTB, Baltimore, MD 21205, USA
* Corresponding author.
*E-mail address:* gsood1@jhmi.edu

Infect Dis Clin N Am 30 (2016) 661–687
http://dx.doi.org/10.1016/j.idc.2016.04.003
0891-5520/16/$ – see front matter © 2016 Elsevier Inc. All rights reserved.

id.theclinics.com

As more health care delivery has shifted from acute care hospitals to outpatient settings and the population ages and more individuals reside in nursing homes, outbreaks are increasingly recognized in alternative settings. The risk factors identified in acute care hospitals are also present in other locations. The entire continuum of health care needs to be considered in assessing the epidemiology of an outbreak.

Outbreaks can be expensive and time-consuming and can cause significant disruptions in health care operations in addition to impacting patient morbidity and mortality. Twelve percent of published outbreaks have led to closures of medical units. The most common pathogens associated with unit closure were not highly resistant organisms but rather, viruses such as influenza and norovirus.[1] Rotavirus and severe acute respiratory syndrome (SARS) were also associated with high closure rates.[1] The greatest challenges in outbreak management are the delay in identification of an outbreak and the delay in determining the source of the outbreak. In 37% of published outbreaks, the source is not identified. When the source is identified, it can be traced back to patients (25.7%), medical equipment or devices (11.9%), the environment (11.6%), and the staff (10.9%).[2] Interestingly, the most common pathogens identified in outbreaks are *Staphylococcus aureus* (14.8%), *Pseudomonas* spp (8.9%), and *Klebsiella* spp (7.1%), and these organisms are rarely associated with unit closures.[2,3]

## APPROACH TO AN OUTBREAK

An outbreak is defined as an increase in events, such as infections or number of organisms above the baseline rate, for a geographic area during a specified period of time. Some experts use a statistical definition. This increase may be a single infection, as in the cases of anthrax, health care–associated *Legionella*, or group A Streptococcal infection, or it may be many infections. The increase may occur over a short period of time or over years and may occur in a single unit or across many hospitals. Evaluating and managing outbreaks can be complex and multifaceted and often multiple steps occur concurrently. In any setting, the investigation should be efficient, thoughtful, and systematic so that appropriate infection prevention processes can be implemented to protect patients and health care personnel (**Box 1**).

Initially, it is important to verify the diagnosis. A varicella rash may be confused with smallpox or a culture may have been misread. Verification may require additional laboratory testing or clinical evaluation. It is, also, essential to communicate with the laboratory to save specimens early on in the investigation. These specimens can be used to identify a common source, trace transmission patterns, or reveal that a perceived outbreak was a cluster of unrelated events. Once the diagnosis has been confirmed, and the laboratory has been notified, a line list is created to describe potential cases with regard to person, place, and time. This is used to help focus the investigation. Simultaneously, it is important to determine if the baseline rate of the organism or infection of interest has changed over time, keeping in mind seasonal variation and comparing equivalent seasons. Such assessments must consider and ensure that other factors are not leading to the newly identified increase to accurately ascertain if there is a "true" increase in the rate of interest. A change in rates could result from altered surveillance definitions (changes in the numerator) or changes in the patient population sampled (changes in the denominator). As this assessment process is occurring, other cases should be identified, which may involve broadening the numbers and types of patients tested.

Once it has been determined that the observed infections represent an increase above baseline, the next step in investigating an outbreak is to create a case definition. This definition should be broad enough to capture any potential cases that may have

---

**Box 1**
**Outbreak investigation**

1. Verify the diagnosis and notify laboratory
2. Determine if this is an outbreak (baseline rates, assess changes in definition and changes in population)
3. Generate an epidemic curve and a line list (describe potential cases person, place, and time)
4. Perform a literature review to guide risk factor assessment
5. Develop a case definition
6. Find cases
7. "Shoe leather epidemiology" talk to staff, evaluate facility structure,
8. Implement appropriate infection-prevention interventions
9. Communicate with hospital leadership, and public relations department and risk department as indicated; involve public health authorities
10. Generate hypothesis and review cases for common epidemiologic links
11. Test the hypothesis (case-controlled evaluation)
12. Perform additional environmental or personnel screening as indicated
13. Evaluate impact of intervention

---

been missed on initial evaluation but not too broad to lose specificity in investigating any important epidemiologic links. Case finding should be performed systematically to avoid bias in data collection. Commonly this requires a review of the literature to understand incubation period, transmission dynamics, and common identified sources of a specific organism or syndrome (**Table 1**). Case definitions may need to be revised in the course of an investigation as new information becomes available. To identify cases, multiple data sources are available, including medical records, microbiology reports, operating room notes, respiratory therapy and procedure logs, or pharmacy records. Once case finding has been performed, generating an epidemic curve, which is a spatial presentation of the number of cases over time, aids in understanding transmission patterns. For example, these data may help differentiate a point source versus ongoing transmission and secondary transmission, and can help in assessing the phase of the epidemic.

These early steps are used to create and test a hypothesis by assessing if the suspected exposure differs in the cases from the uninfected patients (controls) to understand the relative contribution of risk factors to the outbreak. Depending on the situation (see **Table 1**), additional testing, such as environmental sampling from the patient's room or equipment, or testing of health care personnel and other patients to understand the extent of the outbreak may be undertaken. The epidemiologic review guides and supplements culture and clinical data in the investigative phase and is later used to evaluate the impact of the control measures implemented on the outbreak.

Importantly and in reality, measures to stop the outbreak are put into place before the hypothesis can be confirmed. In such situations, a line list of the cases with a list of possible exposures is used to simultaneously investigate epidemiologic links between cases and to implement control measures, such as changing a practice, enhancing a practice like hand hygiene, altering the number of personnel, enhancing isolation practices, testing personnel or patients, or closing a unit. These interventions should be

**Table 1**
Outbreak organisms

| Organism, Type of Infection(s) Associated with Outbreak, Process | Common Reservoirs | Potential Sources and/or Sites Associated with Outbreaks | Method of Detection: P = Patients, E = Environmental Source | Comments |
|---|---|---|---|---|
| *Acinetobacter* species Wounds, bloodstream and respiratory tract Infection and/or colonization | Wounds, genitourinary tract (GU), peri-rectal (PR) area, skin | Instrumentation, burns, trauma, surgery, respiratory equipment, gloves, parenteral nutrition, water | P = micro cultures E = surface swabs and culture of potentially implicated items | Intensive care units, patients returning from war zones; immunocompromised population Contaminates the environment extensively and can be difficult to eradicate |
| Adenovirus Epidemic keratoconjunctivitis (EKC); disseminated infection, cystitis | Oral pharyngeal secretions, urine | Equipment (tonometers) and health care workers | P = viral cultures, PCR E = not known to be useful | Ophthalmology patients, NICU patients, immunocompromised patients |
| *Aspergillus* spp Bloodstream, lower respiratory tract Infection and/or colonization | Air, dust, mold | Building demolition, renovation or construction sites, ventilation systems, dust-generating activities | P = microbiologic clinical (micro) cultures E = air sampling, surface samples | Often pathogenic in immunocompromised populations, and premature infants Can see increases with floods, severe weather events such as hurricanes |
| *Burkholderia cepacia* Bloodstream Infection and/or colonization | Oropharynx, skin | Water, contaminated solutions and skin disinfectants, contaminated equipment | P = micro cultures, stool E = cultures of potentially implicated items | Disinfectants (especially those containing iodine), water, solutions |
| *Candida* species Bloodstream | Skin (intertriginous areas) | Hands, onycholysis, devices | P = micro cultures E = cultures of hands and nail beds | Immunocompromised population at increased risk |

| | | | P = micro cultures<br>E = cultures of potentially implicated items/personnel | NICU patients at risk |
|---|---|---|---|---|
| *Campylobacter fetus* | Gastrointestinal | Food | P = micro cultures<br>E = cultures of potentially implicated items/personnel | NICU patients at risk |
| *Enterobacter* species<br>Urinary tract, bloodstream<br>Infection and colonization | PR, bloodstream, wounds | Contaminated IV fluids, total parenteral nutrition<br>Hands/dermatitis | P = micro cultures<br>E = cultures of potentially implicated items | Intensive care units, reuse of calibrated pressure transducers |
| *Enterococcus faecalis* and faecium (*Enterococcus* or Group D)<br>Neonatal sepsis, cystitis, bacteremia<br>Infection and/or colonization with resistant strains (VRE) | GU, PR, Gastrointestinal (GI) tract | Neonates/surgical patients/transplant patients | P = stool, peri-rectal vaginal cultures; hand cultures<br>E = used for vancomycin-resistant strains, primarily surface samples | Vancomycin resistant strains (VRE) do contaminate the environment and hands of health care personnel; environmental cultures are not used for susceptible strains |
| *Escherichia coli*<br>Epidemic diarrhea, wounds and surgical incisions, urinary tract, bloodstream, neonatal sepsis or meningitis<br>Infection | GI tract, skin, wounds | Equipment or fluids contaminated with organisms from lower GI tract, contaminated fluids | P = micro cultures, stool<br>E = cultures of potentially implicated items | Very common normal flora |
| *E coli* O157:H7 and other hemorrhagic species<br>Diarrhea and hemorrhagic colitis<br>Infection | GI tract of animals | Contaminated water, and foods (meat, salads) | P = micro cultures<br>E = cultures of potentially implicated items | Hemolytic uremic syndrome and thrombotic thrombocytopenic purpura are sequelae, high mortality among elderly and extremely young, cross contamination described |
| Hepatitis A<br>Infection | Liver, stool, blood | Hands/foods, transfusion | P = micro cultures<br>E = not known to be useful, cultures of potentially implicated personnel | Cross contamination described |

(continued on next page)

**Table 1**
*(continued)*

| Organism, Type of Infection(s) Associated with Outbreak, Process | Common Reservoirs | Potential Sources and/or Sites Associated with Outbreaks | Method of Detection: P = Patients, E = Environmental Source | Comments |
|---|---|---|---|---|
| Hepatitis B Infection | Liver, blood, and sterile body fluids | Blood and secretions, transfusions, improperly cleaned equipment, poor infection control practices | P = serology<br>E = not known to be useful, cultures of potentially implicated personnel | Patients with diabetes, on dialysis, patients in psychiatric units |
| Hepatitis C Infection | Liver, blood, and sterile body fluids | Blood and secretions, transfusions, improperly cleaned equipment, multidose vials, poor infection-control practices | P = serology<br>E = not known to be useful although recently integrated into an outbreak investigation, cultures of potentially implicated personnel | Patients on dialysis, patients in psychiatric units |
| Herpes virus infection<br>Skin, pneumonia, mucosal surfaces<br>Infection and/or colonization | Skin, saliva | Patients and health care workers | P = micro cultures<br>E = not known to be useful | Outbreaks reported when patients shed or with lesions in health care workers |
| *Klebsiella pneumoniae*<br>Urinary tract, pneumonia, bloodstream and neonatal infections<br>Infection and/or colonization | PR, nares, mouth, wounds, skin, blood | Urinary catheters, hand lotions, contaminated fluids, ventilators, eczema Foodborne outbreaks recently reported | P = micro cultures<br>E = cultures of potentially implicated items | Can be resistant to extended beta lactamases and carbapenemase; cross contamination described; rarely contaminates the environment |
| *Legionella pneumophila* and other species<br>Pneumonia Infection | Water | Potable water, air conditioning units, cooling towers, ice machines, construction | P = micro cultures<br>E = cultures of potentially implicated items/personnel | Can be associated with intense media scrutiny; 1 health care–associated case should trigger an investigation |

| | | | | |
|---|---|---|---|---|
| *Listeria monocytogenes*<br>Bloodstream and central nervous system infections<br>Infection | Food | Contaminated foods | P = micro cultures<br>E = cultures of potentially implicated items | Immunocompromised and mother-infant pairs at highest risk |
| *Mycobacterium tuberculosis*<br>Respiratory<br>Infection | Lungs, can disseminate | Airborne, improperly cleaned equipment | P = culture and PCR<br>E = not known to be useful, cultures of potentially implicated personnel | Health care transmission suggests poor infection control |
| Nontuberculous mycobacteria<br>(*Mycobacterium avium*, *Mycobacterium gordonae*)<br>Respiratory, skin, bloodstream<br>Infection and/or colonization | Lungs, skin | Contaminated water, improperly cleaned and sterilized equipment | P = micro cultures<br>E = cultures of potentially implicated items | Associated with pseudo-outbreaks<br>Reuse of improperly cleaned dialyzers, contaminated ice machines and other equipment |
| *Pseudomonas aeruginosa*<br>Burns, wounds, urinary tract, pneumonia<br>Infection and/or colonization | Gastrointestinal tract | Ventilators, whirlpools, sitz baths, solutions (mouthwash), any other water sources | P = micro cultures, stool, cultures of potentially implicated items<br>E = cultures of potentially implicated items | Primarily seen in immunocompromised patients and can be normal flora |
| *Ralstonia pickettii*<br>Bloodstream | Skin, oropharynx, blood | Water including sterile, skin disinfectants, incubator water baths | P = micro cultures, stool<br>E = cultures of potentially implicated items | Deliberate contamination of sterile fluids has been reported<br>Neonates and immunocompromised hosts |
| *Salmonella* species<br>GI infections, bloodstream<br>Infection and/or colonization | GI and biliary tract | Contaminated food, dairy, eggs/poultry, contaminated blood products | P = stool, blood cultures<br>E = not known to be useful | Not normal flora, cross contamination reported |

*(continued on next page)*

**Table 1**
*(continued)*

| Organism, Type of Infection(s) Associated with Outbreak, Process | Common Reservoirs | Potential Sources and/or Sites Associated with Outbreaks | Method of Detection:<br>P = Patients,<br>E = Environmental Source | Comments |
|---|---|---|---|---|
| *Serratia marcescens*<br>Urinary tract, bloodstream, respiratory<br>Infection and/or colonization | GI and GU | Solutions, inhalation therapy equipment, disinfectants, plasma, EDTA collection tubes, air conditioning vents, improperly cleaned equipment, chlorhexidine | P = micro cultures<br>E = cultures of potentially implicated items | Cross contamination well described, reuse of calibrated pressure transducers |
| *Staphylococcus aureus* includes methicillin-resistant strains<br>Surgical site, bloodstream<br>Infection and or colonization | Human skin, anterior nares, skin, throat and upper respiratory tract, rarely rectal | Nasal/skin carriage in health care workers<br>Increased nurse-to-patient ratios | P = microbiologic cultures<br>E = hand and anterior nares cultures; rarely environmental cultures are indicated including settle plates if looking for a cloud spreader | Usually associated with surgical site and bloodstream infections, molecular and genotypic typing can determine whether there is a point source or technical problems. Point source can be from a carrier and would require cultures of staff and other patients; technical failures can lead to rhinovirus infection may be a risk factor, cross contamination well described for human shedding |

| Organism/Infection | Reservoir | Tests | Comments |
|---|---|---|---|
| *Staphylococcus* species (coagulase negative) Blood | Human skin | P = microbiologic cultures E = not known to be useful | Pathogenic in immunocompromised hosts and premature infants; commonly a contaminant |
| *Streptococcus pyogenes* (Group A) Deep wounds or intra-abdominal abscess, bloodstream infections | Upper respiratory tract, perianal area (rectum and vagina) | P = wound, stool cultures E = settle plates | Not commonly normal flora; threshold for a health care–associated investigation: 1 case |
| Varicella infections Skin, respiratory Disseminated or localized infection | Secretions and skin lesions | P = viral cultures, PCR or serology E = not known to be useful | Children and immunocompromised patients at risk Unvaccinated exposed can develop disease |
| *Yersinia enterocolitica* Bloodstream, GI tract | GI tract | P = micro cultures E = cultures of potentially implicated items | — |

*Abbreviations:* IV, intravenous; NICU, neonatal intensive care unit; PCR, polymerase chain reaction; PFGE, pulse field gel electrophoresis.

performed thoughtfully and through multidisciplinary groups representing all of the vested parties.

Communication is a critical part of an outbreak investigation. It is essential to keep hospital or entity leadership informed of findings and interventions in a timely and regular manner. It is helpful to include the legal team to advise on medico-legal issues. Communication outside the institution can be challenging and is best handled by an experienced individual who is credible, respected, and can speak to the issues and offer reassurance when appropriate. It also may be necessary and useful to communicate with the local health department depending on the specifics of the outbreak.

## PSEUDO-OUTBREAKS

Pseudo-outbreaks are defined as an increase in identified organisms but without evidence of infection. Sometimes, these can be difficult to distinguish from "true" clusters or outbreaks. Because pseudo-outbreaks generally represent contamination, identification of the source is important to prevent inappropriate treatment and additional testing in patients who do not have a true infection. Between 1965 and 2010, 72 clusters of pseudobacteremia have been published, 22 cases of pseudomeningitis, and 49 cases of pseudopneumonia. Pseudo-infections most commonly present as pseudobacteremias. Pseudobacteremias occur in the setting of contaminated culture media, contaminated antiseptics, contaminated blood culture vials, or inadequate disinfection of the analyzer. Although less common, pseudomeningitis has significant sequelae and has been due to contamination of procedure kits or culture media. Pseudopneumonia was most often due to mycobacterial species and was most often related to bronchoscopy.[4]

## LABORATORY AND TESTING

The expertise and collaboration of the laboratory is critical in the investigation of an outbreak.[5] As noted previously, it is essential to notify the microbiology laboratory of a potential outbreak and ask personnel to save any potentially related specimens. Laboratory testing plays an important role in outbreak investigation. The microbiology laboratory often identifies unusual organisms or clusters of the same organism and notifies the infection prevention department.

Microbiologic and molecular testing is continually evolving. In the past, determining relatedness of organisms was dependent on phenotypic methods. These methods include biotyping, which is the identification of genus and species or organisms, comparison of antibiotic susceptibility patterns, serotyping, and phage typing.[6,7] Serotyping involves the use of antibodies to bind antigens on the bacterial surface and phage typing assesses the sensitivity of the bacteria to various bacteriophage viruses.[8,9] Biotyping and antibiotic susceptibility testing are inexpensive and readily available in most clinical laboratories, but all of these phenotypic methods are limited in their sensitivity.

Over the past decade, many new genotypic approaches have become available and accessible and have allowed for greater resolution of specific strains. Plasmid typing was one of the first genotypic techniques used to type bacterial strains. Plasmids are extracted and a comparison of the number and types of plasmids is performed. The sensitivity of this technique can be enhanced by using restriction endonucleases. This method is time-consuming and is limited in its ability to discriminate strain relatedness in some organisms because plasmids can be mobile between species. Still this process may aid in the evaluation of a specific plasmid or transposon outbreak, which is suspected when different strains present with a similar resistance profiles.[6,8–10]

Pulse field gel electrophoresis (PFGE) has been considered the gold standard for molecular typing. Bacterial DNA is extracted and subsequently cleaved by specific restriction endonucleases, which are then separated in an agarose gel by a shifting electric field creating a pattern of bands known as restriction fragment length polymorphisms (RFLP), which can be used to compare strains.[9,11] A large proportion of the bacterial genome is assessed using this method, and there have been international fingerprinting databases that allow for standardized comparisons.[7-9,11] Ribotyping uses a similar process with more frequent cutting restriction endonucleases. After electrophoresis, the gel can be blotted onto a nitrocellulose or nylon membrane and a labeled DNA or RNA probe can be hybridized to the bacterial DNA. When rRNA is used as the probe, this technique is referred to as ribotyping.[8,9] Virtually all bacteria can be ribotyped, as this gene is highly conserved, but this process is less able to discriminate between strains than PFGE.[8,9,12]

DNA microarray hybridization is another way to type bacterial strains. In this process, DNA probes are attached to a surface and the DNA of the bacteria is isolated, labeled, and then hybridized with the DNA probes to be analyzed. This approach also allows for the detection of plasmids.[11]

More recently, polymerase chain reaction (PCR) techniques have been used to amplify certain DNA segments. Random amplification of polymorphic DNA (RAPD), also known as arbitrarily primed PCR (AP-PCR), uses primers that are specific to the bacterial strain, but not directed at specific sequences. This is a process that allows for multiple mismatches, so as to amplify DNA segments, which are then placed in agarose gel and electrophoresed. This process has been used frequently in outbreak investigations, as it is relatively easy to perform and fast, yet there is significant interlaboratory and intralaboratory variability with this technique.[6,9,11] Repetitive element PCR (rep-PCR) is similar to the RAPD process, but uses specific primers and more stringent amplification process. This process has been semiautomated in commercial machines.[11]

PCR can be used to amplify and sequence a specific gene as in the case of *emm* gene in group A streptococcus, or the protein A gene (*spa*) in *S aureus*. This process is referred to as single locus sequence typing (SLST).[7,9,11] In multilocus sequence typing (MLST), several specific housekeeping genes are amplified and sequenced. Each unique sequence is assigned a number and a sequence type (ST) is determined.[7,9,11] The most significant advantage of this method is standardization. It is, however, an expensive modality.

Optical mapping imbeds bacterial genomic DNA in agarose, which is then stretched in a microfluidic device. Restriction endonucleases are used to digest the bacterial DNA, which is stained with fluorescent dye and visualized by fluorescence microscopy. In this process, the individual genes remain in the order they are seen in vivo. A genomic optimal map can be created using specialized software. This technique is evolving, but its use is limited by cost and the need for specialized equipment.[11]

Whole genomic sequencing (WGS) is the newest tool in outbreak investigation in which the entire genome is sequenced.[11] This technique is becoming much more affordable, making it a viable option for outbreak investigation.[7,11] WGS has been used in outbreak investigations and has uncovered clusters of genetically related organisms that were unnoticed by phenotypic analysis alone,[13] has helped define previously unrecognized transmission patterns as in the case of klebsiella pneumoniae carbapenemase at the National Institutes of Health,[14] and has also shown that organisms, specifically *Clostridium difficile* and *S aureus*, thought to be related, were, in fact, genetically distinct.[15,16]

## SOURCES
### Health Care Personnel

Health care personnel have been implicated in the transmission of gram-negative pathogens; respiratory pathogens, such as influenza, respiratory syncytial virus (RSV), pertussis, severe acute respiratory syndrome (SARS), and Middle East respiratory syndrome coronavirus (MERS-CoV); and gastrointestinal pathogens, such as *Salmonella* spp, Norovirus, and *C difficile*.[17] The most common source in these outbreaks is contact transmission, which is most often related to poor compliance with hand hygiene practices.[2] Artificial nails, rings, and dermatitis can reduce the effectiveness of appropriate hand hygiene practices and have been associated with outbreaks.[18] Rings and artificial nails are associated with higher rates of gram-negative carriage.[18] *Streptococcus pyogenes* has been associated with throat, rectal, and vaginal carriage and with outbreaks.[19] Health care personnel have been implicated as the primary source in fewer than 10% of *S pyogenes* nosocomial outbreaks, but 60% of health care personnel have been found to carry an outbreak strain.[20] *S aureus* has a predilection for the anterior nares and outbreaks have been associated with caregivers who are carriers.[21] This is discussed in more detail as follows.

### Hospital Environment

The hospital environment has been increasingly linked to acquisition of organisms, especially *C difficile*, Norovirus, and multidrug-resistant organisms. Health care personnel frequently touch patients and room surfaces. In one study, 93 contact episodes were identified in 1 hour in medical, surgical, and neurosurgical units.[22] Contacts with the patient environment result in a 52% transfer rate of *S aureus*, vancomycin-resistant *Enterococcus* (VRE), and gram-negative bacilli, which is similar to the rate of transfer after touching patients.[23] These organisms persist in the environment and can persist on hands of health care personnel for several hours.[24]

It can be difficult to implicate environmental surfaces alone as a cause for transmission of infection, because of the uncertainly of the role of the many concurrent confounding variables. Nonetheless, most experts acknowledge the role of the environment in outbreaks. In a prospective cohort study in an intensive care unit, Hardy and colleagues[25] demonstrated that 11.5% of newly colonized patients become colonized with an environmental strain of methicillin-resistant *S aureus* (MRSA). Data from several studies show that colonization of a room from a prior occupant increases the risk that the new occupant will be colonized by 1.5-fold to 3.3-fold.[23] This association has been described with *Acinetobacter*, *C difficile*, *Pseudomonas*, VRE, and MRSA.[23] This risk can be mitigated through thorough cleaning, use of appropriate disinfectants, good compliance with cleaning protocols, and the use of no-touch technologies, such as hydrogen peroxide vapor.[23]

### Waterborne Sources

Over the past century, better public water sanitation methods have reduced community-onset waterborne illness.[26] Nevertheless, outbreaks persist in hospital settings due to complex and antiquated water systems, and poor understanding of the risks to patients. Many organisms have been implicated in both pseudo and true waterborne outbreaks. Geography, weather, and infrastructure influence the types of organisms seen in waterborne outbreaks. The most commonly reported waterborne infection in North America is *Legionella*.[27] Between 2011 and 2012, the Centers for Disease Control and Prevention waterborne illness surveillance system identified drinking water as a cause of 66% of water-related outbreaks and in 26%

of these, the cause was *Legionella*. Other implicated organisms were *Shiga*-toxin producing *Escherichia coli*, *Shigella*, and *Pantoea agglomerans*.[28]

The transmission of waterborne pathogens to patients is likely related to build up of biofilm in plumbing structures, which are then dislodged into the water supply through increased use or construction. Patients may become exposed to the contaminants through showering, bathing, or drinking water or ice or through equipment that is rinsed in contaminated potable water. Not only is this contaminated water in direct contact with patients, but also with the environment and health care personnel, both of which can serve as fomites for transmission.[29]

*Legionella* infections garner significant media attention, yet they are relatively rare. In the United States, there were only 3000 cases in 2009 and 3500 cases in 2005 and 2006.[30,31] Furthermore, only 4% of these infections were associated with outbreaks.[30] *Legionella* presents as a nonspecific pneumonia and requires a specific antigen test for diagnosis and is therefore likely underdiagnosed as a cause of nosocomial pneumonia.[32] Although cooling towers and air conditioning units have been implicated as a common source for this organism, potable water, including hospital ice machines, account for most cases.[33]

## Legionella spp

*Legionella* spp can be detected in 40% of freshwater samples by culture and in 90% by PCR.[34] It is particularly well adapted to cause infections in hospital settings. This organism thrives in water temperatures at 35°C and most organisms are found within biofilms rather than in free-flowing water, making it particularly difficult to disinfect plumbing and the associated contaminated biofilm.[34] A variety of disinfection methods have been used, including copper-silver ionization, chlorine dioxide, monochloramine, ultraviolet (UV) light, and hyperchlorination.[35]

Atypical mycobacteria have a predilection for water and frequently colonize potable water due to their ability to form biofilm. These organisms are difficult to culture, but modern techniques have demonstrated their importance in both outbreaks and pseudo-outbreaks, as discussed later in this article. Multiples species have been reported with *Mycobacteria mucogenicum*, *Mycobacterium gordonae*, *Mycobacterium simiae*, *Mycobacterium fortuitum*, and *Mycobacterium chelonae*.[29,36] These organisms have been shown to be responsible for both outbreaks and pseudo outbreaks, including in outpatient settings. Outbreaks have been traced to hospital water, dialysis water, fountains, ice machines, and hospital water supplies and disinfectant trays.[37]

Gram-negative organisms are emerging as important pathogens that can contaminate the water supply. Gram-negative organisms were reported in 79% of samples from 6 hospitals.[38] *Pseudomonas* from contaminated water in intensive care unit (ICU) settings have been linked by molecular testing to patient strains and to endoscope outbreaks.[29,39,40] In one of these outbreaks, Bukholm and colleagues[39] demonstrated that samples obtained from patients in an ICU were genetically identical (amplified fragment length polymorphisms) to water samples in the same ICU. Other organisms that have contaminated water-based supplies and equipment include *Pseudomonas* spp, *Ralstonia* spp, *Serratia* spp, *Aeromonas* spp, *Burkholderia* spp, *Acinetobacter* spp, and *Klebsiella* spp.[29] These organisms have been associated with outbreaks traced to contaminated ventilators, sitz baths, distilled water, pulsed lavage equipment, incubators, and hand creams.[36] Most recently and worrisome, Walsh and colleagues[41] described the contamination of the environmental water supply in India with the carbapenem-resistant New Delhi Metallobetalactamases (NDM-1) strains.

Other unusual organisms may be associated with waterborne outbreaks. One of the great controversies surrounds the importance of water as a source of fungi, such as *Aspergillus* spp., *Exophiala jeanselmei*, and *Fusarium* spp.[29] Norovirus also has rarely been linked to health care–associated outbreaks and traced to water sources.[42]

## ORGANISMS
### Nontuberculous Mycobacteria

Nontuberculous mycobacteria (NTM) are ubiquitous in the environment in water and soil and can inhabit the health care environment.[43] Clinical infections peak in the late summer and early fall.[44] Health care–associated mycobacterial infections are almost exclusively due to rapid-growing NTM. These organisms have caused pseudo-outbreaks and outbreaks due to their predilection to contaminate water and are increasingly recognized as common causes of outbreaks. Most reported infections are related to surgical site infections and postinjection abscesses, as well as catheter-associated infections and cosmetic procedures.[37] Contamination of bronchoscopes and respiratory specimens are common causes of pseudo-outbreaks.[43]

The 2 most common surgeries associated with NTM infections have been cardiac surgeries and cosmetic surgeries.[43] An early cardiac surgery outbreak was attributed to infected porcine valves.[43] In subsequent cardiac surgery outbreaks it was difficult to identify a source until a postoutbreak analysis using more advanced laboratory methods typed mycobacterial species from previous outbreaks and found that in at least one outbreak, the mycobacteria isolated in the operating room could be traced to the water bath used in cardiac surgery and back to municipal tap water.[43] NTM outbreaks in cardiac surgery were significantly reduced after 1989, presumably due to the elimination of tap water and ice in the operating room.[37] A recent outbreak of *Mycobacterium chimaera* in cardiac surgery was traced a contaminated heater-cooler device that aerosolized the organism.[45]

In addition, other water-related mycobacterial outbreaks have been seen in hospital settings. Ice machines and hospital water have been the sources of outbreaks in susceptible patients.[43] Dialysis infections have also been caused by atypical mycobacteria.[43]

Augmentation mammography and other cosmetic surgeries are also a common procedure associated with rapid-growing NTM outbreaks.[43] The source has not been identified in most of these outbreaks, although the infections cluster around a particular plastic surgeon's practice suggesting a local environmental source.[46] Most (90%) of the sporadic cases were seen in Texas, North Carolina, and Florida.[46,47] In one particularly interesting case, 8 patients undergoing plastic surgery developed *M chelonae* infection attributed to dilution of gentian violet for marking with distilled water instead of alcohol.[48]

Atypical mycobacteria have been associated with mesotherapy and liposuction, including in medical tourists, and a surprising number of outbreaks have been related to tattoos.[37] There have been several outbreaks related to eye surgery,[43] including one recent outbreak implicating the humidifier in the room.[49]

### Acinetobacter spp

*Acinetobacter* is one of the gram-negative organisms that is commonly seen in the setting of outbreaks. *Acinetobacter* genus consists of many different species and many of these species are found in soil and water, and in 40% of healthy humans, 17% of fresh fruits and vegetables, and in 21% of human body lice.[50] *Acinetobacter baumannii* is the most frequent cause of outbreaks and is rarely isolated from the environment in nonoutbreak settings.[50] *Acinetobacter* resist desiccation and can survive for prolonged periods of time in hospital environments.[50] They also acquire resistance genes quickly, thus contributing to the importance of this species in nosocomial infections and outbreaks.[51] *Acinetobacter* has the largest known resistance island harboring 45 resistance genes acquired from *Pseudomonas*, *Salmonella*, and *Escherichia*, reflecting the species propensity to collect resistance genes.[52]

From 1977 to 2000, 51 outbreaks due to *Acinetobacter* spp. were reported, 29 (56%) involved respiratory infections and 22 (43%) were nonrespiratory sites, most commonly bloodstream and wound infection or simply colonization. In 26 (51%) of these outbreaks, a contaminated common source was found in respiratory equipment, humidifiers, and patient bedding.[53]

Because of its ability to survive in the environment, *Acinetobacter* frequently contaminates gowns and gloves used for isolation in health care settings.[54] Airborne dissemination of *Acinetobacter* has also been described.[55]

## Pseudomonas spp

*Pseudomonas* is another gram-negative genus that is commonly a cause of health care–associated infections and outbreaks. Although *Pseudomonas* can cause infections in a variety of settings, it is commonly associated with immunocompromised hosts and ICU settings.[56] *Pseudomonas* spp infections can be difficult to treat due to the many antibiotic resistance mechanisms in this organism[56] and it can also develop resistance to biocides. Several outbreaks have been traced to contaminated benzalkonium chloride, povidone-iodine, and chlorhexedine.[56,57]

This organism can survive in hospital environments for extended periods of time and has been found in potable water, sinks, ultrasound gel, salads (up to $10^3$ colony-forming units), skin creams, blood products, hemodialysis machines, and linens.[58,59] Outbreaks have been described in neonatal ICUs, hematology and oncology units, and other ICUs associated with a variety of sources and with various *Pseudomonas* spp.[59]

Health care personnel, family members, and visitors generally do not carry the organism, and transmission in health care settings is primarily linked to contaminated fomites, the environment, contaminated substances, or from patient-to-patient via contaminated hands.[56]

## Carbapenem-Resistant Enterobacteriaceae

Carbapenem resistance among gram-negative organisms is an important and emerging phenomenon and occurs by a variety of mechanisms, including chromosomal resistance (increase in amp C production), plasmid and mobile element–mediated resistance, and porin mutations.[60]

Importantly, resistance genes that are coded on plasmids are readily transmissible across species.[60] Using whole genomic sequencing, Conlan and colleagues[61] found horizontal transfer of carbapenem resistance among different species in the actual hospital environment.

Since carbapenemase resistance pattern was identified in 2001, other problematic strains such as NDM have emerged and the prevalence of carbapenem-resistant Enterobacteriaceae (CREs) in the United States has increased from 1.2% to 4.2%.[62] Interestingly this increase is largely fueled by clonal spread of a single clone of *Klebsiella* spp: ST258.[60] Infection with these organisms is challenging to treat and is independently associated with increased mortality.[60]

Many CRE outbreaks are associated with asymptomatic carriers and transmission from environmental sources, such as endoscopes and sinks.[63] Transmission is often silent and 50% of colonized patients are not detected through clinical cultures alone and these asymptomatic carriers may be responsible for spread in health care settings.[63] Asymptomatic carriers are thought to be one of the mechanisms of spread in a 2012 NDM outbreak.[64] In another 18-person outbreak investigated using whole-genomic sequencing, complex and multiple modalities of transmission of CREs in the hospital were found and linked to asymptomatic carriers and environmental reservoirs.[14]

Various bundled interventions have been used to stop transmission in these acute outbreak settings, including increased compliance with hand hygiene, contact precautions, use of cohorting, enhanced environmental cleaning, active surveillance, and chlorhexidine bathing.[65]

### S aureus Including Methicillin-Resistant S aureus

S aureus is the second most common organism causing health care–associated infections[66] and the most common cause of published outbreak investigations.[2] Both methicillin-sensitive S aureus (MSSA) and MRSA carriage can be associated with deviations in practice, like poor hand hygiene compliance, overcrowding, and contact with human carriers.[21]

Approximately 33% of the US population is colonized with MSSA and 2% of the general population is colonized with MRSA, and colonization with either organism increases the risk of invasive infection (http://www.cdc.gov/mrsa/tracking/index. html).[67] Overall, 4.6% (0%–40%) of health care personnel carry MRSA.[21] The primary ecologic niche is the anterior nares, although the skin, and perineum also can be colonized.[21] Although poor infection control practices are risk factors for acquisition of S aureus among health care personnel, good infection control practices do not fully prevent health care personnel carriage and transmission.[21]

Most nasal carriers do not disperse S aureus or cause outbreaks, but nasal carriers can cause airborne dispersal in the presence of an upper respiratory infection or skin lesions, known as "cloud dispersal."[68] Health care personnel are uncommonly the source of S aureus outbreaks. Among 191 MRSA outbreaks from 1966 to 2005, health care personnel were the source in 11 (5.8%), and in 8 (72%) of these, the implicated individual had either an upper respiratory infection, dermatitis, or skin infection.[69] In combined endemic and outbreak situations, 106 studies evaluated transmission from health care personnel to patients and found clear evidence of transmission in 27 (25.6%) studies and probable transmission in another 52 (49.1%) studies.[21] Due to the high prevalence of colonization in health care personnel, it is important to link epidemiologic findings with molecular typing to determine the source and appropriately decolonize the individual.[21] Because of the sensitivity and personal guilt associated with S aureus carriage and transmission to patients, the process requires extreme confidentiality and a thoughtful and caring approach.

The environment is also a potential source for MRSA outbreaks. Patient room environment is also colonized with MRSA in 73% of infected patient rooms and 65% of colonized patient rooms and can be a reservoir for outbreaks.[70] The higher the burden of S aureus in their nares, the more likely the person will shed organisms and have higher degrees of environmental contamination.[71]

### Fungus and Mold, Including Aspergillus

Mold infections cause significant morbidity and mortality in high-risk patients, especially those with impaired granulocyte dysfunction or immature or altered skin (ie, extreme prematurity or burns). Mold species are found throughout the health care environment and similar to other organisms, multiple studies have shown concordance between clinical isolates and environmental genotypes, highlighting the role of the environment in acquisition of these organisms.[72] Aspergillus spp outbreaks are the best described of these organisms. *Aspergillus* has been associated with at least 60 outbreaks in health care settings.[72–74] Fifty percent of outbreaks have been attributed to construction, renovation, or demolition, and virtually all outbreaks are ultimately attributable to airborne dissemination from primary sources.[74] Fungal outbreaks have been associated with distribution of organisms through nearby construction, vacuum cleaning, contaminated carpet, contaminated air ducts, humidifiers, fireproofing material, rotting wood cabinets, and dressings, in-hospital plants, and tape.[72]

Installation of high-efficiency particle (HEPA) filtration has shown to be instrumental in prevention and abatement of fungal environmental contamination and clinical outbreaks.[73] However, sealing and repairing leaky or open windows, assessing water leaks in ceilings, maintaining appropriate air pressure relationships in patient care areas, and dust removal remain key strategies to prevent and abate fungal outbreaks occurring in the presence of HEPA filtration.[72,74]

Weather may play a significant role in fungal outbreaks. Several studies have documented seasonal variation of fungal spores with higher levels in the fall; however, these results are inconsistent and indoor samples do not correlate with outdoor samples.[75,76] The seasonal variation in the prevalence of *Aspergillus* spores inside a hospital has been associated with rainfall and internal relative humidity and temperature.[76]

Severe weather events such as floods and hurricanes have been associated with outbreaks of bacterial and fungal diseases. Most of these investigations have focused on bacterial pathogens.[77] Flooding in Thailand has been associated with fungal outbreaks and pseudo-outbreaks.[77] The 2005 tsunami in Sri Lanka resulted in an outbreak of *Aspergillus* meningitis due to contaminated supplies from poor postflooding storage.[78]

### Respiratory Infections

Respiratory infections are one of the most common types of infections encountered in the health care setting, and their importance and impact in this setting is being increasingly recognized. Most of these infections are transmitted by large droplets, but in some settings and situations, aerosolization is an important mode of transmission. Respiratory infections account for a large number of hospital admissions and hospital complications and can be a frequent reason to close a hospital unit, which disrupts hospital processes. Annual seasonal increases of respiratory infections during respiratory virus seasons can also lead to outbreaks within the health care setting. Viruses account for the largest proportion of identified pathogens (22%) in hospitalized patients with respiratory infections.[79] Of these, influenza A and B account for the largest proportion in patients older than 65 years and RSV is a significant pathogen in children and immunosuppressed patients.[80] Many outbreaks and sporadic cases have been attributed to influenza.[81] Attack rates in outbreak settings are as high as 55% among health care personnel and 37% of patents.[82] Health care personnel vaccinations are the mainstay of prevention for influenza and may reduce the incidence of nosocomial influenza.[83]

More recently, SARS and MERS coronaviruses have been reported in health care settings. Risk factors for transmission of these viruses include aerosol-generating procedures and failure to comply with recommended infection-control practices for contact and droplet precautions.[84] Both of these infections are associated with higher mortality rates and dramatic illness in health care providers and patients.[84]

Pertussis is a bacterial disease that has caused outbreaks in primarily pediatric health care settings.[85] There is significant morbidity and mortality in young unvaccinated infants.[85] These outbreaks can be difficult to manage due to the long latency period of pertussis, the infectiousness of the organism, and the activities and care rendered in pediatric settings.[85] In one report, a single case cost $75,000 to manage.[86] Pertussis cases have increased over the past 10 years,[87] and outbreaks are likely to increase due to the decreased immunogenicity of the acellular vaccine compared with the whole cell vaccine.[88]

Emerging respiratory viruses, like SARS and MERS coronavirus, and vaccine-preventable diseases, like pertussis and measles, continue to provide unique challenges in identification, diagnosis, control, and transmission.

### Gastrointestinal Infections

Gastroenteritis infections are common, and in settings in which rotavirus vaccine is available, norovirus is the leading cause of gastroenteritis epidemics across various health care settings and also in long-term care facilities, cruise ships, schools, and recreational activities. In a retrospective review of 90 outbreaks reported to health departments, 96% of nonbacterial gastroenteritis cases were ultimately attributed to norovirus.[89] Norovirus is a resilient, round virus that is spread through fecal oral contamination even before infected patients are symptomatic. It requires a low inoculum of virus to cause disease and can persist in the environment for days to weeks. Additionally, the virus has a high rate of genetic mutation, and host immunity is transient, making humans continually susceptible hosts. These factors lead to secondary attack rates of 30%.[90] Cleaning of environmental surfaces with hypochlorite can reduce the attack rate for norovirus.[91] Infection control interventions that work in this setting include restricting movement, screening staff and visitors and isolating those that are ill, enhanced cleaning and improved compliance, hand hygiene.[91]

*C difficile* is the most common pathogen identified in health care–associated infections in North America.[66] It is identified in the stool of 25% of hospitalized patients and in 2% to 3% of healthy adults.[92] To develop *C difficile* disease, 2 steps are needed: acquisition of the pathogen and alteration of gastrointestinal microbiome primarily through antibiotic use. Patients with active disease shed up to 100 million *C difficile* spores per gram of stool; hence, the organism has a predilection for the hospital environment and 20% to 51% of hospital room surfaces are contaminated in rooms of patients with active *C difficile* infection.[93] Hand of health care personnel are easily contaminated by spores after examining patients or even through contact of the patient's environment.[94] Daily cleaning reduces the risk of hand contamination.[95] Having a previous room occupant or roommate with diagnosed *C difficile* disease increased the risk the current occupant developing *C difficile* infection.[23] These data suggest an important role of the environment in the development of *C difficile* infection.

However, our understanding of *C difficile* epidemiology has evolved with the use of better laboratory tests, including whole genomic sequencing. Interestingly, despite the heavy and frequent environmental contamination with *C difficile*, only 25% of health care–acquired *C difficile* can be epidemiologically and genetically traced to another symptomatic contact, reemphasizing the importance of combined antimicrobial stewardship and infection-prevention strategies to prevent outbreaks.[96]

Gastroenteritis is extremely common in resource-limited settings, yet precious little is known about the pathogens in these settings. Organisms such as rotavirus, *Salmonella*, and enterotoxigenic *E coli* should be considered in these settings.[97]

## HIGH-RISK SETTINGS
### Neonatal Intensive Care Unit

The neonatal ICU (NICU) is unique environment with significant risks for outbreaks. Studies evaluating the unique physical environment in the NICU demonstrate the importance of the facility design, and in fact, temporary facilities have been shown to have a higher rate of infection.[98] Modeling pathogen transmission in a NICU surrogate DNA demonstrated very rapid spread throughout the NICU.[99] In addition, neonates are particularly vulnerable to health care–associated infections. The prevalence of these infections is 5% to 24%; higher in premature infants than full-term infants.[100] Neonates have immature immune systems, require multiple invasive devices, and have multiple contacts with health care personnel.[100] For these reasons, NICUs account for 38% of ICU outbreaks and 18% of all published outbreaks.[101] The source of these outbreaks was identified in only 51% of outbreaks.[101] *Klebsiella*, *S aureus*, *Serratia* spp, and *Enterobacter* spp are the most common organisms identified. Patients were the source of 20% of outbreaks, contaminated equipment accounted for 12%, personnel were the source in 11%, and the environment contributed to 9%.[101]

Viral infections, including rotavirus (23%), RSV (17%), enterovirus (15%), and hepatitis A (11%) have been increasingly recognized as important pathogens among infants hospitalized in NICU settings.[102] Unsurprisingly, patients and personnel accounted for the source of transmission in 50% and 8% of viral outbreaks, respectively.[101]

*S aureus* and MRSA outbreaks are commonly reported in this unique setting.[101] Intravenous fluid may be a significant risk factor in this setting. Because of the common use of intravenous lipids, this is one of the settings in which *Malassezia furfur* is commonly seen.[103] Additionally, in resource-limited settings, bloodstream infection outbreaks with gram-negative organisms may be traced to poor sterile practices associated with mixing intravenous medications.[104–106]

Multiple interventions have been used to control outbreaks in this setting, most commonly reinforcing hand hygiene practices, active surveillance of patients, barrier precautions, and cohorting. Personnel screening was performed in 44% of outbreaks, most commonly associated with *S aureus* and modifications of care and equipment were implemented in 39% of NICU outbreaks.[101]

### Endoscopes and Endoscopy Suites

As biomedical engineering in health care grows, more complex medical devices are being used to treat patients. These devices are increasingly recognized as sources of organisms that can be transmitted from patient to patient. Several studies have shown a high contamination rate, 1% to 2% to 50% to 60%, depending on sampling method in appropriately cleaned and disinfected endoscopes, highlighting the challenges with new technology.[107] The high rate of microbiological contamination may be in part due to the high prevalence of biofilms seen on endoscopes.[108]

Between 1966 and 2004, 19 reports of gastrointestinal endoscopy–related outbreaks were published. More than 90% of outbreaks linked to bronchoscopes and gastrointestinal endoscopes could have been prevented by better cleaning and disinfection processes.[109] Endoscopes have complex channels that make them difficult to clean properly.[110] *Pseudomonas* and multidrug-resistant *Klebsiella* spp and NTM have been associated with several outbreaks in which the cause was related to insufficient reprocessing.[109] A recent highly publicized outbreak of NDM-producing CRE resulted in 29 cases of colonization or infection in which no lapses in reprocessing were noted, suggesting that usual cleaning methods may not be effective in sterilizing complicated endoscopes with multiple moving pieces.[111] Similarly, an outbreak involving 32 cases of an AmpC-producing carbapenem-resistant *E coli* with 7 deaths was related to damaged endoscopes.[112,113]

Despite these reports and other challenges with determining how to safely reprocess endoscopes of all types, manual cleaning remains the cornerstone of practice and can reduce the bioburden in colonoscopes up to 5 logs.[110] These recent outbreaks highlight the difficulties and cleaning and disinfecting new and important technologies with designs that do not lend themselves to the current processes.

### Transplant Units

Infections are the leading cause of death in solid organ transplantation.[114] The first 30 days after transplantation are associated with procedure and health care–associated infections and are overwhelmingly due to bacterial infections.[114] Bloodstream infections are highest during the first month and then sharply decline after this period.[115] Multidrug-resistant organisms, particularly *Enterococcus* and gram-negative organisms, are frequent causes of infection in solid organ transplant patients.[116] Respiratory viruses, such as influenza, RSV, adenovirus, and rhinovirus, are common reasons for medical consultation and hospitalization in transplant patients. These viruses are more likely to cause lower lung involvement compared with healthy hosts, with relatively high mortality rates and can cause outbreaks in this patient population.[117]

Hematopoietic stem cell transplants are life-saving procedures for patients with leukemia and lymphoma. These procedures involve host bone marrow ablation, which results in profound immunosuppression until the autologous (host) or allogeneic (donor) bone marrow engrafts. Engraftment can take several weeks.[118] Gram-positive infections (20%–30%), gram-negative infections (5%–10%), *C difficile* (5%–10%), and respiratory viruses (15%) are the most common causes of infection in the preengraftment period.[118] The hospital environment poses significant risks to patients in this vulnerable time period. In addition, transmission from hands of health care personnel, and sources such as creams, mouthwash, sitz baths, and sinks, have been associated with infections in these patients.[119]

### SUMMARY

Outbreaks should be considered in any health care delivery site and can encompass a variety of pathogens and vectors of transmission. Epidemiologic and laboratory diagnostic tools can help guide a systematic investigation; however, often multiple steps occur simultaneously in the complex situations.

Many interventions have been used to abort an ongoing outbreak. Most significantly, it is important to ensure that basic infection prevention practices, such as hand hygiene and isolation, are in place and that health care personnel are compliant with these practices. Beyond this, prevention strategies need to be tailored to the epidemiologic findings, the organism, and the patients. The goal is to remove the offending source and protect patients and health care personnel.

Enhanced patient screening and surveillance are implemented 54% of the time, personnel screening in 38% of outbreaks, isolation or cohorting in 32%, enhanced or revised sterilization or disinfection practices in 24%, modification of care or equipment in 23%, increased use of protective clothing in 19%, and ward closure in 11%.[2] In most situations, these interventions are applied in combination and simultaneously, as there are limited data to empirically guide management.

Epidemiologic data are important tools in identifying potential sources and guiding additional testing. It is important to quickly implement reasonable prevention strategies, and communicate to leadership and public health authorities while refining further investigations. The goal is to abort further transmission or harm and provide a safe atmosphere for patient care while protecting the health care personnel and the institution. This harmonious balance requires engagement of all of the vested parties and access to necessary resources.

## REFERENCES

1. Hansen S, Stamm-Balderjahn S, Zuschneid I, et al. Closure of medical departments during nosocomial outbreaks: data from a systematic analysis of the literature. J Hosp Infect 2007;65(4):348–53.
2. Gastmeier P, Stamm-Balderjahn S, Hansen S, et al. How outbreaks can contribute to prevention of nosocomial infection: analysis of 1,022 outbreaks. Infect Control Hosp Epidemiol 2005;26(4):357–61.
3. Gastmeier P, Stamm-Balderjahn S, Hansen S, et al. Where should one search when confronted with outbreaks of nosocomial infection? Am J Infect Control 2006;34(9):603–5.
4. Cunha CB, Cunha BA. Pseudoinfections and pseudo-outbreaks. In: Mayhall CG, editor. Hospital epidemiology and infection control. 4th edition. Baltimore (MD): Lippincott Williams & Wilkins; 2012. p. 142–53.
5. Pfaller MA, Herwaldt LA. The clinical microbiology laboratory and infection control: emerging pathogens, antimicrobial resistance, and new technology. Clin Infect Dis 1997;25(4):858–70.
6. Weber S, Pfaller MA, Herwaldt LA. Role of molecular epidemiology in infection control. Infect Dis Clin North Am 1997;11(2):257–78.
7. MacCannell D. Bacterial strain typing. Clin Lab Med 2013;33(3):629–50.
8. Tenover FC, Arbeit RD, Goering RV. How to select and interpret molecular strain typing methods for epidemiological studies of bacterial infections: a review for healthcare epidemiologists. Molecular Typing Working Group of the Society for Healthcare Epidemiology of America. Infect Control Hosp Epidemiol 1997; 18(6):426–39.
9. Singh A, Goering RV, Simjee S, et al. Application of molecular techniques to the study of hospital infection. Clin Microbiol Rev 2006;19(3):512–30.
10. John JF, Twitty JA. Plasmids as epidemiologic markers in nosocomial gram-negative bacilli: experience at a university and review of the literature. Rev Infect Dis 1986;8(5):693–704.
11. Sabat AJ, Budimir A, Nashev D, et al. Overview of molecular typing methods for outbreak detection and epidemiological surveillance. Euro Surveill 2013;18(4): 20380.
12. Bingen EH, Denamur E, Elion J. Use of ribotyping in epidemiological surveillance of nosocomial outbreaks. Clin Microbiol Rev 1994;7(3):311–27.
13. Harris SR, Cartwright EJP, Török ME, et al. Whole-genome sequencing for analysis of an outbreak of methicillin-resistant *Staphylococcus aureus*: a descriptive study. Lancet Infect Dis 2013;13(2):130–6.
14. Snitkin ES, Zelazny AM, Thomas PJ, et al. Tracking a hospital outbreak of carbapenem-resistant *Klebsiella pneumoniae* with whole-genome sequencing. Sci Transl Med 2012;4(148):148ra16.
15. Eyre DW, Golubchik T, Gordon NC, et al. A pilot study of rapid benchtop sequencing of *Staphylococcus aureus* and *Clostridium difficile* for outbreak detection and surveillance. BMJ Open 2012;2(3) [pii:e001124].
16. Koser CU, Holden MT, Ellington MJ, et al. Rapid whole-genome sequencing for investigation of a neonatal MRSA outbreak. N Engl J Med 2012;366(24): 2267–75.
17. Huttunen R, Syrjänen J. Healthcare workers as vectors of infectious diseases. Eur J Clin Microbiol Infect Dis 2014;33(9):1477–88.
18. Boyce JM, Pittet D, Healthcare Infection Control Practices Advisory Committee, Society for Healthcare Epidemiology of America, Association for Professionals in

Infection Control, Infectious Diseases Society of America, Hand Hygiene Task Force. Guideline for hand hygiene in health-care settings: recommendations of the Healthcare Infection Control Practices Advisory Committee and the HIC-PAC/SHEA/APIC/IDSA Hand Hygiene Task Force. Infect Control Hosp Epidemiol 2002;23(12 Suppl):S3–40.

19. Kolmos HJ, Svendsen RN, Nielsen SV. The surgical team as a source of postoperative wound infections caused by *Streptococcus pyogenes*. J Hosp Infect 1997;35(3):207–14.

20. Daneman N, McGeer A, Low DE, et al. Hospital-acquired invasive group a streptococcal infections in Ontario, Canada, 1992-2000. Clin Infect Dis 2005; 41(3):334–42.

21. Albrich WC, Harbarth S. Health-care workers: source, vector, or victim of MRSA? Lancet Infect Dis 2008;8(5):289–301.

22. Cheng VC, Chau PH, Lee WM, et al. Hand-touch contact assessment of high-touch and mutual-touch surfaces among healthcare workers, patients, and visitors. J Hosp Infect 2015;90(3):220–5.

23. Otter JA, Yezli S, French GL. The role played by contaminated surfaces in the transmission of nosocomial pathogens. Infect Control Hosp Epidemiol 2011; 32(7):687–99.

24. Kampf G, Kramer A. Epidemiologic background of hand hygiene and evaluation of the most important agents for scrubs and rubs. Clin Microbiol Rev 2004;17(4): 863–93.

25. Hardy KJ, Oppenheim BA, Gossain S, et al. A study of the relationship between environmental contamination with methicillin-resistant *Staphylococcus aureus* (MRSA) and patients' acquisition of MRSA. Infect Control Hosp Epidemiol 2006;27(2):127–32.

26. Centers for Disease Control and Prevention (CDC). Control of infectious diseases. MMWR Morb Mortal Wkly Rep 1999;48(29):621–9.

27. Craun GF, Brunkard JM, Yoder JS, et al. Causes of outbreaks associated with drinking water in the United States from 1971 to 2006. Clin Microbiol Rev 2010;23(3):507–28.

28. Beer KD, Gargano JW, Roberts VA, et al. Surveillance for Waterborne Disease Outbreaks Associated with Drinking Water - United States, 2011-2012. MMWR Morb Mortal Wkly Rep 2015;64(31):842–8.

29. Anaissie EJ, Penzak SR, Dignani MC. The hospital water supply as a source of nosocomial infections: a plea for action. Arch Intern Med 2002;162(13):1483–92.

30. Centers for Disease Control and Prevention (CDC). Legionellosis: United States, 2000-2009. MMWR Morb Mortal Wkly Rep 2011;60(32):1083–6.

31. Joseph CA, Ricketts KD, European Working Group for Legionella Infections. Legionnaires disease in Europe 2007-2008. Euro Surveill 2010;15(8):19493.

32. Cunha BA, Burillo A, Bouza E. Legionnaires' disease. Lancet 2016;387(10016): 376–85.

33. Sabria M, Yu VL. Hospital-acquired legionellosis: solutions for a preventable infection. Lancet Infect Dis 2002;2(6):368–73.

34. Fields BS, Benson RF, Besser RE. Legionella and Legionnaires' disease: 25 years of investigation. Clin Microbiol Rev 2002;15(3):506–26.

35. Lin YE, Stout JE, Yu VL. Controlling *Legionella* in hospital drinking water: an evidence-based review of disinfection methods. Infect Control Hosp Epidemiol 2011;32(2):166–73.

36. Ferranti G, Marchesi I, Favale M, et al. Aetiology, source and prevention of waterborne healthcare-associated infections: a review. J Med Microbiol 2014; 63(Pt 10):1247–59.

37. Brown-Elliott BA, Wallace RJ Jr. Nontuberculous mycobacteria. Hospital epidemiology and infection control. Philadelphia: Lippincott Williams & Wilkins; 2012. p. 594–610.

38. Stojek NM, Szymanska J, Dutkiewicz J. Gram-negative bacteria in water distribution systems of hospitals. Ann Agric Environ Med 2008;15(1):135–42.

39. Bukholm G, Tannaes T, Kjelsberg AB, et al. An outbreak of multidrug-resistant *Pseudomonas aeruginosa* associated with increased risk of patient death in an intensive care unit. Infect Control Hosp Epidemiol 2002;23(8):441–6.

40. Muscarella LF. Contribution of tap water and environmental surfaces to nosocomial transmission of antibiotic-resistant *Pseudomonas aeruginosa*. Infect Control Hosp Epidemiol 2004;25(4):342–5.

41. Walsh TR, Weeks J, Livermore DM, et al. Dissemination of NDM-1 positive bacteria in the New Delhi environment and its implications for human health: an environmental point prevalence study. Lancet Infect Dis 2011;11(5):355–62.

42. Schvoerer E, Bonnet F, Dubois V, et al. A hospital outbreak of gastroenteritis possibly related to the contamination of tap water by a small round structured virus. J Hosp Infect 1999;43(2):149–54.

43. Phillips MS, von Reyn CF. Nosocomial infections due to nontuberculous mycobacteria. Clin Infect Dis 2001;33(8):1363–74.

44. El Helou G, Viola GM, Hachem R, et al. Rapidly growing mycobacterial bloodstream infections. Lancet Infect Dis 2013;13(2):166–74.

45. Sax H, Bloemberg G, Hasse B, et al. Prolonged outbreak of *Mycobacterium chimaera* infection after open-chest heart surgery. Clin Infect Dis 2015;61(1): 67–75.

46. Clegg HW, Foster MT, Sanders WE Jr, et al. Infection due to organisms of the *Mycobacterium fortuitum* complex after augmentation mammaplasty: clinical and epidemiologic features. J Infect Dis 1983;147(3):427–33.

47. Wallace RJ Jr, Steele LC, Labidi A, et al. Heterogeneity among isolates of rapidly growing mycobacteria responsible for infections following augmentation mammaplasty despite case clustering in Texas and other southern coastal states. J Infect Dis 1989;160(2):281–8.

48. Safranek TJ, Jarvis WR, Carson LA, et al. *Mycobacterium chelonae* wound infections after plastic surgery employing contaminated gentian violet skin-marking solution. N Engl J Med 1987;317(4):197–201.

49. Edens C, Liebich L, Halpin AL, et al. *Mycobacterium chelonae* eye infections associated with humidifier use in an outpatient LASIK clinic–Ohio, 2015. MMWR Morb Mortal Wkly Rep 2015;64(41):1177.

50. Peleg AY, Seifert H, Paterson DL. *Acinetobacter baumannii*: emergence of a successful pathogen. Clin Microbiol Rev 2008;21(3):538–82.

51. Fournier PE, Richet H. The epidemiology and control of *Acinetobacter baumannii* in health care facilities. Clin Infect Dis 2006;42(5):692–9.

52. Fournier PE, Vallenet D, Barbe V, et al. Comparative genomics of multidrug resistance in *Acinetobacter baumannii*. PLoS Genet 2006;2(1):e7.

53. Villegas MV, Hartstein AI. Acinetobacter outbreaks, 1977-2000. Infect Control Hosp Epidemiol 2003;24(4):284–95.

54. Morgan DJ, Liang SY, Smith CL, et al. Frequent multidrug-resistant *Acinetobacter baumannii* contamination of gloves, gowns, and hands of healthcare workers. Infect Control Hosp Epidemiol 2010;31(7):716–21.

55. Rock C, Harris AD, Johnson JK, et al. Infrequent air contamination with *Acinetobacter baumannii* of air surrounding known colonized or infected patients. Infect Control Hosp Epidemiol 2015;36(7):830–2.
56. Stosor V, Hauser AR, Flaherty JP. Nonfermentative gram-negative bacilli. In: Mayhall CG, editor. Hospital epidemiology and infection control. 4th edition. Baltimore (MD): Lippincott Williams & Wilkins; 2012. p. 521–35.
57. Weber DJ, Rutala WA, Sickbert-Bennett EE. Outbreaks associated with contaminated antiseptics and disinfectants. Antimicrobial Agents Chemother 2007; 51(12):4217–24.
58. Morrison AJ, Wenzel RP. Epidemiology of infections due to *Pseudomonas aeruginosa*. Rev Infect Dis 1984;6(Suppl 3):S627–42.
59. Kerr KG, Snelling AM. *Pseudomonas aeruginosa*: a formidable and ever-present adversary. J Hosp Infect 2009;73(4):338–44.
60. Gupta N, Limbago BM, Patel JB, et al. Carbapenem-resistant Enterobacteriaceae: epidemiology and prevention. Clin Infect Dis 2011;53(1):60–7.
61. Conlan S, Thomas PJ, Deming C, et al. Single-molecule sequencing to track plasmid diversity of hospital-associated carbapenemase-producing Enterobacteriaceae. Sci Transl Med 2014;6(254):254ra126.
62. Centers for Disease Control Prevention (CDC). Vital signs: carbapenem-resistant Enterobacteriaceae. MMWR Morb Mortal Wkly Rep 2013;62(9):165–70.
63. Temkin E, Adler A, Lerner A, et al. Carbapenem-resistant Enterobacteriaceae: biology, epidemiology, and management. Ann N Y Acad Sci 2014;1323:22–42.
64. Epson EE, Pisney LM, Wendt JM, et al. Carbapenem-resistant *Klebsiella pneumoniae* producing New Delhi metallo-beta-lactamase at an acute care hospital, Colorado, 2012. Infect Control Hosp Epidemiol 2014;35(4):390–7.
65. Munoz-Price LS, Quinn JP. Deconstructing the infection control bundles for the containment of carbapenem-resistant Enterobacteriaceae. Curr Opin Infect Dis 2013;26(4):378–87.
66. Magill SS, Edwards JR, Bamberg W, et al. Multistate point-prevalence survey of health care-associated infections. N Engl J Med 2014;370(13):1198–208.
67. Wertheim HFL, Melles DC, Vos MC, et al. The role of nasal carriage in *Staphylococcus aureus* infections. Lancet Infect Dis 2005;5(12):751–62.
68. Sherertz RJ, Reagan DR, Hampton KD, et al. A cloud adult: the *Staphylococcus aureus*-virus interaction revisited. Ann Intern Med 1996;124(6):539–47.
69. Vonberg RP, Stamm-Balderjahn S, Hansen S, et al. How often do asymptomatic healthcare workers cause methicillin-resistant *Staphylococcus aureus* outbreaks? A systematic evaluation. Infect Control Hosp Epidemiol 2006;27(10): 1123–7.
70. Dancer SJ. Importance of the environment in methicillin-resistant *Staphylococcus aureus* acquisition: the case for hospital cleaning. Lancet Infect Dis 2008;8(2):101–13.
71. Livorsi DJ, Arif S, Garry P, et al. Methicillin-resistant *Staphylococcus aureus* (MRSA) nasal real-time PCR: a predictive tool for contamination of the hospital environment. Infect Control Hosp Epidemiol 2015;36(1):34–9.
72. Weber DJ, Peppercorn A, Miller MB, et al. Preventing healthcare-associated *Aspergillus* infections: review of recent CDC/HICPAC recommendations. Med Mycol 2009;47(Suppl 1):S199–209.
73. Kanamori H, Rutala WA, Sickbert-Bennett EE, et al. Review of fungal outbreaks and infection prevention in healthcare settings during construction and renovation. Clin Infect Dis 2015;61(3):433–44.

74. Vonberg RP, Gastmeier P. Nosocomial aspergillosis in outbreak settings. J Hosp Infect 2006;63(3):246–54.

75. Panackal AA, Li H, Kontoyiannis DP, et al. Geoclimatic influences on invasive aspergillosis after hematopoietic stem cell transplantation. Clin Infect Dis 2010;50(12):1588–97.

76. Cavallo M, Andreoni S, Martinotti MG, et al. Monitoring environmental *Aspergillus* spp. contamination and meteorological factors in a haematological unit. Mycopathologia 2013;176(5–6):387–94.

77. Apisarnthanarak A, Warren DK, Mayhall CG. Healthcare-associated infections and their prevention after extensive flooding. Curr Opin Infect Dis 2013;26(4): 359–65.

78. Gunaratne PS, Wijeyaratne CN, Chandrasiri P, et al. An outbreak of *Aspergillus* meningitis following spinal anaesthesia for caesarean section in Sri Lanka: a post-tsunami effect? Ceylon Med J 2006;51(4):137–42.

79. Jain S, Self WH, Wunderink RG, et al. Community-acquired pneumonia requiring hospitalization among U.S. adults. N Engl J Med 2015;373(5):415–27.

80. Gaunt ER, Harvala H, McIntyre C, et al. Disease burden of the most commonly detected respiratory viruses in hospitalized patients calculated using the disability adjusted life year (DALY) model. J Clin Virol 2011;52(3):215–21.

81. Evans ME, Hall KL, Berry SE. Influenza control in acute care hospitals. Am J Infect Control 1997;25(4):357–62.

82. Horcajada JP, Pumarola T, Martinez JA, et al. A nosocomial outbreak of influenza during a period without influenza epidemic activity. Eur Respir J 2003;21(2): 303–7.

83. Ahmed F, Lindley MC, Allred N, et al. Effect of influenza vaccination of healthcare personnel on morbidity and mortality among patients: systematic review and grading of evidence. Clin Infect Dis 2014;58(1):50–7.

84. Suwantarat N, Apisarnthanarak A. Risks to healthcare workers with emerging diseases: lessons from MERS-CoV, Ebola, SARS, and avian flu. Curr Opin Infect Dis 2015;28(4):349–61.

85. Maltezou HC, Ftika L, Theodoridou M. Nosocomial pertussis in neonatal units. J Hosp Infect 2013;85(4):243–8.

86. Calugar A, Ortega-Sanchez IR, Tiwari T, et al. Nosocomial pertussis: costs of an outbreak and benefits of vaccinating health care workers. Clin Infect Dis 2006; 42(7):981–8.

87. Centers for Disease Control Prevention (CDC). Pertussis–United States, 2001-2003. MMWR Morb Mortal Wkly Rep 2005;54(50):1283–6.

88. Sheridan SL, Frith K, Snelling TL, et al. Waning vaccine immunity in teenagers primed with whole cell and acellular pertussis vaccine: recent epidemiology. Expert Rev Vaccines 2014;13(9):1081–106.

89. Fankhauser RL, Noel JS, Monroe SS, et al. Molecular epidemiology of "Norwalk-like viruses" in outbreaks of gastroenteritis in the United States. J Infect Dis 1998;178(6):1571–8.

90. Robilotti E, Deresinski S, Pinsky BA. Norovirus. Clin Microbiol Rev 2015;28(1): 134–64.

91. Greig JD, Lee MB. A review of nosocomial norovirus outbreaks: infection control interventions found effective. Epidemiol Infect 2012;140(7):1151–60.

92. Carroll KC, Bartlett JG. Biology of *Clostridium difficile*: implications for epidemiology and diagnosis. Annu Rev Microbiol 2011;65:501–21.

93. Barbut F. How to eradicate *Clostridium difficile* from the environment. J Hosp Infect 2015;89(4):287–95.

94. Otter JA, Yezli S, Salkeld JA, et al. Evidence that contaminated surfaces contribute to the transmission of hospital pathogens and an overview of strategies to address contaminated surfaces in hospital settings. Am J Infect Control 2013;41(5 Suppl):S6–11.
95. Kundrapu S, Sunkesula V, Jury LA, et al. Daily disinfection of high-touch surfaces in isolation rooms to reduce contamination of healthcare workers' hands. Infect Control Hosp Epidemiol 2012;33(10):1039–42.
96. Eyre DW, Cule ML, Wilson DJ, et al. Diverse sources of *C. difficile* infection identified on whole-genome sequencing. N Engl J Med 2013;369(13):1195–205.
97. Lanata CF, Fischer-Walker CL, Olascoaga AC, et al. Global causes of diarrheal disease mortality in children <5 years of age: a systematic review. PLoS One 2013;8(9):e72788.
98. Von Dolinger de Brito D, de Almeida Silva H, Jose Oliveira E, et al. Effect of neonatal intensive care unit environment on the incidence of hospital-acquired infection in neonates. J Hosp Infect 2007;65(4):314–8.
99. Oelberg DG, Joyner SE, Jiang X, et al. Detection of pathogen transmission in neonatal nurseries using DNA markers as surrogate indicators. Pediatrics 2000;105(2):311–5.
100. Curtis C, Shetty N. Recent trends and prevention of infection in the neonatal intensive care unit. Curr Opin Infect Dis 2008;21(4):350–6.
101. Gastmeier P, Loui A, Stamm-Balderjahn S, et al. Outbreaks in neonatal intensive care units—they are not like others. Am J Infect Control 2007;35(3):172–6.
102. Civardi E, Tzialla C, Baldanti F, et al. Viral outbreaks in neonatal intensive care units: what we do not know. Am J Infect Control 2013;41(10):854–6.
103. Devlin RK. Invasive fungal infections caused by *Candida* and *Malassezia* species in the neonatal intensive care unit. Adv Neonatal Care 2006;6(2):68–77 [quiz: 8–9].
104. De Smet B, Veng C, Kruy L, et al. Outbreak of *Burkholderia cepacia* bloodstream infections traced to the use of Ringer lactate solution as multiple-dose vial for catheter flushing, Phnom Penh, Cambodia. Clin Microbiol Infect 2013; 19(9):832–7.
105. Kimura AC, Calvet H, Higa JI, et al. Outbreak of *Ralstonia pickettii* bacteremia in a neonatal intensive care unit. Pediatr Infect Dis J 2005;24(12):1099–103.
106. Macias AE, Munoz JM, Galvan A, et al. Nosocomial bacteremia in neonates related to poor standards of care. Pediatr Infect Dis J 2005;24(8):713–6.
107. Ofstead CL, Wetzler HP, Doyle EM, et al. Persistent contamination on colonoscopes and gastroscopes detected by biologic cultures and rapid indicators despite reprocessing performed in accordance with guidelines. Am J Infect Control 2015;43(8):794–801.
108. Pajkos A, Vickery K, Cossart Y. Is biofilm accumulation on endoscope tubing a contributor to the failure of cleaning and decontamination? J Hosp Infect 2004; 58(3):224–9.
109. Seoane-Vazquez E, Rodriguez-Monguio R, Visaria J, et al. Exogenous endoscopy-related infections, pseudo-infections, and toxic reactions: clinical and economic burden. Curr Med Res Opin 2006;22(10):2007–21.
110. Rutala WA, Weber DJ. ERCP scopes: what can we do to prevent infections? Infect Control Hosp Epidemiol 2015;36(6):643–8.
111. Epstein L, Hunter JC, Arwady MA, et al. New Delhi metallo-beta-lactamase-producing carbapenem-resistant *Escherichia coli* associated with exposure to duodenoscopes. JAMA 2014;312(14):1447–55.

112. Wendorf KA, Kay M, Baliga C, et al. Endoscopic retrograde cholangiopancreatography-associated AmpC *Escherichia coli* outbreak. Infect Control Hosp Epidemiol 2015;36(6):634–42.

113. Ross AS, Baliga C, Verma P, et al. A quarantine process for the resolution of duodenoscope-associated transmission of multidrug-resistant *Escherichia coli*. Gastrointest Endosc 2015;82(3):477–83.

114. Singh N, Limaye AP. Infections in solid-organ transplant recipients. In: Bennett JE, Dolin R, Blaser MJ, editors. Mandell, Douglas, and Bennett's principles and practice of infectious diseases. 8th edition. Philadelphia: Churchill Livingstone Elsevier; 2015. p. 3440–52.

115. Al-Hasan MN, Razonable RR, Eckel-Passow JE, et al. Incidence rate and outcome of gram-negative bloodstream infection in solid organ transplant recipients. Am J Transplant 2009;9(4):835–43.

116. Cervera C, van Delden C, Gavaldà J, et al. Multidrug-resistant bacteria in solid organ transplant recipients. Clin Microbiol Infect 2014;20(Suppl 7):49–73.

117. Manuel O, López-Medrano F, Keiser L, et al. Influenza and other respiratory virus infections in solid organ transplant recipients. Clin Microbiol Infect 2014; 20(Suppl 7):102–8.

118. Young J-AH, Weisdorf DJ. Infections in recipients of hematopoietic stem cell transplants. In: Bennett JE, Dolin R, Blaser MJ, editors. Mandell, Douglas, and Bennett's principles and practice of infectious diseases. 8th edition. Philadelphia: Churchill Livingstone Elsevier; 2015. p. 3425–39.

119. Paitoonpong L, Neofytos D, Cosgrove SE, et al. Infection prevention and control in hematopoietic stem cell transplant patients. In: Mayhall CG, editor. Hospital epidemiology and infection control. 4th edition. Baltimore (MD): Lippincott Williams & Wilkins; 2012. p. 837–71.

# Water Safety and Legionella in Health Care

## Priorities, Policy, and Practice

Shantini D. Gamage, PhD, MPH[a,b,*], Meredith Ambrose, MHA[a],
Stephen M. Kralovic, MD, MPH[a,b,c], Gary A. Roselle, MD[a,b,c]

## KEYWORDS

- Water-associated infections • Health care premise plumbing • Water safety plans
- Risk assessment • Legionella prevention

## KEY POINTS

- Water has extensive uses in health care, and therefore there are multiple considerations for preventing water-associated infections in these settings.
- Although the health care setting is increasingly recognized as an important contributor to the burden of water-associated infections in the United States, especially those caused by opportunistic premise plumbing pathogens, health care–associated infections from water pathogens remain underappreciated. Many health care facilities do not have specific plans to address their prevention.
- The risk for water-associated infections in health care, such as Legionella, and triggers for control are building specific, and require individualized assessments related to multiple factors to determine prevention strategies.
- There are multiple, often competing, priorities regarding water in health care buildings, such as preventing pathogen growth and transmission, avoiding scald injury, reducing energy usage and costs, promoting conservation, and maintaining water security. Focusing on 1 aspect without consideration for the others could result in unintended consequences, such as water-associated infections.
- Effective water safety in health care requires a coordinated, multidisciplinary approach inclusive of facility administration, facilities management staff (eg, engineering), and clinical staff (eg, infection prevention and control, infectious diseases) for control of pathogens in the environment.

Disclosure: The authors have nothing to disclose.
[a] National Infectious Diseases Service, Specialty Care Services, Patient Care Services, Veterans Health Administration, Department of Veterans Affairs (VA), 810 Vermont Avenue, NW, Washington, DC 20420, USA; [b] Division of Infectious Diseases, Department of Internal Medicine, University of Cincinnati College of Medicine, 3230 Eden Avenue, Cincinnati, OH 45267, USA; [c] Medical Service, Cincinnati VA Medical Center, 3200 Vine Street, Cincinnati, OH 45220, USA
* Corresponding author. 205 West 4th Street, Suite 1020, Cincinnati, OH 45202.
E-mail address: Shantini.Gamage@va.gov

Infect Dis Clin N Am 30 (2016) 689–712
http://dx.doi.org/10.1016/j.idc.2016.04.004
0891-5520/16/$ – see front matter Published by Elsevier Inc.

id.theclinics.com

## INTRODUCTION

The treatment of drinking water by municipalities to reduce infectious diseases is one of the major public health accomplishments of the twentieth century in the developed world.[1] Now, more than a century from its first implementation in the United States, drinking water that is safe from pathogens is largely taken for granted. In addition, although the regulatory and oversight authority of public water utilities in the United States does not generally include premise plumbing (ie, water distribution within buildings and property lines), little consideration is given for water safety and quality in the potable water distribution system of buildings. Outbreaks caused by deficiencies in federally regulated public water utilities have decreased, but outbreaks associated with premise plumbing have increased,[2] indicating both the lack of attention to infectious disease transmission from this source and the missed opportunity for directed prevention.

Several pathogens related to water have been implicated in causing disease in humans, with varying routes of exposure (**Fig. 1**).[3,4] An important distinction, especially when considering the control of these pathogens, is the nature of their association with water[5]:

- Water based: pathogens that naturally inhabit water and grow in water systems (eg, *Legionella* species that cause legionnaires' disease [LD])
- Waterborne: pathogens that do not replicate in water but can be transmitted by water, often as a result of fecal contamination (eg, *Escherichia coli* that cause gastroenteritis)
- Water related: pathogens that are associated with a vector that requires water for part of its life cycle (eg, dengue virus transmitted by mosquitoes)

In the United States, waterborne pathogens in drinking water are controlled by biocide treatment before distribution to customers (eg, buildings); organizations supplying the water are responsible for monitoring contaminants, including indicators of waterborne (ie, fecal) pathogens. In contrast, water-based pathogens are found in low numbers in natural bodies of water, and treatment plants do not specifically target or monitor levels. These pathogens, notably *Legionella* species, *Pseudomonas aeruginosa*, and nontuberculous mycobacteria (NTM), can grow in building water distribution systems; they are associated with free-living amoeba and/or biofilms, both of which can offer protection to the pathogens from disinfecting biocides in the water system.[4,6] Water-based pathogens have been referred to as opportunistic premise plumbing pathogens, and the significance of their ecology for persistence and control in buildings has recently been reviewed.[5,7]

This article mainly focuses on water-based pathogens; those that can multiply in building water distribution systems and for which primary prevention activities at the building level may be appropriate. From the many recent reviews on these pathogens and their management in health care settings,[4,6–13] it now seems clear that increased actions regarding premise water distribution system safety are warranted, although they are not often prioritized.

## WATER IN THE HEALTH CARE SETTING AND PATHOGENS

Health care facility water distribution systems are complex given the variation in building and campus sizes, health care delivery goals, and facility operations with variable water demands within the system. All of these factors can influence premise plumbing pathogen growth and persistence, sometimes in competing ways. In addition, different health care settings (eg, acute care hospitals, long-term care facilities)

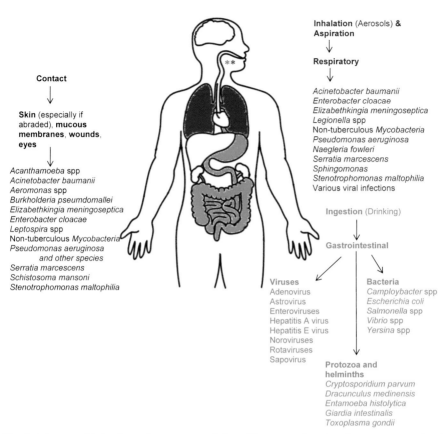

**Fig. 1.** Water and infectious disease transmission. Water-associated pathogens categorized by routes of transmission. Asterisks indicate upper respiratory (*blue*) and upper gastrointestinal (*green*) tracts. (*Data from* Exner M, Kramer A, Lajoie L, et al. Prevention and control of health care-associated waterborne infections in health care facilities. Am J Infect Control 2005;33(5 Suppl 1):S26–40; and Williams MM, Armbruster CR, Arduino MJ. Plumbing of hospital premises is a reservoir for opportunistically pathogenic microorganisms: a review. Biofouling 2013;29(2):147–62.)

have varying infrastructures, operational requirements, and patient populations that contribute to environmental pathogen growth and infection.

Experience from decades of outbreak control and water management in health care highlights the importance of understanding characteristics that may promote premise plumbing pathogen growth on a building-specific level.[14–18] However, health care facility water safety is often overlooked when it comes to risk management efforts. The necessity of and ability to implement prevention practices are not the same in all situations. The assessment of risks and need for actions are likely to change over time, requiring continual vigilance. The different water management priorities in the health care setting and considerations for prevention of water-associated health care–associated infections (HAIs) are discussed here. In addition, although facilities management has the responsibility to maintain water systems, awareness by clinical staff of these priorities and risks provides a critical interface between building operations and patient safety.

### Water Management Priorities

#### Safety

At present, water safety associated with premise plumbing pathogens largely focuses on measures to prevent growth of *Legionella*. The primary mechanisms for microbial control in health care facility water distribution systems are maintenance of inhibitory water temperatures and implementation of remedial actions when indicated. The US Centers for Disease Control and Prevention (CDC) recommends the following actions for routine prevention of microbial contamination[19]:

- Hot water storage tanks should be set to 60°C (140°F).[20]
- Hot water should constantly recirculate in patient care areas. Maintain hot water temperatures at the return at the highest temperature allowable by state regulations or code, preferably at least 51°C (124°F); if a temperature greater than or equal to 51°C is allowed, consider engineering options such as thermostatic mixing valves at the tap to minimize scald risk.[20]
- If hot water temperatures are not allowed to be at least 51°C (eg, codes that limit hospital water to 41°C–49°C [105°F–120°F] or nursing care facility water to 35°C–43°C [95°F–110°F]), periodic actions to minimize *Legionella* growth should be followed.[19]
- Maintain cold water temperature less than 20°C (68°F).[20]

Some guidance bodies recommend assessment of disinfectant levels[21,22] in the water distribution system, and this may be particularly important if circulating hot water temperatures are lower than recommended to suppress pathogen growth (discussed later).

#### Distribution and quality

Health care facilities are responsible for infrastructure and maintenance of water systems for the distribution of potable and nonpotable water for various uses. Potable water, processed to be safe for consumption per US Environmental Protection Agency regulations, is provided by local water utilities or on-site treatment facilities. Further processing may occur at the building for purposes such as supplementary disinfection, water softening, and water heating for provision of hot water. In addition to providing water for consumption, potable water in health care is used for showering/bathing, hand hygiene, toilets, emergency systems (emergency showers, eye washes, fire sprinklers), housekeeping, sterile processing, and other water uses in patient care (**Table 1**). Some considerations for potable water distribution and prevention of premise plumbing pathogen growth include:

**Water stagnation in pipes** Slow or nonmoving water in hospital plumbing can be caused by dead legs, intermittent use of areas, or low water usage. Stagnation can lead to biofilm formation, lower levels of inhibitory controls (ie, hot water, disinfectant), and promote pathogen growth. In addition, pathogens can grow in the low-oxygen environment in stagnant water.[6] Flushing programs that periodically flow water through outlets to reduce persistent standing water may reduce the risk of pathogen growth.[17,21,23]

**Disinfectant residual** The disinfectant residual is "the net amount of a chemical disinfectant remaining in the treated water after chemical demand exerted by the water is satisfied."[22] Depending on various factors, such as water age and distribution system organic and inorganic load, water may have little to no disinfectant residual by the time it is delivered from the treatment plant to the health care campus (the point where the premise begins), or from that point to patient care/residential buildings and the end points where users access it. The use of supplemental disinfection systems to provide additional chemical treatment, such as chlorine, copper and silver ions, chlorine dioxide, or monochloramine, to enhance disinfectant residual levels in health care water distribution systems has been evaluated.[24,25] Accordingly, some health care systems

**Table 1**
**Water uses in health care settings and infection risks**

| Water Use | Infection Risks and/or Considerations | Case/Outbreak Example | References |
|---|---|---|---|
| Hydrotherapy | Aerosolization of contaminated water; water stagnation caused by intermittent use; contaminated pumps and hoses; insufficient cleaning and disinfection | Outbreak of pseudomonas folliculitis among patients and staff who used a swimming pool in a physiotherapy unit | 74 |
| Ice from plumbed ice machines | Aspiration risk; cold water in piping can become warmed by heat from condenser and/ or compressor; water stagnation when not in use; charcoal filter colonized by bacteria; lack of routine maintenance, cleaning, and disinfection | Legionellosis from aspiration of water from ice chips | 75,76 |
| Food preparation | Appropriate washing and disinfection procedures; use of sterilizers | Outbreak of *P aeruginosa* infection in a neonatal intensive care unit was linked to the feeding bottle preparation room | 77 |
| Dialysis | Chemical or bacterial contamination, or modifications to potable water system (eg, supplementary treatment) can affect dialysis water Dialysis water must meet specific ANSI/AAMI/ISO requirements to prevent illness as a result of contaminants in the water (eg, endotoxin, disinfection byproducts) | Outbreak of *Mycobacterium chelonae abscessus* at a hemodialysis outpatient clinic caused by use of high-flux dialyzers that were manually reprocessed | 78,79 |
| Pharmacy: medication preparation | Water for pharmaceutical use should meet drinking-water standards. Water used for specific pharmaceutical purposes (eg, water for injections, water for compounding) should meet pharmacopoeial specifications for chemical and microbiological purity | Outbreak of *Exophiala jeanselmei* fungemia, most likely linked to deionized water from the hospital pharmacy for preparation of antiseptic solutions | 80,81 |

(*continued on next page*)

**Table 1**
**(continued)**

| Water Use | Infection Risks and/or Considerations | Case/Outbreak Example | References |
|---|---|---|---|
| Dental unit waterlines | Aerosolization of contaminated water; water stagnation; plastic tubing conducive to biofilm and bacterial growth; water temperatures in ranges that allow bacterial growth; patient oral microorganisms can contaminate the unit during procedure<br>The CDC recommends that water used as a coolant/irrigant in nonsurgical dental procedures should meet standards for safe drinking-water quality | LD from contaminated dental unit water lines | 82,83 |
| Respiratory equipment (eg, nebulizers, continuous positive airway pressure devices) | Bacterial growth in devices without sufficient maintenance and cleaning; aerosolization of contaminated water<br>Use sterile water only; follow CDC guidelines for cleaning/disinfecting equipment | P aeruginosa infection caused by contaminated nebulizers | 84 |
| Heater-cooler devices | Aerosolization of contaminated water from the device's exhaust vent<br>The US Food and Drug Administration recommends the use of sterile or filtered water and other practices to reduce risk to patients | Nontuberculous mycobacterium infections diagnosed in cardiothoracic surgery patients | 85,86 |

*Abbreviations:* AAMI, Association for the Advancement of Medical Instrumentation; ANSI, American National Standards Institute; ISO, International Organization for Standardization.

have included assessment of disinfectant residual and consideration for implementing supplementary systems as a component of primary prevention for *Legionella* control.[23,26–28] Regardless of the type of system installed, all require routine monitoring and maintenance to ensure optimal and sustained operations.

**Water temperature** As with disinfectant residual, numerous factors could influence whether or not the hot water temperature at the point of use is at a level inhibitory to *Legionella* ($\geq 51^\circ$C [124$^\circ$F]) or other pathogens, including water stagnation (especially if the hot water system is not recirculating) and complex infrastructure that does not support delivery of hot water to points remote from hot water generation.[29] However, even when the distribution system is fully capable of delivering hot water, preventing scald injury is also a priority.

**The balance between scald prevention and microbial control** It is not possible to simultaneously prevent the risk of scald injury and ensure inhibition of some pathogens (eg, *Legionella*) by hot water at the point where the end user contacts the water. Patients in hospitals and residents in long-term care facilities are at heightened risk for scald injury.[30] Different local regulations or building codes may require reduced hot water temperatures delivered to end users in these settings, often in the optimal water temperature range for pathogen growth. What often ensues is the reduction of the hot water temperature at the point of generation (eg, hot water tank) to a level lower than the recommended 60°C (140°F) to ensure distribution at a safe temperature. Although this can allow compliance with anti-scald regulations, it turns the hot water distribution system into an environment conducive to pathogen growth, and low hot water temperature has contributed to proliferation of *Legionella*[29] and outbreaks of disease.[24] As recommended in guidance,[19,20] a more balanced approach to mitigate both risks in health care settings would be the installation of thermostatic mixing valves or anti-scald devices as close to the end points of use as possible to permit circulating hot water at higher temperatures throughout most of the distribution system.

**Thermostatic mixing valves/anti-scald devices** Installation of these devices at outlets to allow for hotter circulating water can help balance scald and infection prevention. However, they permit the water in the piping distal to the device to be at a temperature conducive to growth of *Legionella* and other pathogens, especially if disinfectant residual is low. Consequently, some have expressed caution for their use and recommend a tiered implementation of the devices based on risk.[31,32] This option may or may not be feasible for all health care systems depending on local requirements and policies. If mixing valves will be used, consider including routine maintenance and cleaning, periodic assessment of the water at distal sites for pathogens (eg, *Legionella*), and/or periodic flushing of chlorinated water through the distribution system.

**Construction activities** As facilities reconfigure the use of existing space or add new construction, plumbing lines may be capped (creating dead legs) or tied into, which affects water use and flow. Construction and renovation can result in the temporary disruption of water circulation in the area and/or changes in water pressure, which could result in descaling of the pipes and contamination of the water with biofilm and microbes.[33,34] High temperatures or chlorine flushing of the affected system is recommended with specific details for the type and extent of decontamination efforts dependent on building and construction characteristics.[20]

**Leaking pipes/condensation** The structural integrity of premise plumbing may be compromised by corrosion (eg, from source water physical parameters, supplementary disinfection) or from damage. Water that leaks from pipes or collects on surfaces from condensation can cause dampness in building materials, resulting in growth of fungi (mold) and bacteria, and subsequently in respiratory illness or infection in building occupants.[35]

**Decorative water features** Ornamental water features, including fountains and water walls, are installed in health care buildings for aesthetics. However, documented outbreaks of disease[36,37] from indoor installations of these features in health care settings substantiate that these indoor decorations are a risk for health care facility occupants and should not be used.[19]

Nonpotable water (process water) is nonconsumable water used for facility utility operations (eg, cooling towers/evaporative condensers, boilers, chilled water for cooling coils, and outdoor decorative fountains). Of particular concern is the transmission of *Legionella* from cooling towers. Because microbes can grow to high concentrations in improperly maintained cooling tower water and then be dispersed by aerosols in cooling tower drift,[38] outbreaks related to cooling towers can result in large numbers of cases in a short period of time. One recent outbreak associated with a newly installed cooling tower in an Ohio long-term care facility resulted in 39 identified cases of LD and 6 deaths.[39] This outbreak shows the importance of several factors: system design for biocide delivery; proper maintenance, monitoring, and documentation of controls; oversight of subcontracted water treatment companies; and placement of the cooling tower away from the building's fresh air intakes. The US Cooling Technology Institute has published a guideline of best practices for the control of *Legionella*.[38]

## Conservation

Conservation pertains to the implementation of water management actions to reduce water use for the purpose of meeting demand, protecting the environment, reducing water and sewer costs, and/or reducing energy consumption. Mechanisms to reduce water usage within health care buildings include the installation of reduced flow faucet/shower fixtures, laminar flow fixtures, faucet aerators, sensor-activated electronic faucets (also installed to reduce cross-contamination of fixtures), and automatic shut-off valves. These devices may promote conditions favorable to pathogen growth, such as water stagnation. One study[40] found that electronic faucets in a hospital were more colonized with *Legionella* than manual faucets. It may be that some types of sensor faucets allow increased growth of *Legionella* on components of the faucet. Because these faucets are at the point of use, further investigation is warranted to understand the risk of these devices for water-based HAIs; nonetheless, both electronic and manual faucets can become contaminated with *Legionella*, and unresolved issues of *Legionella* in the water distribution system may be the underlying factor that needs addressing.

## Emergency water supply (water security)

A consistent water supply is critical for hospital operations and patient care. Interruptions to the water supply can result from several factors, including water utility service failures, power failures, natural disasters, construction damage, or terrorism, with the water supply compromised for hours to days. The Centers for Medicare and Medicaid Services and accreditation by The Joint Commission (TJC) require health care facilities to assess the capability to provide utilities for at least 96 hours in facility emergency/preparedness plans.[41] One option for maintaining water security is to hold a supply of water on site in storage tanks capable of providing sufficient water for critical operations for a period of time. Prolonged storage of water may result in bacterial (and pathogen) growth, especially if there is loss of disinfection residual. Depletion of disinfection residual in storage tanks can be accelerated if organic sediment and biological growth are present. Therefore, storage tanks should be on a routine monitoring, cleaning/maintenance, and usage/flushing program to assess and ensure water quality and safety.

## Water-based Health Care–associated Infections

HAIs account for a substantial burden of infectious diseases in the United States.[42] Increasingly, human pathogens transmitted in the health care setting by water are being recognized for their contribution to the burden of HAIs. For example, the proactive installation of point-of-use filters on the outlets of a transplant unit to prevent water-related infections in patients in the absence of a known outbreak resulted in a decrease in HAIs in these patients over a 9-month period, suggesting that water is a routine source of infection.[43]

Review articles have summarized key pathogens associated with premise plumbing, including *Legionella* species, NTMs, *P aeruginosa*, *Acanthamoeba*, gram-negative bacilli, and fungi.[4–7,11,13] **Table 2** lists some of these pathogens that are of particular concern in health care. Incidences for these infections in the United States are included when available, but the proportion of these that are attributable to water exposure as opposed to other mechanisms is largely unknown.

*Health care–associated infections and Legionella*
*Legionella* bacteria cause LD, a type of pneumonia, and Pontiac fever, a milder non-pneumonia illness, collectively known as legionellosis. Occurrence of legionellosis in the United States has been increasing,[44] but attribution of these infections to specific settings is not reported and the burden of health care–associated (HCA) legionellosis in the United States is not well characterized. Estimates from hospital studies suggest that 10% to 40% of hospital-acquired pneumonias are LD[45]; similar estimates for long-term care facilities are not available.[46,47] Regardless, *Legionella* is a pathogen with recognized association with both hospital and long-term care water systems. The most recent surveillance report of drinking-water outbreaks from the US Waterborne Disease and Outbreak Surveillance System substantiates health care as increasingly important in contributing to LD burden: 67% of *Legionella* outbreaks (14 out of 21) in 2011 to 2012 occurred in health care facilities, and 86% of outbreak-associated deaths (12 out of 14) were cases associated with these settings.[2]

LD is an acute-onset pneumonia with an estimated mortality of 5% to 30%.[48] Patients in health care settings are considered to be at high risk for LD because of comorbidities, compromised immune function, and/or very young or advanced age.[19,49] Clinically, LD is indistinguishable from other pneumonias and requires specific testing to confirm diagnosis. The *Legionella* urine antigen test, which targets detection of disease caused by *Legionella pneumophila* serogroup 1, is the primary LD diagnostic test used in the United States. Microbiological culturing of respiratory specimens, if available, can detect other *Legionella* species and serogroups as well as provide a clinical isolate for comparison with environmental *Legionella* isolates by molecular methods. However, pneumonia is often treated empirically with antibiotics, in alignment with current professional guidance.[50,51] A retrospective review of LD cases at one hospital found that 41% (15 out of 37) did not meet the guideline's criteria for *Legionella* testing of community-acquired pneumonia.[52] Not diagnosing LD can result in lack of recognition of environmental health care exposure, and a missed opportunity for an epidemiologic investigation and water system remediation to prevent further cases. Accordingly, CDC guidance recommends a high index of suspicion for LD in patients with health care–associated pneumonia (HAP) and subsequent epidemiologic and environmental investigations if HCA LD occurs.[19,49] In the United States, per revised CDC reporting guidelines,[53] association of a case of legionellosis with health care exposure is temporal according to the following criteria:

- Definitely HCA: patient was hospitalized or a resident of a long-term care facility for the entire 10 days before onset
- Possibly HCA: patient had exposure to a health care facility for a portion of the 10 days before onset
- Not HCA: no exposure to a health care facility in the 10 days before onset

Clinicians at any health care facility with a case of HCA LD should have heightened awareness for LD in other patients with HAP or if an environmental investigation reveals *Legionella* in the facility water system.[19,23,49]

**Table 2**
**Select water-associated pathogens in the health care setting**

| Pathogen | Diseases | Cases in United States | Modes of Exposure | Resistance to Chlorine[a] | Comments | References |
|---|---|---|---|---|---|---|
| Legionella species | LD (an acute pneumonia); Pontiac fever | 5166 reported cases (2014) 8000–18,000 estimated cases requiring hospitalization per year | Inhalation or aspiration In general, not transmitted person to person | ++ Some resistance reported; increased resistance when inside amoeba (up to 50 ppm) | Approximately 90% of LD cases reported in United States are caused by Legionella pneumophila; LD attack rate approx. 5%; seasonal variation; reportable disease Water-based pathogen; replicates within amoeba; optimal growth in warm water (32.2°C–40.6°C [90°F–105°F]); associated with biofilm in pipes; cases in health care setting from many types of exposures, including showers, ice machines, respiratory devices, and decorative fountains | 87–89 |
| NTM; eg, Mycobacterium avium-intracellulare complex, M chelonae, Mycobacterium fortuitum, Mycobacterium chimaera) | Pulmonary disease; cervical lymphadenitis (children); skin/ soft tissue infection; disseminated infection | Estimated 86,244 cases of pulmonary NTM disease in 2010, and predicted 181,037 cases in United States in 2014 | Inhalation or aspiration; ingestion; direct inoculation No person-to-person transmission | ++++ Concern that chlorine (and chloramine) treatment of drinking-water systems to control Legionella enriches for NTMs | Opportunistic pathogens, especially affecting immunocompromised persons; slowly progressive disease that can become chronic and/or disseminated; slight, elderly women identified as a risk group; not reportable Water-based pathogen; associated with biofilm in pipes | 90 |

| Organism | Types of infection/disease | Burden of disease | Mode of transmission | | Comments | References |
|---|---|---|---|---|---|---|
| *Stenotrophomonas maltophilia* | Bacteremia; catheter-related infection; pneumonia; skin/soft tissue infection; ophthalmic infections | — | Inhalation or aspiration; contact | +/++ | Opportunistic gram-negative pathogen, especially affecting immunocompromised persons; resistant to multiple antibiotics; not reportable Water-based pathogen; isolated from hospital tap water during case investigations | 5 |
| *P aeruginosa* | Urinary tract infections; respiratory infections; dermatitis; soft tissue infections; bacteremia; bone and joint infections; gastrointestinal infections | ~51,000 US HAIs per year; >6000 of these are multidrug-resistant infections and ~400 deaths per year (CDC, 2013) ~1400 deaths from waterborne nosocomial pneumonia | Inhalation; contact; direct wound inoculation | ++/+++ | Outbreaks linked to hospital water; burden of disease associated with health care water distribution systems is unknown; not reportable Water-based pathogen; grows in a highly structured biofilm; inhibitory to amoeba | 8,91,92 |
| *Acinetobacter* spp | Pneumonia; bacteremia; intracranial infections (associated with trauma or neurosurgical procedures); device-associated infections; skin/soft tissues | ~1500 US HAIs from 2009–2010 in 2039 US hospitals; estimated to have 7300 cases with 500 deaths/y in United States with drug-resistant *Acinetobacter* spp | Inhalation and aspiration; contact; contaminated surfaces; inoculation | ++ | Ubiquitous in the environment; nearly a quarter of healthy adults may show colonization; seasonal occurrence; in general, not reportable unless associated with outbreaks; nearly 2 out of 3 health care-associated cases with multidrug resistance present | 93–95 |

*(continued on next page)*

**Table 2**
**(continued)**

| Pathogen | Diseases | Cases in United States | Modes of Exposure | Resistance to Chlorine[a] | Comments | References |
|---|---|---|---|---|---|---|
| Other gram-negative pathogens: Enterobacteriaceae such as *E coli*, *Klebsiella* spp | Pneumonia; bloodstream infections; wound infections; secondary urinary tract infections; diarrhea | ~140,000 US health care–associated Enterobacteriaceae infections (CDC, 2009–2010) | Person-to-person contact; contact with contaminated surfaces; inhalation | + | Waterborne pathogens; burden of disease associated with health care water distribution systems is unknown; outbreaks have been associated with drinking water; in general, not reportable | 95 |

[a] Relative chlorine resistance for comparison; + least resistant, ++++ most resistant.
*Adapted from* Pruden A, Edwards MA, Falkingam JO. State of the science and research needs for opportunistic pathogens in premise plumbing. Dever (CO): Water Research Foundation; 2013. Available at: http://www.waterrf.org/PublicReportLibrary/4379.pdf. Accessed December 17, 2015.

### Legionella in health care building water distribution systems

Numerous reports and outbreak investigations substantiate that hospital and long-term care water distribution systems can be colonized with *Legionella*,[24,54–56] although the link of the environmental isolates to the cases may not always be definitively established. Less clear is the number of health care buildings in the United States colonized with *Legionella* species, or the extent and frequency of colonization, because standardized routine testing is not done; results, if such testing occurs, are not reportable and often not published. It has been described that 12% to 70% of hospitals are colonized with *Legionella*,[57] although higher rates have been reported.[58]

At present in the United States, there is no standard public health recommendation, or consensus, on the routine testing of health care facility potable water for *Legionella* in the absence of a case or outbreak investigation. Differing opinions exist among experts on whether it should be done[47,48] and, if so, how to interpret the data for risk mitigation. Key issues include:

- The *Legionella* species on which to focus for detection (ie, *L pneumophila* serogroup 1, all *L pneumophila*, or all *Legionella* species). Although *L pneumophila* serogroup 1 is the predominant cause of LD in the United States, other species and serogroups are pathogenic, especially in immunocompromised patients.
- The reliability of *Legionella* concentration detected. Variability in the ability of laboratories to consistently determine concentration has been reported.[59]
- The sampling protocol to be used (eg, volume of water, procedure for collecting the samples, location of samples, limit of detection) to correlate with building risk.
- The triggers to use for initiation of corrective actions. The CDC position is that there is no known safe level of *Legionella* in building water systems and recommends attempts to reduce *Legionella* to undetectable levels if routine testing is done.[19,60] Other guidance is to use *Legionella* concentration[21,61] or a percentage of positive outlets[62] to initiate corrective actions. The US Veterans Health Administration HCA LD Prevention Directive[23] is an example of a policy that attempts to address all *Legionella*-positive outlets, following the recommendations of the CDC and other external stakeholders. However, achieving sustained, undetectable levels of *Legionella* in many buildings is unlikely and of unknown necessity in all situations. Other health care organizations have adopted the use of *Legionella* concentration[63] or percentage of positive outlets[17] as thresholds to trigger actions.

Environmental and epidemiologic data suggest that *Legionella* can be present in hospital premise plumbing with an absence of cases.[28] The infectious dose, pathogen virulence, transmission potential, and host susceptibility all likely play roles in determining whether cases will occur, and research into these areas is critical for developing evidence-based policies and consensus. With the current state of knowledge, the most informative uses of environmental *Legionella* data are validation of control effectiveness, verification of remedial actions, and trend analysis of positive areas in order to ascertain changing risks. Because of the challenges in interpretation and use of environmental *Legionella* data,[60] the CDC makes no recommendation for routine environmental testing for *Legionella* except for transplant units or protective environments; the focus instead is on testing of HAP cases for LD to indicate a potential environmental issue.[19,49] However, if the risk of *Legionella* in water is that there is no known safe level, routine surveillance for the hazard to determine whether controls are effective can be informative for avoiding cases.[64] Accordingly, several other countries have included routine *Legionella* testing as a component of health care building water safety[48] and some US health care systems have included this testing as a validation that engineering controls are inhibiting *Legionella* growth.[17,23]

### The unapparent or creeping outbreak

The general situation in many health care facilities is that HAPs are empirically treated without LD diagnostic testing; HCA LD when it is recognized is considered to be a sporadic case; linking of the case to the facility is not undertaken or definitive; and/or the presence of *Legionella* in the water distribution system is not known. Because *Legionella* bacteria can persist in building water distribution systems for many years,[55,56] especially in the absence of effective controls, these sporadic HCA LD cases can occur over a prolonged period of time: an unapparent or creeping outbreak. **Table 3** lists examples of slowly progressing or recurrent outbreaks of LD, and it is clear that this is not a new concept.[65–67] Sporadic cases are often considered to be isolated incidences and the connection that a continued source of a preventable HAI exists is not made; several of the long-term transmissions of *Legionella* noted in

**Table 3**
**The unapparent or creeping outbreak: examples of long-term association of LD cases with buildings**

| Location | Type of Building | Reported Years of Cases[a] | Number of Cases[b] (Reported Cause) | References |
|---|---|---|---|---|
| Los Angeles, CA | Hospital | 1977–1982 | 219 nosocomial cases (*L pneumophila* sg 1; *L pneumophila* spp; *Legionella* species unnamed) | 96 |
| Innsbruck, Austria | Hospital | 1985–1993 | 14 nosocomial cases (*L pneumophila* sg 1) | 65 |
| Arizona | Hospital | 1987–1996* | 16 definite nosocomial cases 9 possible nosocomial cases (*L pneumophila* sg 1; other *L pneumophila* spp) | 66,97 |
| Ohio | Hospital | 1989–1996* | 9 definite nosocomial cases 29 possible nosocomial cases (*L pneumophila* sg 1) | 97 |
| Connecticut | Hospital | 1990–1994* | 12 definite nosocomial cases 14 possible nosocomial cases (*L pneumophila* sg 1) | 67 |
| Pittsburgh, PA | Long-term care facility | 1995–1997 | 6 nosocomial cases (*L pneumophila* sg 1; other *L pneumophila* spp) | 98 |
| Kuopio, Finland | Hospital | 1995–1998 | 3 laboratory-confirmed cases 2 suspect cases (*L pneumophila* sg 5) | 55 |
| Las Vegas, NV, USA | Condominium complex | 2001–2008* | 16 laboratory-confirmed cases 19 probable cases (*L pneumophila* sg 1) | 99 |
| Ocean City, MD | Hotel | 2003–2004* | 7 laboratory-confirmed cases 1 possible case (*L pneumophila* sg 1) | 100 |
| Pittsburgh, PA | Hospital | 2011–2012* | 5 definite HCA cases 17 probable HCA cases (*L pneumophila* sg 1) | 18 |
| Brisbane, Australia | Hospital | 2011–2013* | 3 nosocomial cases (*L pneumophila* sg 1) | 101 |

[a] Years with an asterisk (*) include reported retrospective case finding.
[b] Terminology used for the types of cases (eg, nosocomial, confirmed, possible) are as reported in each reference.

the table were discovered on retrospective case findings and suggest missed opportunities for interventions. This contention holds regardless of whether or not the cases are caused by the same strain of *Legionella* over time because intervention to control *Legionella* on first recognition of HCA LD cases can prevent growth of other strains as well. Furthermore, earlier intervention for a creeping outbreak may avoid a later spike in cases that seems to be a de novo outbreak.[18] The creeping outbreak of other opportunistic premise plumbing pathogens is also possible.[68] As with *Legionella*, multiple outbreaks caused by different strains is possible,[69] but early recognition of one environmental transmission may inform actions that prevent other cases.

## BUILDING WATER SAFETY PLANS

A building water safety plan is a mechanism for implementing a program for the methodical assessment and management of risks in the building water distribution system. The World Health Organization (WHO) has published guidance on the implementation of water safety plans for buildings, indicating that this process is the "most effective means of consistently ensuring the safety of drinking-water supplies."[14] These plans promote the identification of risks and implementation of actions for their control; this is a good practice for infection control programs for prevention of HAIs in general but with specific considerations for water safety responsibilities because the implementation of controls is usually based in facilities management functions and not clinical care functions. Components of a comprehensive water safety program include formation of a team and development of a plan that addresses (1) description of the water systems, (2) identification of hazards (eg, water-based pathogens), (3) risk assessment and prioritization, (4) identification and implementation of control measures, (5) definition of corrective actions, and (6) verification of the implementation of the program. **Table 4** lists some of the decision points to consider when developing a facility water safety plan.

In the United States, there is no requirement by regulatory or accreditation bodies for health care facilities to have specific, written water safety plans to control pathogens in accordance with the components advocated by WHO. Instead, for TJC accreditation, facilities are to maintain water systems to minimize pathogenic agents as a component of the actions to reduce risks in facility utility systems.[48,70] It is unknown how many hospitals in the United States have written water safety plans, or even targeted plans to control *Legionella*. Often, such plans are implemented after a crisis; an outbreak occurs or an adverse litigation is filed. This situation is caused in part by HCA water-based infections being considered to be rare among the HAIs, which provides a false sense of security that there is no risk; prevention is not considered necessary until cases occur. However, a proactive plan to control an environmental hazard and prevent illness in patients is in alignment with the general prioritization of HAI prevention. Furthermore, many of the controls for prevention of water-associated pathogens are general good practice for management of water systems.[14]

### The Team Approach

An important component for effective water safety in health care is the establishment of a multidisciplinary team of facility experts and stakeholders. Although health care facilities typically have infection control committees and/or environment of care committees that may address water safety, a dedicated water safety committee can focus on the various water management priorities in the health care setting. Furthermore, this committee can foster routine and targeted communication between facilities management and clinical staff on the implementation of actions (and, importantly,

**Table 4**
**Examples of decision points for health care facility water safety plans**

| Component | Decision Points |
|---|---|
| Decision making | Involvement of facility leadership<br>Institute a water safety committee<br>Key stakeholders and responsibilities (eg, engineering, infection prevention and control)<br>Prioritization of actions |
| Scope | Potable and/or process water<br>Water safety focus and/or other water priorities (eg, water security, conservation)<br>Special water uses to be included (eg, dialysis, dental)<br>Microbiological focus or all-hazards approach (eg, chemical, scald injury)<br>   For microbiological component: *Legionella* focus or other potential water pathogens as well<br>Types of buildings included (eg, inpatient facilities, outpatient clinics, long-term care facilities/residential buildings, administrative buildings) |
| Management plan | Knowledge and understanding<br>Water distribution system infrastructure (eg, schematic diagrams)<br>   Education and training of staff; competency requirements<br>Risk assessment mechanism and criteria<br>Selection of controls (eg, water temperature, disinfection residual)<br>   Prevention of scald injury<br>   Mechanism to ensure implementation of controls<br>Determination of necessity for supplementary disinfectant treatment system and, if so, which one<br>   Ensure appropriate permits if necessary<br>Triggers for remedial action<br>Remedial actions that will be taken to mitigate risk<br>Safety considerations<br>   Patients and residents<br>   Employees |
| Data collection | Surveillance for disease: which infections, if any, and tracking mechanism (clinical validation of prevention efforts)<br>Monitoring of engineering controls: which ones (if any), mechanism, and frequency<br>Environmental testing for hazards: which ones (if any), mechanism, and frequency (environmental validation of prevention efforts) |

follow-up) and discussion of physical (eg, control monitoring), environmental (eg, *Legionella* testing), and clinical (eg, case surveillance) data for trending of integrated information over time. **Box 1** lists some of the facility stakeholders for consideration of membership on the committee, depending on the types of buildings, patient care services offered, and scope of the water safety plan. Notably, unlike public water utilities that have persons with expertise in water system operations, maintenance, and chemistry on staff, health care facilities typically do not have staff with these specific proficiencies even though implementation of controls and remediation can be complex. Education and training for staff competency in water systems is critical, whether for implementation of engineering controls or for informed interaction with subcontracted water management companies.

### Legionella Prevention Plans

With the increasing incidence of legionellosis in the United States, the growing appreciation for *Legionella* transmission in health care settings, and the attention on

---

**Box 1**
**Stakeholders in water safety at the health care facility: potential members for a water safety committee**

Facility leadership
  Administrative and/or clinical

Engineering/facilities management
  Plumbing shop

Infectious diseases

Infection Prevention and Control

Pathology and laboratory medicine

Hemodialysis

Dental

Safety/industrial hygiene

Central supply

Occupational health

Public affairs

Labor partners

---

*Legionella* from recent prominent outbreaks,[18,39,71,72] there is continued, robust discussion on the state of the art in understanding *Legionella* ecology, control, and prevention policies in acute care hospitals and long-term care facilities.[9,10,47,48,73]

The recently published American National Standards Institute/American Society of Heating, Refrigerating, and Air-conditioning Engineers (ASHRAE) "Standard 188-2015, Legionellosis: Risk Management for Building Water Systems,"[22] is the first standard of its kind in the United States and is in alignment with the general principles of the WHO water safety plan guidance. It contains a normative annex specifically addressing requirements for health care facilities, including guidance for the membership of the designated team and the components of risk management plans. Even facilities that do not meet the criteria for compliance (eg, some long-term care facilities) can use the document to guide policy development. In contrast with the United States, several other countries have instituted recent national public health guidance or policy for the primary prevention of LD, which have been reviewed and compared.[9,47]

Risk factors for the occurrence of HCA LD have been described previously and include patient susceptibility, potential for exposure of occupants to *Legionella* in water through the water distribution system or from devices, and ability to implement controls to suppress *Legionella* growth in the water distribution system.[4,11,19,49] Because the relationship between *Legionella* in the water system and the occurrence of cases is not well understood, risk of *Legionella* in water systems, and decision points for assessment and control (see **Table 4**), should be ascertained on a building-specific level. For example, a critical indication of risk is whether there have been any HCA LD cases associated with the building in the past. This information indicates whether a strain of *Legionella* in the water system is capable of causing disease, can grow to levels at the infectious dose, and has been transmitted to building occupants. *Legionella* can persist in water distribution systems for decades, so a facility that experienced previous HCA LD cases should be vigilant in implementation of controls to avoid future cases.[18]

## SUMMARY: THE FUTURE OF WATER SAFETY IN HEALTH CARE IN THE UNITED STATES

Although there are many gaps in knowledge regarding water safety in premise plumbing, it is clear that more active approaches to water safety in US health care settings will continue to evolve with regard to microbial pathogens. The WHO and ASHRAE publications and the international efforts to address *Legionella* prevention in the health care setting show the increasing importance of this topic. To promote the development of evidence-based recommendations, more research and reporting on opportunistic premise plumbing pathogens and disease incidence will be necessary. Consensus on risk assessment and prevention of these pathogens, while balancing the different water system priorities in the health care setting, can bolster actions. In the interim, protection of patients and residents from water-based pathogens must still be prioritized; the unique nature of each individual building and its water distribution systems necessitates that a knowledgeable, multidisciplinary cadre of personnel in health care settings do risk evaluations and assessments to best identify strategies for risk mitigation.

## REFERENCES

1. Centers for Disease Control and Prevention (CDC). Ten great public health achievements – United States, 1900–1999. MMWR Morb Mortal Wkly Rep 1999;48(12):241–3.
2. Beer KD, Gargano JW, Roberts VA, et al. Surveillance for waterborne disease outbreaks associated with drinking water – United States, 2011-2012. MMWR Morb Mortal Wkly Rep 2015;64(31):842–8.
3. Exner M, Kramer A, Lajoie L, et al. Prevention and control of health care-associated waterborne infections in health care facilities. Am J Infect Control 2005;33(5 Suppl 1):S26–40.
4. Williams MM, Armbruster CR, Arduino MJ. Plumbing of hospital premises is a reservoir for opportunistically pathogenic microorganisms: a review. Biofouling 2013;29(2):147–62.
5. Ashbolt NJ. Environmental (saprozoic) pathogens of engineered water systems: understanding their ecology for risk assessment and management. Pathogens 2015;4(2):390–405.
6. Falkinham JO, Pruden A, Edwards M. Opportunistic premise plumbing pathogens: increasingly important pathogens in drinking water. Pathogens 2015; 4(2):373–86.
7. Falkinham JO 3rd, Hilborn ED, Arduino MJ, et al. Epidemiology and ecology of opportunistic premise plumbing pathogens: *Legionella pneumophila*, *Mycobacterium avium*, and *Pseudomonas aeruginosa*. Environ Health Perspect 2015; 123(8):749–58.
8. Anaissie EJ, Penzak SR, Dignani MC. The hospital water supply as a source of nosocomial infections: a plea for action. Arch Intern Med 2002;162(13):1483–92.
9. Bilinski P, Holownia P, Parafinska K, et al. Managing water safety in healthcare. Part 1—strategies and approaches for waterborne pathogen control. Ann Agric Environ Med 2012;19(3):395–402.
10. Bilinski P, Holownia P, Wojtyla C, et al. Managing water safety in healthcare. Part 2—practical measures and considerations taken for waterborne pathogen control. Ann Agric Environ Med 2012;19(4):619–24.
11. Decker BK, Palmore TN. Hospital water and opportunities for infection prevention. Curr Infect Dis Rep 2014;16(10):432.

12. Ferranti G, Marchesi I, Favale M, et al. Aetiology, source and prevention of waterborne healthcare-associated infections: a review. J Med Microbiol 2014; 63:1247–59.

13. Spagnolo AM, Orlando P, Perdelli F, et al. Hospital water and prevention of waterborne infections. Rev Med Microbiol 2016;27(1):25–32.

14. World Health Organization. Water safety in buildings. 2011. Available at: http://apps.who.int/iris/bitstream/10665/76145/1/9789241548106_eng.pdf. Accessed January 7, 2016.

15. Marchesi I, Cencetti S, Marchegiano P, et al. Control of *Legionella* contamination in a hospital water distribution system by monochloramine. Am J Infect Control 2012;40(3):279–81.

16. Marchesi I, Ferranti G, Bargellini A, et al. Monochloramine and chlorine dioxide for controlling *Legionella pneumophila* contamination: biocide levels and disinfection by-product formation in hospital water networks. J Water Health 2013; 11(4):738–47.

17. Krageschmidt DA, Kubly AF, Browning MS, et al. A comprehensive water management program for multicampus healthcare facilities. Infect Control Hosp Epidemiol 2014;35(5):556–63.

18. Demirjian A, Lucas CE, Garrison LE, et al. The importance of clinical surveillance in detecting legionnaires' disease outbreaks: a large outbreak in a hospital with a *Legionella* disinfection system—Pennsylvania, 2011–2012. Clin Infect Dis 2015;60(11):1596–602.

19. Sehulster L, Chinn RYW. Guidelines for environmental infection control in healthcare facilities. Recommendations of CDC and the Healthcare Infection Control Practices Advisory Committee (HICPAC). MMWR Morb Mortal Wkly Rep 2003; 52(RR10):1–42.

20. American Society of Heating, Refrigerating and Air-conditioning Engineers, Inc. (ASHRAE). Guideline 12–2000. Minimizing the risk of legionellosis associated with building water systems. 2000.

21. Health Protection Surveillance Centre. National Guidelines for the Control of Legionellosis in Ireland, 2009. Report of Legionnaires' Disease Subcommittee of the Scientific Advisory Committee. 2009. Available at: https://www.hpsc.ie/A-Z/Respiratory/Legionellosis/Publications/File,3936,en.pdf. Accessed January 16, 2016.

22. ASHRAE. ANSI/ASHRAE Standard 188-2015. Legionellosis: risk management for building water systems. 2015.

23. Veterans Health Administration (VHA). Prevention of healthcare-associated *Legionella* disease and scald injury from potable water distribution system. Washington, DC: VHA directive 1061; 2014. Available at: http://www.va.gov/vhapublications/ViewPublication.asp?pub_ID=3033. Accessed January 8, 2016.

24. Kool JL, Bergmire-Sweat D, Butler JC, et al. Hospital characteristics associated with colonization of water systems by *Legionella* and risk of nosocomial legionnaires' disease: a cohort study of 15 hospitals. Infect Control Hosp Epidemiol 1999;20(12):798–805.

25. Lin YE, Stout JE, Yu VL. Controlling *Legionella* in hospital drinking water: an evidence-based review of disinfection methods. Infect Control Hosp Epidemiol 2011;32(2):166–73.

26. Zhang Z, McCann C, Hanrahan J, et al. *Legionella* control by chlorine dioxide in hospital water systems. J Am Water Works Assoc 2009;101(5):117–27.

27. Casini B, Buzzigoli A, Cristina ML, et al. Long-term effects of hospital water network disinfection on *Legionella* and other waterborne bacteria in an Italian university hospital. Infect Control Hosp Epidemiol 2014;35(3):293–9.

28. Stout JE, Yu VL. Experiences of the first 16 hospitals using copper-silver ionization for *Legionella* control: implications for evaluation of other disinfection modalities. Infect Control Hosp Epidemiol 2003;24(8):563–8.

29. Alary M, Joly JR. Factors contributing to the contamination of hospital water distribution systems by legionellae. J Infect Dis 1992;165:565–9.

30. Hartley D, McCarthy A, Greenwood JE. Water temperature from hot water outlets in a major public hospital: how hot is our water? Eplasty 2011;11:e49.

31. Makin T, Tench K. Examining "risks" of overspecifying TMVs. Health Estate 2014; 68(5):39–44.

32. Armstrong C. Preventing scalding/controlling *Legionella*. Health Estate 2015; 69(5):53–9.

33. Mermel LA, Josephson SL, Giorgio CH, et al. Association of legionnaires' disease with construction: contamination of potable water? Infect Control Hosp Epidemiol 1995;16(2):76–81.

34. Health Canada, Centre for Infectious Disease Prevention and Control. Construction-related nosocomial infections in patients in health care facilities: decreasing the risk of aspergillus, *Legionella* and other infections. Can Commun Dis Rep 2001;27(Suppl 2). i–x, 1–42, i–x, 1–46.

35. National Institute for Occupational Safety and Health. Preventing occupational respiratory disease from exposure caused by dampness in office buildings, schools and other nonindustrial buildings. Cincinnati (OH): DHHS (NIOSH); 2012. Publication no. 2013-102. Available at: http://www.cdc.gov/niosh/docs/2013-102/pdfs/2013-102.pdf. Accessed January 12, 2016.

36. Palmore TN, Stock F, White M, et al. A cluster of cases of nosocomial legionnaires disease linked to a contaminated hospital decorative water fountain. Infect Control Hosp Epidemiol 2009;30(8):764–8.

37. Haupt TE, Heffernan RT, Kazmierczak JJ, et al. An outbreak of legionnaires disease associated with a decorative water wall fountain in a hospital. Infect Control Hosp Epidemiol 2012;33(2):185–91.

38. Cooling Technology Institute. Legionellosis. Guideline: best practices for control of *Legionella*. 2008. Available at: http://www.cti.org/downloads/WTP-148.pdf. Accessed July 3, 2015.

39. Quinn C, Demirjian A, Watkins LF, et al. Legionnaires' disease outbreak at a long-term care facility caused by a cooling tower using an automated disinfection system – Ohio, 2013. J Environ Health 2015;78(5):8–13.

40. Sydnor ER, Bova G, Gimburg A, et al. Electronic-eye faucets: *Legionella* species contamination in healthcare settings. Infect Control Hosp Epidemiol 2012; 33(3):235–40.

41. CDC and American Water Works Association. Emergency water supply planning guide for hospitals and health care facilities. Atlanta (GA): US Department of Health and Human Services; 2012. Available at: http://www.cdc.gov/healthywater/pdf/emergency/emergency-water-supply-planning-guide.pdf. Accessed January 11, 2016.

42. Klevens RM, Edwards JR, Richards CL, et al. Estimating health care-associated infections and deaths in U.S. Hospitals, 2002. Public Health Rep 2007;122(2): 160–6.

43. Cervia JS, Farber B, Armellino D, et al. Point-of-use water filtration reduces healthcare-associated infections in bone marrow transplant recipients. Transpl Infect Dis 2010;12:238–41.

44. Adams D, Fullerton K, Sharp P, et al. Summary of notifiable infectious diseases and conditions – United States, 2013. MMWR Morb Mortal Wkly Rep 2015; 62(53):1–119.

45. Seenivasan M, Yu VL, Muder RR. Legionnaires' disease in long-term care facilities: overview and proposed solutions. J Am Geriatr Soc 2005;53(5):875–80.

46. Yu VL, Stout JE. Legionellosis in nursing homes and long-term care facilities: what the Slovenian experience can teach us. Scand J Infect Dis 2012;44(9): 716–9.

47. Barker KA, Whitney EA, Blake S, et al. A review of guidelines for the primary prevention of legionellosis in long-term care facilities. J Am Med Dir Assoc 2015; 16(10):832–6.

48. Parr A, Whitney EA, Berkelman RL. Legionellosis on the rise: a review of guidelines for prevention in the United States. J Public Health Manag Pract 2015; 21(5):E17–26.

49. Tablan OC, Anderson LJ, Besser R, et al. Guidelines for preventing health-care–associated pneumonia. Recommendations of CDC and the Healthcare Infection Control Practices Advisory Committee. MMWR Morb Mortal Wkly Rep 2004; 53(RR03):1–36.

50. American Thoracic Society and Infectious Diseases Society of America. Guidelines for the management of adults with hospital-acquired, ventilator-associated, and healthcare-associated pneumonia. Am J Respir Crit Care Med 2005;171(4): 388–416.

51. Mandell LA, Wunderink RG, Anzueto A, et al. Infectious Diseases Society of America/American Thoracic Society consensus guidelines on the management of community-acquired pneumonia in adults. Clin Infect Dis 2007;44(Suppl 2): S27–72.

52. Hollenbeck B, Dupont I, Mermel LA. How often is a work-up for *Legionella* pursued in patients with pneumonia? A retrospective study. BMC Infect Dis 2011; 11:237.

53. CDC. Legionellosis case report form. CDC document 52.56(E), OMB No. 0920–0728. 2014. Available at: http://www.cdc.gov/Legionella/downloads/case-report-form.pdf. Accessed September 10, 2015.

54. Goetz AM, Stout JE, Jacobs SL, et al. Nosocomial legionnaires' disease discovered in community hospitals following cultures of the water system: seek and ye shall find. Am J Infect Control 1998;26:6–11.

55. Perola O, Kauppinen J, Kusnetsov J, et al. Nosocomial *Legionella pneumophila* serogroup 5 outbreak associated with persistent colonization of a hospital water system. APMIS 2002;110(12):863–8.

56. Scaturro M, Dell'Eva I, Helfer F, et al. Persistence of the same strain of *Legionella pneumophila* in the water system of an Italian hospital for 15 years. Infect Control Hosp Epidemiol 2007;28:1089–92.

57. Lin YE, Vidic RD, Stout JE, et al. *Legionella* in water distribution systems. J Am Water Works Assoc 1998;90(9):112–22.

58. Stout JE, Muder RR, Mietzner S, et al. Role of environmental surveillance in determining the risk of hospital-acquired legionellosis: a national surveillance study with clinical considerations. Infect Control Hosp Epidemiol 2007;28(7): 818–24.

59. Lucas CE, Taylor TH Jr, Fields BS. Accuracy and precision of *Legionella* isolation by US laboratories in the ELITE program pilot study. Water Res 2011; 45(15):4428–36.

60. Garrison LE, Lucas CE, Demirjian A, et al. Reply to Gamage, et al. Clin Infect Dis 2015;61(9):1488.

61. Occupational Safety & Health Administration (OSHA). OSHA Technical manual, section III: Chapter 7. Legionnaire's disease. January 20, 1999.5.

62. Squier CL, Stout JE, Krsytofiak S, et al. A proactive approach to prevention of health care-acquired legionnaires' disease: the Allegheny County (Pittsburgh) experience. Am J Infect Control 2005;33(6):360–7.

63. Dyck A, Exner M, Kramer A. Experimental based experiences with the introduction of a water safety plan for a multi-located university clinic and its efficacy according to WHO recommendations. BMC Public Health 2007;7:34.

64. Gamage SD, Kralovic SM, Roselle GA. The case for routine environmental testing for *Legionella* bacteria in healthcare facility water distribution systems-reconciling CDC position and guidance regarding risk. Clin Infect Dis 2015; 61(9):1487–8.

65. Prodinger WM, Bonatti H, Allerberger F, et al. *Legionella* pneumonia in transplant recipients: a cluster of cases of eight years' duration. J Hosp Infect 1994;26(3):191–202.

66. Kool JL, Fiore AE, Kioski CM, et al. More than 10 years of unrecognized nosocomial transmission of legionnaires' disease among transplant patients. Infect Control Hosp Epidemiol 1998;19(12):898–904.

67. Lepine LA, Jernigan DB, Butler JC, et al. A recurrent outbreak of nosocomial legionnaires' disease detected by urinary antigen testing: evidence for long-term colonization of a hospital plumbing system. Infect Control Hosp Epidemiol 1998; 19(12):905–10.

68. Guyot A, Turton JF, Garner D. Outbreak of *Stenotrophomonas maltophilia* on an intensive care unit. J Hosp Infect 2013;85(4):303–7.

69. Alfieri N, Ramotar K, Armstrong P, et al. Two consecutive outbreaks of *Stenotrophomonas maltophilia* (*Xanthomonas maltophilia*) in an intensive-care unit defined by restriction fragment-length polymorphism typing. Infect Control Hosp Epidemiol 1999;20(8):553–6.

70. The Joint Commission. Environment of care standard. EC.02.05.01. E-edition, 2016.

71. CDC. Keeping cool under pressure: NYC legionnaires' disease outbreak, summer 2015. Public Health Matters Blog. 2015. Available at: http://blogs.cdc.gov/publichealthmatters/2015/09/keeping-cool-under-pressure-nyc-legionnaires-disease-outbreak-summer-2015/. Accessed January 16, 2016.

72. Illinois Department of Public Health. Legionnaires' disease outbreak at Illinois veterans' home – Quincy update. 2015. Available at: http://dph.illinois.gov/news/legionnaires%E2%80%99-disease-outbreak-illinois-veterans%E2%80%99-home-quincy-update. Accessed 1/16/2016.

73. Pruden A, Edwards MA, Falkinham JO. State of the science and research needs for opportunistic pathogens in premise plumbing. Denver (CO): Water Research Foundation; 2013. Available at: http://www.waterrf.org/PublicReportLibrary/4379.pdf. Accessed December 17, 2015.

74. Schlech WF, Simonsen N, Sumarah R, et al. Nosocomial outbreak of *Pseudomonas aeruginosa* folliculitis associated with a physiotherapy pool. CMAJ 1986;134(8):909–13.

75. Graman PS, Quinlan GA, Rank JA. Nosocomial legionellosis traced to a contaminated ice machine. Infect Control Hosp Epidemiol 1997;18(9):637–40.
76. Bencini MA, Yzerman EPF, Koornstra RHT, et al. A case of legionnaires' disease caused by aspiration of ice water. Arch Environ Occup Health 2005;60(6): 302–6.
77. Sánchez-Carrillo C, Padilla B, Marin M, et al. Contaminated feeding bottles: The sources of an outbreak of *Pseudomonas aeruginosa* infections in a neonatal intensive care unit. Am J Infect Control 2009;37:150–4.
78. Association for the Advancement of Medical Instrumentation. Dialysate for hemodialysis. ANSI/AAMI RD52:2004.
79. Lowry PW, Beck-Sague CM, Bland LA, et al. *Mycobacterium chelonae* infection among patients receiving high-flux dialysis in a hemodialysis clinic in California. J Infect Dis 1990;161(1):85–90.
80. World Health Organization (WHO). WHO good manufacturing practices: water for pharmaceutical use. WHO Technical Report Series, No. 970. 2012. Annex 2. Available at: http://apps.who.int/medicinedocs/documents/s19832en/s19832en.pdf. Accessed January 14, 2016.
81. Nucci M, Akiti T, Barreiros G, et al. Nosocomial outbreak of *Exophiala jeanselmei* fungemia associated with contamination of hospital water. Clin Infect Dis 2002; 34(11):1475–80.
82. Ricci ML, Fontana S, Pinci F, et al. Pneumonia associated with a dental unit waterline. Lancet 2012;379:684.
83. Centers for Disease Control and Prevention. Guidelines for infection control in dental health-care settings—2003. MMWR Morb Mortal Wkly Rep 2003; 52(RR-17):1–61. Available at: http://www.cdc.gov/mmwr/preview/mmwrhtml/rr5217a1.htm.
84. Cobben NA, Drent M, Jonkers M, et al. Outbreak of severe *Pseudomonas aeruginosa* respiratory infections due to contaminated nebulizers. J Hosp Infect 1996;33:63–70.
85. Sax H, Bloemberg G, Hasse B, et al. Prolonged outbreak of *Mycobacterium chimaera* infection after open-chest heart surgery. Clin Infect Dis 2015;61(1): 67–75.
86. US Food and Drug Administration. Nontuberculous mycobacterium infections associated with heater-cooler devices: FDA safety communication. Available at: http://www.fda.gov/MedicalDevices/Safety/AlertsandNotices/ucm466963.htm. Accessed October 15, 2015.
87. Centers for Disease Control and Prevention. Final 2014 reports of nationally notifiable infectious diseases. MMWR Morb Mortal Wkly Rep 2015;64(36):1019–33. Available at:http://www.cdc.gov/mmwr/preview/mmwrhtml/mm6436a8.htm?s_cid=mm6436a8_w.
88. Marston BJ, Plouffe JF, File TM Jr, et al. Incidence of community-acquired pneumonia requiring hospitalization. Results of a population-based active surveillance study in Ohio. The Community-Based Pneumonia Incidence Study Group. Arch Intern Med 1997;157(15):1709–18.
89. Cunha BA, Burillo A, Bouza E. Legionnaires' disease. Lancet 2015;387(10016): 376–8.
90. Strollo SE, Adjemian J, Adjemian MK, et al. The burden of pulmonary nontuberculous mycobacterial disease in the United States. Ann Am Thorac Soc 2015; 12(10):1458–64.

91. Jeffries JMC, Cooper T, Yam T, et al. *Pseudomonas aeruginosa* outbreaks in the neonatal intensive care unit – a systematic review of risk factors and environmental sources. J Med Microbiol 2012;61:1052–61.

92. Hunter PR. National disease burden due to waterborne transmission of nosocomial pathogens is substantially overestimated. Arch Intern Med 2003;163(16):1974.

93. Sievert DM, Ricks P, Edwards JR, et al. Antimicrobial-resistant pathogens associated with healthcare-associated infections: summary of data reported to the National Health Safety Network at the Centers for Disease Control and Prevention, 2009-2010. Infect Control Hosp Epidemiol 2013;34(1):1–14.

94. Karumanthil DP, Yin HB, Kollanoor-Johny A, et al. Effect of chlorine exposure on the survival and antibiotic gene expression of multidrug resistant *Acinetobacter baumannii* in water. Int J Environ Res Public Health 2014;11(2):1844–54.

95. Centers for Disease Control and Prevention. Antibiotic resistance threats in the United States, 2013. Available at: http://www.cdc.gov/drugresistance/threat-report-2013/pdf/ar-threats-2013-508.pdf. Accessed January 18, 2016.

96. Edelstein PH, Nakahama C, Tobin JO, et al. Paleoepidemiologic investigation of legionnaires disease at Wadsworth Veterans Administration hospital by using three typing methods for comparison of legionellae from clinical and environmental sources. J Clin Microbiol 1986;23(6):1121–6.

97. Kioski C, Cage G, Johnson B, et al. Sustained transmission of nosocomial legionnaires disease – Arizona and Ohio. MMWR Morb Mortal Wkly Rep 1997;46(19):416–21.

98. Stout JE, Brennen C, Muder RR. Legionnaires' disease in a newly constructed long-term care facility. J Am Geriatr Soc 2000;48(12):1589–92.

99. Silk BJ, Moore MR, Bergtholdt M, et al. Eight years of legionnaires' disease transmission in travelers to a condominium complex in Las Vegas, Nevada. Epidemiol Infect 2012;140:1993–2002.

100. Goeller D, Blythe D, Davenport M, et al. Legionnaires disease associated with potable water in a hotel – Ocean City, Maryland, October 2003–February 2004. MMWR Morb Mortal Wkly Rep 2005;54(07):165–8.

101. Bartley PB, Ben Zakour NL, Stanton-Cook M, et al. Hospital-wide eradiation of a nosocomial *Legionella pneumophila* serogroup 1 outbreak. Clin Infect Dis 2016;62(3):273–9.

# Prevention by Design

## Construction and Renovation of Health Care Facilities for Patient Safety and Infection Prevention

Russell N. Olmsted, MPH, CIC

### KEYWORDS

- Construction • Health care facilities • Risk assessment
- Waterborne and airborne pathogen • Health care design • Ventilation • Water quality
- Operating room design

### KEY POINTS

- Outbreaks of disease are associated with construction and renovation when planning and risk mitigation are ignored or not effective.
- The infection control risk assessment (ICRA) and mitigation recommendations are essential components of infection prevention and patient safety programs.
- Infection preventionists/health care epidemiologists should be aware of and have access to the guidelines for design and construction of health care facilities developed by the Facility Guidelines Institute as well as other applicable requirements enforced by the authority having jurisdiction that applies to their local affiliates.
- Infection preventionists/health care epidemiologists can inform and proactively assist multidisciplinary teams involved in construction and renovation but this needs to be part of the project as early as possible in its inception to ensure the protection of patients, personnel, and visitors.
- Policies and procedures that address ICRA, safe work practices, training, monitoring, contingencies, and authority should be established and made operational.

In Jules Verne's[1] 1879 novel, "The Begum's Millions" ("Les Cinq Cents Millions de la Bégum" in French), one of the main characters, Dr Sarrasin, inherits a large fortune and sets out to create a utopian model city. He desires that this new city address unsanitary conditions evident in his native country, France. Of note, his designs include a preference that health care is delivered in the home. Recognizing that an acute care hospital would still be needed, he specified that this be limited to 20 to 30 beds per

Clinical Intelligence, Unified Clinical Organization, Trinity Health, Mailstop W3B, 20555 Victor Parkway, Livonia, MI 48152, USA
E-mail address: olmstedr@trinity-health.org

Infect Dis Clin N Am 30 (2016) 713–728
http://dx.doi.org/10.1016/j.idc.2016.04.005
0891-5520/16/$ – see front matter © 2016 Elsevier Inc. All rights reserved.

ward but that each room be a single-patient room with attached bathroom. In addition, the structure was to be disposable (meaning made of pinewood) with no carpet or wallpaper and incinerated at the end of the year of use. This article shows that Verne was prescient in that many of these design elements, except for the disposable nature of the built environment, have been incorporated into contemporary guidelines.

## INTRODUCTION

The built environment encompasses a broad range of physical design elements, including spaces for care of patients, support services, electronics, and major technical equipment; building systems that provide air and water; and surfaces and finishes. This spectrum of spaces and surfaces collectively is referred as the environment of care (EOC). In general, these are less frequently a source of microorganisms causing health care–associated infection (HAI) compared with other sources, such as the patient's endogenous microflora, especially when an invasive device is present, or a surgical procedure.[2] Carriage of microbes on hands of health care personnel (HCP) also is a more likely mechanism of exposure to potential pathogens. Even so, the proportional contribution of the EOC as a reservoir of pathogens is estimated at 20%.[3] Over the past several years there have been several studies showing that the EOC is a significant source of multidrug-resistant organisms (MDROs), *Clostridium difficile*, and norovirus.[4] In addition, investigation of the role of the EOC has found that admission to a patient room previously occupied by a patient with an MDRO or *C difficile* is a risk factor for their acquisition by the next occupant.[5]

Specific pathogens can suggest an environmental source; for example, from demolition of drywall or gaps in maintenance of key mechanical systems, which include *Aspergillus* spp, *Fusarium* spp, *Rhizopus* spp, *Bacillus cereus*, *Legionella* spp, a wide range of gram-negative bacteria, and nontuberculous mycobacteria.[2] When HAIs are caused by opportunistic pathogens it is important to apply key principles such as chain of transmission and the following criteria to determine whether reservoirs are present in the environment and to help guide implementation of mitigation strategies, if applicable.

## CRITERIA FOR EVALUATING THE STRENGTH OF EVIDENCE FOR ENVIRONMENTAL SOURCES OF INFECTION

1. The organism can survive after inoculation onto the fomite.[2]
2. The organism can be cultured from in-use fomites.
3. The organism can proliferate in or on the fomite.
4. Some measure of acquisition of infection cannot be explained by other recognized modes of transmission.
5. Retrospective case-control studies show an association between exposure to the fomite and infection.
6. Prospective case-control studies may be possible when more than 1 similar type of fomite is in use.
7. Prospective studies allocating exposure to the fomite to a subset of patients show an association between exposure and infection.
8. Decontamination of the fomite results in the elimination of infection transmission.

Annual spend on construction or renovation of health care facilities is approximately $40 billion.[6] Because cost of construction per square meter ranges from $4300 to $12,920, there has been some modulation in the build of larger inpatient rooms.[7] A large proportion of current construction projects therefore involve a shift toward construction of outpatient facilities. A recent survey of providers found that the types of outpatient projects include ambulatory surgery centers (48%), freestanding imaging (23%), health system–branded clinics in retail space (23%), health system–branded general medicine and family care in the community (53%), immediate care facilities (49%), medical office buildings (60%), and telehealth (23%).[7] This finding reflects the general direction toward home-based and ambulatory-based care delivery with an emphasis on population health and value-based purchasing.

Disturbance of the EOC, especially from construction, renovation, or remediation, can result in exposure of patients and personnel to microorganisms present in air, water, or on surfaces. Other maintenance activities, such as repair and remediation work (eg, installing wiring for new information systems, removing old sinks, and repairing elevator shafts) can also disrupt and release contaminants. Aging equipment, deferred maintenance, and natural disasters provide additional mechanisms for the entry of environmental pathogens into high-risk patient-care areas.

To mitigate contamination of patient-care areas several infection preventionists developed the use of infection control risk assessment (ICRA).[8] ICRA is a process that begins during planning and design of construction and renovation to ensure that elements of infection prevention are incorporated into the project. It includes strategies such as physical barriers to contain and confine dust, soil, and contaminants (eg, fungal spores) that may be released into the air during demolition, once construction begins. Use of an ICRA has been incorporated into design standards as well as Healthcare Infection Control Practices Advisory Committee guidelines that address construction and renovation.

## OVERVIEW OF DISEASE TRANSMISSION RISKS FROM THE BUILT ENVIRONMENT
### Air as a Reservoir of Health Care–associated Infections

Although the percentage of HAIs directly related to construction is unknown, the morbidity, mortality, and costs of mitigation of these preventable infections are considerable. The mechanism of exposure of patients to airborne pathogens during construction is often from disturbance of building materials or surfaces that have been contaminated; for example, intrusion of water onto drywall substrate where fungal spores are present. Demolition of these substrates releases bursts of spores into the air and, if not contained and removed, can result in exposure of occupants.

Vonberg and Gastmeier[9] reviewed outbreaks of infection caused by *Aspergillus* spp and found that almost half were associated with construction or renovation in hospitals. In addition, they identified that the infective dose of invasive pulmonary aspergillosis in immunocompromised patients can be as low as 1 colony forming unit/$m^3$. This finding highlights the critical need for isolation and containment of construction activities from other occupied spaces.

Patient populations at increased risk of fungal infection and that are exposed to contaminated airborne spores include those undergoing hematopoietic stem cell or solid organ transplant, undergoing chemotherapy for conditions such as leukemia, in receipt of high-dose steroid therapy, the critically ill, neonates, those undergoing cardiac surgery, and those with chronic lung disease.

Kanamori and colleagues[10] recently reevaluated disease outbreaks from airborne fungal spores associated with construction. They found it encouraging that since 2010 there have been fewer reports of outbreaks. Although not necessarily a direct causal relationship, this points to the efficacy of ICRA in mitigating transmission and protecting patients, personnel, and visitors in facilities that have ongoing construction or renovation. Their search of the literature found 28 construction-associated outbreaks between 1976 and 2014, *Aspergillus* spp being the most common pathogen, and a predominance of pulmonary infection with attributable mortality approaching 60%.

### Water as a Reservoir of Health Care–associated Infections

The spectrum of microorganisms present in water is broad and includes gram-negative bacteria (eg, legionellae and *Pseudomonas* spp), nontuberculous mycobacteria, protozoa, and fungi.[2] Potable water provided by municipal water authorities must meet federal standards for drinking water and these are enforced by the US Environmental Protection Agency.[11] Water supplied to the health care facility is then distributed through an extensive network of plumbing to fixtures such as handwashing stations, ice machines, medical equipment (eg, automated endoscope reprocessors), and utility systems. This distribution network readily supports development of biofilm, and the microbial contaminants embedded in this matrix of extracellular polymeric substances, mainly composed of exopolysaccharides, proteins, and nucleic acids, protects microorganisms from disinfectants that are otherwise effective against planktonic forms.[12] Stagnant water in this network, often from renovation of areas in the facility that has resulted in redundant lengths of pipework that are left in place and capped, also enhances development of biofilm. In addition, disruption of water utility systems during construction or renovation can disrupt biofilm and release contaminants into the water delivery network, posing a possible risk to patients, including those far away from the work area.

A recent, extensive review of waterborne disease outbreaks found that the more susceptible patient populations, such as the critically ill, neonates, transplant recipients, surgical patients, and those with hematological disease, are often the sentinel signal of a new cluster.[13] Of late the types of devices and architectural features that were a source of infections are growing in complexity. This article discusses these outbreak investigations and emphasizes the need to be vigilant for their detection and mitigation.

> …Waterborne healthcare-associated outbreaks and infections continue to occur and were mostly associated with well-recognized water reservoirs as previously described. Moreover, recent studies document electronic faucets (P. aeruginosa, Legionella, M. mucogenicum), decorative water wall fountains (Legionella), and heater-cooler devices used for cardiac surgery (M. chimaera) as water reservoirs…[13]

There are some landmark investigations of waterborne disease outbreaks worth highlighting because these investigations have informed guidelines for construction and renovation in the United States.

## HANDWASHING STATION DESIGN

Hand hygiene is the foundation of infection prevention and control. The 2 primary methods HCP use to clean their hands are alcohol-based hand rub (ABHR) or soap and water and a handwashing station. Hota and colleagues[14] reported an outbreak of *Pseudomonas aeruginosa* infections that, ironically, centered on handwashing stations in intensive care units (ICUs) and transplant units. The outbreak unit featured single-occupancy patient rooms with convenient access to a handwashing station near the entrance in each for use by HCP. Biofilm within the drains of these were identified as the source and the sink design included a shallow basin with the faucet spout directly over the drain. This arrangement resulted in splashes of water contaminated with *P aeruginosa* out of the drain contaminating surfaces near the sink, including a medication preparation area and the patient bed. Interventions to mitigate contamination from sinks included a physical barrier between the sink and adjacent countertops, offset of the faucet spout so it did not discharge directly into the drain, and lower water pressure. The lessons from this outbreak have been incorporated into guidelines published by the Facility Guidelines Institute (FGI).[15] Key design features in current FGI guidelines include:

- Basins that reduce the risk of splashing and are made of porcelain, stainless steel, or other solid surface material
- Basin size of no less than 929.08 cm$^2$ (144 square inches) with 22.86 cm$^2$ (9 square inches) width or length
- Sealed to prevent water intrusion into supporting cabinet, wall, and countertop
- Discharge of water from faucet spout is at least 25.4 cm (10 inches) above the bottom of the basin and avoids dropping directly into the drain
- Water pressure in station fixture is regulated
- Allows controls for sink fixture to be wrist blade, single lever, or sensor activated

**WATER FEATURE: NOT ALLOWED**

Decorative water features have been a popular element of design. However, there have been 2 recent outbreaks of legionnaires' disease associated with these. The first involved 2 patients with extended hospital stay preparing for stem cell transplant for treatment of leukemia.[16] Investigation identified a decorative water fountain as the source; of note, testing of water identified a diverse range of other microorganisms in addition to *Legionella pneumophila* serogroup 1. This fountain had been turned off for several months and the investigators commented that stagnation in the water circulation conduits likely promoted development of biofilm.

Haupt and colleagues[17] investigated a cluster of legionnaires' disease associated with a decorative water wall that was installed in a public corridor near the main entrance lobby of a community hospital. Eight cases were detected and the only common risk factor was visiting the hospital where this feature was in use; most patients simply walked through the lobby past the water wall. *L pneumophila* serogroup 1 was detected from the water in this fountain despite adherence with the manufacturer's instructions for cleaning and maintenance. This incident and other evidence has led the FGI to state that, "unsealed, open water features are not permitted."[15]

## Inpatient Rooms, Surfaces, and Finishes

The microbiome of the inpatient room has undergone renewed appreciation following a considerable body of evidence that finds significant risk of acquisition of pathogens such as MDROs or *C difficile* related to infection or colonization in the room's prior occupant, for as long as 3 weeks.[5] However, this contamination can be removed with attention and focus on thorough cleaning and disinfection of surfaces in rooms that are touched with high frequency, combined with real-time feedback.[18,19]

The evidence that MDROs can persist in the environment for a prolonged time, as described earlier, in combination with the observed efficiency of cross-transmission of these in multibed rooms, has led to a preference for single-patient rooms. This design also enhances safety related to a variety of other potential harms, supports patient privacy, and lessens disruption from ambient noise.[20] By contrast, the lack of spatial separation between patients in multibed rooms or wards has been associated with increased risk of respiratory viral infections and bacterial infection when patient with similar devices are in the same room.[21,22] Other investigators identified a temporal association between fewer bloodstream infections, detection of MDROs, and prevalence of antibiotic resistance with redesign of patient-care units from open wards to single-patient rooms.[23]

Studies of cross-transmission of microorganisms in health care facilities have identified that surfaces nearer to patients are more likely to be contaminated. Further, patients with acute infection, especially when symptoms result in contamination of the immediate environment with body fluids containing the pathogen (eg, diarrhea), result in higher microbial burden on environmental surfaces.[5] This finding is particularly true of norovirus, for which studies find that person-to-person transmission depends on close or direct contact as well as short-range aerosol exposures. Also, experience with control of outbreaks of norovirus highlight the need to clean and disinfect frequently touched surfaces (eg, patient and staff bathrooms, utility rooms, tables, chairs, commodes, computer keyboards and mice, and items in close proximity to symptomatic patients).[24]

## STRATEGIES AND DESIGN ELEMENTS TO SUPPORT INFECTION PREVENTION

The FGI guidelines serve as a foundational resource for the design of health care facilities.[15] They are used as a basis for regulation and a national standard in 42 states as well as being cited by the Joint Commission, the Department of Housing and Urban Development, and the Indian Health Service as normative, national standards. The guidelines are consensus-based and developed by the Health Guidelines Revision Committee and are updated every 4 years. The 2014 guidelines include 2 separate standards, one for hospitals and outpatients and the other for residential health, care, and support facilities. Importantly, they provide minimum design standards; not necessarily parameters that involve daily operations of facilities. Many of the elements discussed later are addressed in these guidelines and readers are referred to this resource for more details.

ICRA is the core framework of design and construction/renovation. It is a component of the overall safety risk assessment called for in the FGI 2014 guidelines. ICRA calls for design recommendations and infection control risk mitigation recommendations (ICRMR) that are applied to the construction project being planned. Key aspects that ICRA needs to address include:

- Design elements that support infection prevention and control
- Proactive planning for mitigating sources of infection both within and external to the construction project that will be affected
- Identify potential risk for transmission of airborne and waterborne pathogens during construction, renovation, and commissioning
- Develop ICRMRs to mitigate identified risks (see Appendix A for a stepwise approach to developing ICRMRs)

There is evidence that an effective ICRA process can prevent HAIs.[25] **Fig. 1** provides examples of effective containment methods.

### Select Elements of Design

#### Heating, ventilation, and air conditioning

Heating, ventilation, and air conditioning (HVAC) is a building system that is designed to provide comfort, support aseptic procedures, remove contaminants from air, and deliver an acceptable indoor air quality. FGI 2014 includes the American Society of Heating, Refrigerating, and Air-conditioning Engineers (ASHRAE) 170 Standard for design of HVAC for health care facilities. This standard provides a wide range of

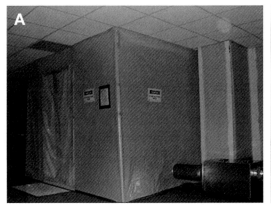
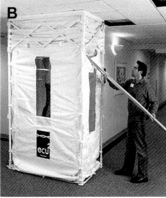
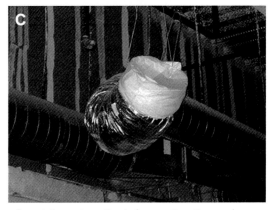

Fig. 1. Examples of containment methods for construction and renovation. (A) One hour, fire-rated, temporary containment wall. (B) Portable environmental containment unit. (C) Protection of new duct work with cover over open end.

parameters for HVAC systems that supply patient-care, procedural (eg, surgery suite), and support areas. Parameters included in ASHRAE 170 include air changes per hour, design temperature and relative humidity ranges, and pressure relationships to adjacent areas.[26]

*Universal or acuity-adaptable and single-occupancy patient-care rooms*
The FGI commissioned a systematic review of available evidence on the value of single-patient rooms[20] that found suggestive, albeit low-quality, evidence that this prevents infection and improves overall patient safety and experience of care. The addition of adaptability of these based on the patient's need also is worth considering. Additional elements for adult ICUs have been described elsewhere and support this need for flexibility to accommodate changes in care practices and advances in technology.[27]

*Airborne-infection isolation room*
Planning for airborne-infection isolation rooms (AIIRs) should be based on the local epidemiology and risk assessment for the prototype airborne disease, tuberculosis. Other diseases in which AIIRs are used include chickenpox and measles, and experience with these can also help inform on location and number of AIIRs for a facility planning team as part of ICRA. There are also procedures that increase the risk of transmission if performed on someone with active pulmonary tuberculosis (eg,

bronchoscopy), and these need to be considered when identifying the optimal number of AIIRs. More recently, emerging and remerging diseases, such as Ebola and Middle East respiratory syndrome coronavirus, have highlighted the need to plan and respond as appropriate, from frontline facilities that receive patients to regional and national emergency preparedness and response. Details of regional facilities designed for definitive treatment of patients with infections such as Ebola are described elsewhere.[28]

### Protective environment room

A protective environment (PE) room is designed to provide a filtered supply of high-efficiency particulate air (HEPA) to rooms used to care for patients who are severely immunocompromised (eg, solid organ transplant patients or allogeneic neutropenic patients). These rooms need to be designed to ensure that rooms are well sealed by maintaining ceilings that are smooth and free of fissures, open joints, and crevices; sealing walls above and below the ceiling; and, once occupied, to monitor for leakage. Additional details are available elsewhere.[2] Recommendations for quality processes to ensure protection of immunocompromised patients during construction have been published.[29]

### Handwashing stations and hand hygiene

Design features were identified earlier in the review of water as a reservoir. Reliable, readily available access to devices and products to use for hand hygiene is the foundation of infection prevention and control. The FGI guidelines include both handwashing stations and proactive planning for placement of dispensers of ABHR that are readily visible to HCP.

### Toilets and disposal of human waste

The move to single-patient rooms has resulted in most rooms having an attached bathroom/shower for use by the patient. For critically ill patients, the ability to use the bathroom is less likely; the exception might be a cardiac ICU. Swing-out or fold-down fixtures (Swivette toilets) should be avoided, because they are prone to mechanical problems and leakage, are difficult to use (especially for the acutely ill), and may not be rated for the bariatric patient population. Alternatives for the ICU population to manage human waste include body fluid disposal systems or plumbed, bedpan flushing/disinfection devices. If planned, it is important for these to be convenient for HCP because there are aesthetic and safety barriers to transport of human waste over long distance. Importantly, fixtures used for disposal of human waste should be limited to that purpose and not used for other activities, such as hand hygiene.

### Surfaces, finishes, and furnishings

The renewed attention on the inanimate environment as a source of pathogens has stimulated interest in strategies that can support infection prevention. There are several antimicrobial treatments that have been applied to inanimate surfaces; nonporous and soft surfaces such as textiles and privacy curtains. The types of antimicrobial treatments include photoreactive substances that release antimicrobials when exposed to natural sunlight, heavy metals like copper and silver, organosilane, triclosan, and quaternary ammonium compound. There is suggestive evidence that many of these can reduce the concentration of microorganisms on environmental surfaces.[30] Direct evidence that these treatments reduce the incidence of HAIs in which transmission from the inanimate EOC is involved is lacking. This lack of evidence reflects the complex environment in an acute care facility given the myriad of sources by which personnel can contaminate their hands (eg, shared equipment) so treating several surfaces in a room may still not be more effective than processes and real-time feedback to personnel who clean and disinfect the built environment. Guidance is available for some of the surfaces and finishes being planned for health care facilities. Highlights of these include[31]:

1. Nonupholstered surfaces should be capable of being easily cleaned; minimize surface joints and seams.
2. Upholstered surfaces used in patient-care areas should be impervious (nonporous); untreated (non–high performance) woven fabrics should not be used. Upholstered surfaces should be durable and resist tearing, peeling, cracking, or splitting; damaged surfaces are more difficult to clean effectively. Upholstered furniture in patient-care areas should be covered with fabrics that are fluid-resistant, nonporous, and can withstand cleaning with hospital-grade disinfectants.

*Floors, walls, and ceilings*
CDC guidelines have identified that, "…Compared to hard-surface flooring, carpeting is harder to keep clean, especially after spills of blood and body substances. It is also harder to push equipment with wheels (eg, wheelchairs, carts, and gurneys) on carpeting…"[2] There are several recommendations on carpeting in these guidelines but a key one is to avoid the use of carpeting in high-traffic zones in patient-care areas or where spills are likely (eg, burn therapy units, operating rooms, laboratories, and ICUs). Walls should be cleanable and able to withstand repeated exposure to chemical surface disinfectants. Ceilings in areas needing special HVAC requirements, such as AIIR, operating room, PE, and so forth, are an important aspect of ensuring that the room envelope is sealed to maintain desired pressurization and contain contaminants. For operating rooms, FGI 2014 guidelines call for a monolithic ceiling as a strategy to facilitate effective envelope seal.

## FUTURE DIRECTIONS FOR HEALTH CARE IN THE UNITED STATES

The FGI convened a futures summit to assist with development of upcoming editions of their guidelines. This summit identified the following trends and needs going forward, and awareness of these is important for infection preventionists and health care epidemiologists in applying relevant infection prevention strategies[32]:

*Trends*

- More health care provided at home
- More access to medical care in the community
- More specialized diagnosis and treatment facilities
- Hospitals provide only for the sickest or those with most complicated needs
- Navigators and health coaches provide assistance to patients, providers, and/or payers
- Increased use of technology for health care monitoring and communication
- Continued government involvement in regulating health care

*Informing Future Guidelines Development*

- Health care will increasingly be provided in outpatient facilities and residential care settings of numerous types.
- Acute care facilities will see slower growth and be focused on providing care to higher-acuity patients with more complex treatment and care needs.
- As a society, the United States needs to encourage development of high-value, high-engagement models of care; how the design of health care facilities can relate to this goal should be considered.

- A 4-year cycle for document development is not optimal for responding to the rapidly changing health care landscape.
- Documents focused on fundamental design requirements are important but do not address complex health care delivery needs. FGI also needs to facilitate development of best practice and alternative concept guidance for health care design.

## RESOURCES FOR DESIGNING IN INFECTION PREVENTION

Scientific studies that inform design of the EOC are challenging. Even so, Zimring and colleagues[33] called for the use of evidence-based design (EBD) to drive design and construction of health care facilities. The steps in the process of EBD include:

1. Framing of goals and models; most recently the emphasis is on patient-centered care
2. Incorporation of health care facility guidelines; for example, FGI
3. Planning and design
4. Operations: daily care delivery issues that may require variation from design parameters; for example, reducing the temperature in the operating room to address comfort of surgeons and perioperative personnel

Other resources are available to improve the effectiveness of the planning and design. These resources include a comprehensive safety risk assessment tool sponsored by the Agency for Healthcare Research and Quality and FGI.[34] Elements of this tool include ICRA, patient handling, medication safety, mitigating risk of patient falls, and security. A manual for incorporating infection prevention into construction projects is also available.[35]

## SUMMARY/DISCUSSION

Infection prevention and control is an essential component of the built environment. When absent or when there are disruptions, risk of exposure of patients and disease outbreaks often result. However, there are well-established, evidence-based guidelines to assist infection preventionists and health care epidemiologists with identifying strategies for prevention in collaboration with the multiple disciplines involved in construction and renovation (EIC 2003[2], FGI 2014[15]). The ICRA remains the keystone of designing in prevention at the inception of a project through the completion and commissioning phases. Future trends in care delivery in the United States are going to have a significant impact on construction and renovation of health care facilities; however, involvement and subject matter expertise provided by infection preventionists/health care epidemiologists will remain a core component into the future.

## REFERENCES

1. Grousset P, Verne J. The begum's fortune (extraordinary voyages #18). In: Evans AB, Luce SL, editors. Middletown (CT): Wesleyan University Press; 2005. p. 262.
2. Centers for Disease Control and Prevention (CDC). Guidelines for environmental infection control in health-care facilities: recommendations of CDC and the Healthcare Infection Control Practices Advisory Committee (HICPAC). MMWR 2003; 52 (No. RR-10): 1–48. Available at: http://www.cdc.gov/hicpac/pdf/guidelines/eic_in_HCF_03.pdf. Accessed January 2, 2016.
3. Weinstein RA. Epidemiology and control of nosocomial infections in adult intensive care units. Am J Med 1991;91(Suppl 3B):179S–84S.

4. Weber DJ, Rutala WA. Understanding and preventing transmission of healthcare-associated pathogens due to the contaminated hospital environment. Infect Control Hosp Epidemiol 2013;34:449–52.
5. Otter JA, Yezli S, Salkeld JA, et al. Evidence that contaminated surfaces contribute to the transmission of hospital pathogens and an overview of strategies to address contaminated surfaces in hospital settings. Am J Infect Control 2013;41(Suppl 5):S6–11.
6. US Department of Commerce. 2016 Construction at $1,140.8 billion annual rate. Available at: https://www.census.gov/construction/c30/pdf/release.pdf. Accessed February 1, 2016.
7. Vesely R, Hoppszallern S, Morgan J. Outpatient facility construction set to grow. Healthcare Facilities Management Magazine. Chicago: American Hospital Association; 2016. Available at: http://www.hfmmagazine.com/display/HFM-news-article.dhtml?dcrPath=/templatedata/HF_Common/NewsArticle/data/HFM/Magazine/2016/feb/hfm-survey-construction-outpatient. Accessed February 25, 2016.
8. Bartley JM. APIC state-of-the-art report: the role of infection control during construction in health care facilities. Am J Infect Control 2000;28:156–69.
9. Vonberg RP, Gastmeier P. Nosocomial aspergillosis in outbreak settings. J Hosp Infect 2006;63:246–54.
10. Kanamori H, Rutala WA, Sickbert-Bennett EE, et al. Review of fungal outbreaks and infection prevention in healthcare settings during construction and renovation. Clin Infect Dis 2015;61:433–44.
11. Environmental Protection Agency (EPA). 2016 U.S. drinking water contaminants – standards and regulations. Available at: https://www.epa.gov/dwstandardsregulations. Accessed January 7, 2016.
12. Walker J, Moore G. *Pseudomonas aeruginosa* in hospital water systems: biofilms, guidelines, and practicalities. J Hosp Infect 2015;89:324–7.
13. Kanamori H, Weber DJ, Rutala WA. Healthcare outbreaks associated with a water reservoir and infection prevention strategies. Clin Infect Dis 2016;62:1–3.
14. Hota S, Hirji Z, Stockton K, et al. Outbreak of multidrug-resistant *Pseudomonas aeruginosa* colonization and infection secondary to imperfect intensive care unit room design. Infect Control Hosp Epidemiol 2009;30:25–33.
15. Facility Guidelines Institute. Guidelines for design and construction of hospitals and outpatient facilities. Dallas (TX): Facility Guidelines Institute, published by the American Society for Healthcare Engineering. Chicago. Available at: http://www.fgiguidelines.org/. Accessed December 15, 2015.
16. Palmore TN, Stock F, White M, et al. A cluster of cases of nosocomial legionnaires disease linked to a contaminated hospital decorative water fountain. Infect Control Hosp Epidemiol 2009;30:764–8.
17. Haupt TE, Heffernan RT, Kazmierczak JJ, et al. An outbreak of legionnaires disease associated with a decorative water wall fountain in a hospital. Infect Control Hosp Epidemiol 2012;33(2):185–91.
18. Datta R, Platt R, Yokoe DS, et al. Environmental cleaning intervention and risk of acquiring multidrug-resistant organisms from prior room occupants. Arch Intern Med 2011;171:491–4.
19. Rupp ME, Fitzgerald T, Sholtz L, et al. Maintain the gain: program to sustain performance improvement in environmental cleaning. Infect Control Hosp Epidemiol 2014;35:866–8.
20. Chaudhury H, Mahmood A, Valente M. The use of single patient rooms versus multiple occupancy rooms in acute care environments. Coalition for Health

Environments Research (CHER). 2005. Available at: https://www.healthdesign.org/sites/default/files/use_of_single_patient_rooms_v_multiple_occ._rooms-acute_care.pdf. Accessed February 4, 2016.

21. Yu IT, Xie ZH, Tsoi KK, et al. Why did outbreaks of severe acute respiratory syndrome occur in some hospital wards but not in others? Clin Infect Dis 2007;44:1017–25.

22. Fryklund B, Haeggman S, Burman LG. Transmission of urinary bacterial strains between patients with indwelling catheters - nursing in the same room and in separate rooms compared. J Hosp Infect 1997;36:147–53.

23. Lazar L, Abukaf H, Sofer S, et al. Impact of conversion from an open ward design paediatric intensive care unit environment to all isolated rooms environment on incidence of bloodstream infections and antibiotic resistance in southern Israel (2000 to 2008). Anaesth Intensive Care 2015;43:34–41.

24. CDC. Guideline for the prevention and control of norovirus gastroenteritis outbreaks in healthcare settings. 2011. Available at: http://www.cdc.gov/hicpac/norovirus/002_norovirus-toc.html. Accessed December 14, 2015.

25. Goebes MD, Baron EJ, Mathews KL, et al. Effect of building construction on *Aspergillus* concentrations in a hospital. Infect Control Hosp Epidemiol 2008;29:462–4.

26. American Society of Heating, Refrigerating and Air-conditioning Engineers (ASHRAE). ANSI/ASHRAE/ASHE Standard 170–2013. Ventilation of health care facilities. Atlanta (GA): ASHRAE.

27. Thompson D, Hamilton K, Cadenhead CD, et al. Guidelines for intensive care unit design. Crit Care Med 2012;40:1586–600.

28. Smith PW, Boulter KC, Hewlett AL, et al. Planning and response to Ebola virus disease: an integrated approach. Am J Infect Control 2015;43:441–6.

29. Chang CC, Ananda-Rajah M, Belcastro A, et al. Consensus guidelines for implementation of quality processes to prevent invasive fungal disease and enhanced surveillance measures during hospital building works, 2014. Intern Med J 2014;44:1389–97.

30. Humphreys H. Self-disinfecting and microbiocide-impregnated surfaces and fabrics: what potential in interrupting the spread of healthcare-associated infection? Clin Infect Dis 2014;58:848–53.

31. Business and Institutional Furniture Manufacturers (BIFMA). Health care furniture design - guidelines for cleanability (BIFMA HCF 8.1–2014). Grand Rapids (MI): BIFMA; 2014. Available at: http://c.ymcdn.com/sites/www.bifma.org/resource/resmgr/standards/BIFMA_CleanGuide_6Oct14.pdf?hhSearchTerms=%228+and+1-2014%22. Accessed December 15, 2015.

32. FGI. The future of health care as predicted using scenario planning. 2015. Available at: http://www.fgiguidelines.org/resource/the-future-of-health-care-as-predicted-using-scenario-planning/. Accessed January 6, 2016.

33. Zimring C, Denham ME, Jacob JT, et al. Evidence-based design of healthcare facilities: opportunities for research and practice in infection prevention. Infect Control Hosp Epidemiol 2013;34:514–6.

34. Center for Health Design. Safety risk assessment for healthcare facility environments. Available at: https://www.healthdesign.org/insights-solutions/safety-risk-assessment-toolkit-pdf-version. Accessed February 4, 2016.

35. Vogel R. Infection prevention manual for construction and renovation. Washington, DC: Association for Professionals in Infection Control & Epidemiology; 2015.

**APPENDIX A: STEPWISE PROCESS FOR INFECTION CONTROL RISK MITIGATION RECOMMENDATIONS FOR CONSTRUCTION AND RENOVATION**

Step 1: using the following table, identify the type of construction project activity (types A–D)

| | |
|---|---|
| Type A | Inspection and noninvasive activities<br>Includes but is not limited to:<br>• Removal of ceiling tiles for visual inspection only; eg, limited to 1 tile per 4.6 m² (50 square feet)<br>• Painting (but not sanding)<br>• Wallcovering, electrical trim work, minor plumbing, and activities that do not generate dust or require cutting of walls or access to ceilings other than for visual inspection |
| Type B | Small-scale, short-duration activities that create minimal dust<br>Includes but is not limited to:<br>• Installation of telephone and computer cabling<br>• Access to chase spaces<br>• Cutting of walls or ceiling where dust migration can be controlled |
| Type C | Work that generates a moderate to high level of dust or requires demolition or removal of any fixed building components or assemblies<br>Includes but is not limited to:<br>• Sanding of walls for painting or wall covering<br>• Removal of floorcoverings, ceiling tiles, and casework<br>• New wall construction<br>• Minor duct work or electrical work above ceilings<br>• Major cabling activities<br>• Any activity that cannot be completed within a single work shift |
| Type D | Major demolition and construction projects<br>Includes but is not limited to:<br>• Activities that require consecutive work shifts<br>• Requires heavy demolition or removal of a complete cabling system<br>• New construction |

Step 2: using the following table, identify the patient risk groups that will be affected. If more than 1 risk group will be affected, select the higher risk group:

| Low Risk | Medium Risk | High Risk | Highest Risk |
|---|---|---|---|
| Office areas | • Cardiology<br>• Echocardiography<br>• Endoscopy<br>• Nuclear medicine<br>• Physical therapy<br>• Radiology/MRI<br>• Respiratory therapy | • Cardiac care unit<br>• Emergency room<br>• Labor and delivery<br>• Laboratories (specimen)<br>• Medical units<br>• Newborn nursery<br>• Outpatient surgery<br>• Pediatrics<br>• Pharmacy<br>• Postanesthesia care unit<br>• Surgical units | • Any area caring for immunocompromised patients<br>• Burn unit<br>• Cardiac catheterization laboratory<br>• Central sterile supply<br>• ICUs<br>• Negative pressure isolation rooms<br>• Oncology<br>• Operating rooms, including cesarean section rooms |

Step 3: match the:

- Patient risk group (low, medium, high, highest) with the planned:
- Construction project type (A, B, C, D) on the following matrix, to find the:
- Class of precautions (I, II, III, or IV) or level of infection control activities required.
- Class I to IV or color-coded precautions are delineated later.

Infection control matrix for class of precautions: construction project by patient risk

| Patient Risk Group | Construction Project Type | | | |
|---|---|---|---|---|
| | TYPE A | TYPE B | TYPE C | TYPE D |
| Low-risk group | I | II | II | III/IV |
| Medium-risk group | I | II | III | IV |
| High-risk group | I | II | III/IV | IV |
| Highest-risk group | II | III/IV | III/IV | IV |

Note: infection control approval is required when the construction activity and risk level indicate that class III or class IV control procedures are necessary.

## Description of required infection control precautions by class

| | During Construction Project | Upon Completion of Project |
|---|---|---|
| Class I | 1. Execute work by methods to minimize raising dust from construction operations<br>2. Immediately replace a ceiling tile displaced for visual inspection | 1. Clean work area upon completion of task |
| Class II | 1. Provide active means to prevent airborne dust from dispersing into atmosphere<br>2. Water mist work surfaces to control dust while cutting<br>3. Seal unused doors with duct tape<br>4. Block off and seal air vents<br>5. Place dust mat at entrance and exit of work area<br>6. Remove or isolate HVAC system in areas where work is being performed | 1. Wipe work surfaces with cleaner/disinfectant<br>2. Contain construction waste before transport in tightly covered containers<br>3. Wet mop and/or vacuum with HEPA filtered vacuum before leaving work area<br>4. Upon completion, restore HVAC system where work was performed |
| Class III | 1. Remove or isolate HVAC system in area where work is being done to prevent contamination of duct system<br>2. Complete all critical barriers (ie, sheetrock, plywood, plastic) to seal area from nonwork area or implement control cube method (cart with plastic covering and sealed connection to work site with HEPA vacuum for vacuuming prior to exit) before construction begins | 1. Do not remove barriers from work area until completed project is inspected by the owner's safety department and infection prevention and control department and thoroughly cleaned by the owner's environmental services department<br>2. Remove barrier materials carefully to minimize spreading of dirt and debris associated with construction<br>3. Vacuum work area with HEPA filtered vacuums |

(continued on next page)

**(continued)**

| During Construction Project | Upon Completion of Project |
|---|---|
| 3. Maintain negative air pressure within work site utilizing HEPA-equipped air filtration units<br>4. Contain construction waste before transport in tightly covered containers<br>5. Cover transport receptacles or carts. Tape covering unless solid lid | 4. Wet mop area with cleaner/disinfectant<br>5. Upon completion, restore HVAC system where work was performed |
| Class IV 1. Isolate HVAC system in area where work is being done to prevent contamination of duct system<br>2. Complete all critical barriers (ie, sheetrock, plywood, plastic) to seal area from nonwork area or implement control cube method (cart with plastic covering and sealed connection to work site with HEPA vacuum for vacuuming prior to exit) before construction begins<br>3. Maintain negative air pressure within work site using HEPA-equipped air filtration units<br>4. Seal holes, pipes, conduits, and punctures<br>5. Construct anteroom and require all personnel to pass through this room so they can be vacuumed using an HEPA vacuum cleaner before leaving work site, or they can wear cloth or paper coveralls that are removed each time they leave work site<br>6. All personnel entering work site are required to wear shoe covers. Shoe covers must be changed each time the worker exits the work area | 1. Do not remove barriers from work area until completed project is inspected by the owner's safety department and infection prevention and control department and thoroughly cleaned by the owner's environmental services department<br>2. Remove barrier material carefully to minimize spreading of dirt and debris associated with construction<br>3. Contain construction waste before transport in tightly covered containers<br>4. Cover transport receptacles or carts. Tape covering unless lid is solid<br>5. Vacuum work area with HEPA filtered vacuums<br>6. Wet mop area with cleaner/disinfectant<br>7. Upon completion, restore HVAC system where work was performed |

Step 4: identify the areas surrounding the project area, assessing potential impact.

| Unit Below | Unit Above | Lateral | Lateral | Behind | Front |
|---|---|---|---|---|---|
| Risk group | Risk group | Risk group | Risk group | Risk group | Risk group |

Step 5: identify specific site of activity; for example, patient rooms, medication room, and so forth.

Step 6: identify issues related to ventilation, plumbing, electrical (in terms of the occurrence of probable outages).

Step 7: identify containment measures, using prior assessment. What types of barriers (eg, solids wall barriers)? Will HEPA filtration be required? (Note: renovation/construction area will be isolated from the occupied areas during construction and will be negative with respect to surrounding areas).

Step 8: consider potential risk of water damage. Is there a risk from the compromising of structural integrity (eg, wall, ceiling, roof)?

Step 9: work hours. Can or will the work be done during non–patient-care hours?

Step 10: do plans allow for an adequate number of isolation/negative airflow rooms?

Step 11: do the plans allow for the required number and type of handwashing sinks?

Step 12: do the infection prevention and control staff agree with the minimum number of sinks for this project? Verify against FGI design and construction guidelines for types and area.

Step 13: do the infection prevention and control staff agree with the plans relative to clean and soiled utility rooms?

Step 14: plan to discuss containment issues with the project team; eg, traffic flow, housekeeping, debris removal (how and when).

# Occupational Health Update

## Focus on Preventing the Acquisition of Infections with Pre-exposure Prophylaxis and Postexposure Prophylaxis

David J. Weber, MD, MPH[a,b,]*, William A. Rutala, PhD, MPH[a,b]

### KEYWORDS

- Occupational health • Health care personnel • Vaccines • Postexposure prophylaxis
- Hepatitis B • Hepatitis C • HIV

### KEY POINTS

- An effective occupational program is a key aspect of preventing the acquisition of an infection by health care providers through pre-exposure assessment of immunity to vaccine-preventable diseases and immediate access to medical evaluation for postexposure prophylaxis (PEP) after exposure to a communicable disease.
- All health care providers should be immune to mumps, measles, rubella, varicella, pertussis, and influenza. Health care providers with the potential for blood or body fluid exposure should also be immune to hepatitis B.
- PEP is available after exposure to several diseases, including hepatitis A, hepatitis B, HIV, measles, pertussis, invasive meningococcal infection, and syphilis.
- Health care personnel (HCP) with certain communicable disease need to be evaluated for work restrictions or furlough.

## INTRODUCTION

Health care is the fastest-growing sector of the US economy, employing more than 18 million persons.[1] HCP face a range of noninfectious hazards on the job, including back injuries, strains and sprains, latex allergy, violence, and stress.[1] HCP are also commonly exposed to infectious agents via sharp injuries (eg, hepatitis C virus [HCV], hepatitis B virus [HBV], and human immunodeficiency virus [HIV]), direct patient

Disclosure Statement: D.J. Weber is a speaker and consultant for Pfizer and Merck.
[a] Hospital Epidemiology, University of North Carolina Health Care, Chapel Hill, NC 27514, USA;
[b] Division of Infectious Diseases, University of North Carolina School of Medicine, Chapel Hill, NC 27599-7030, USA
* Corresponding author. University of North Carolina, 2163 Bioinformatics, CB #7030, Chapel Hill, NC 27599-7030.
E-mail address: dweber@unch.unc.edu

Infect Dis Clin N Am 30 (2016) 729–757
http://dx.doi.org/10.1016/j.idc.2016.04.008
0891-5520/16/$ – see front matter © 2016 Elsevier Inc. All rights reserved.

id.theclinics.com

care (eg, respiratory viruses, gastrointestinal pathogens, and pertussis), and the contaminated environment (eg, *Clostridium difficile*). Cases of nonfatal occupational injury and illness among HCP are among the highest of any industry sector.[1] The risks and methods preventing occupational acquisition of infection by HCP have been reviewed.[2–7] Minimizing the risk of disease acquisition is based on 6 key recommended practices: (1) proper training of HCP at initiation of health care practice and annually (eg, infection control practices and sharp injury prevention); (2) immunity to vaccine-preventable diseases[2,6,8–11]; (3) evaluation of HCP who were exposed to communicable diseases for receipt of PEP[2,12–14]; (4) adherence to standard precautions when providing patient care,[15] especially the performance of appropriate hand hygiene before and after patient care[16–18]; (5) rapid institution of appropriate isolation precautions for patients with a known or suspected communicable disease[15,19,20]; and (6) proper use of personal protective equipment, such as masks, N95 respirators, eye protection, and gowns when caring for patients with potentially communicable diseases.[15,21] Prevention of laboratory-acquired infection requires adherence to recommended administrative protocols (eg, no eating, drinking, or smoking in areas where microbiologic or pathologic samples are processed), engineering controls (eg, containment hoods), personal protective equipment (eg, N95 masks when culturing *Mycobacterium tuberculosis*), and appropriate immunizations.[22,23]

## DEFINITIONS

HCP refers to all paid and unpaid persons providing services in health care settings who have the potential for exposure to patients and/or infectious materials, including body substances, contaminated medical supplies and equipment, contaminated environmental surfaces, or contaminated air. These HCP may include but are not limited to those listed in **Box 1**. In general, HCP who have regular or frequent contact with patients, body fluids, or specimens have a higher risk of acquiring or transmitting infections than do HCP who have only brief contact with patients and their environment (eg, beds, food trays, and medical equipment). All HCP who work within the confines of a health care facility, however should be covered by the occupational health service (OHS) and receive appropriate screening and pre-exposure prophylaxis even if they do not provide direct patient care because they frequently interact with HCP providing direct care and are, therefore, at risk for acquiring or transmitting infectious pathogens.

---

**Box 1**
**Health care personnel whose care should be covered by an occupational health service**

- Emergency medical service personnel
- Nurse and nursing assistants
- Physicians and dentists
- Technicians
- Therapists (eg, occupational health, physical, and respiratory care)
- Pharmacists
- Students and trainees
- Contractual staff not employed by the health care facility
- Persons not directly involved in patient care (eg, clerical, dietary, housekeeping, laundry, security, maintenance, administrative, billing, volunteers, laboratory, and mortuary)

Health care settings refers to locations where health care is provided and includes, but is not limited to, facilities that provide acute care, long-term care, assisted living, rehabilitation, home health, dialysis, and ambulatory surgery. It also includes vehicles that transport patients (eg, ambulances, medical helicopters, and planes).

Occupational health programs refer to formal, well-designed, organized plans that provide OHSs to HCP. Most commonly, OHSs are provided onsite within the health care facility in which HCP are performing patient care but may also be provided offsite. Occupational health programs should include a variety of activities designed to minimize the risk for HCP to acquire an infectious disease, to evaluate HCP with a potential exposure to a communicable disease, and to evaluate HCP with a communicable disease (**Box 2**).

Occupational health programs should be aware of appropriate guidelines from the Centers for Disease Control and Prevention and professional organizations. They should adhere to appropriate state and federal laws and regulations. Specific regulations promulgated by the US Occupational Health and Safety Administration (OSHA) related to HCP include Bloodborne Pathogens (1910.1030)[24] and Tuberculosis/Respiratory Protection (1910.134).[25] The federal Needlestick Safety and Prevention Act (HR 5178), which was enacted in 2000, requires the use of safety engineered devices whenever possible to reduce the likelihood of sharp injuries.[26]

## PRE-EXPOSURE SCREENING AND IMMUNIZATIONS
### Pre-exposure Screening

All new HCP should undergo a new personnel orientation. As part of the orientation process, new HCP should undergo screening and education directed at reducing the risk of acquisition of infection diseases by health care providers (see **Box 2**). All information obtained should be entered into an electronic database.

### Immunizations

General recommendations regarding vaccination of HCP have been published by the Centers for Disease Control and Prevention (CDC),[2] the Advisory Committee on Immunization Practices (ACIP),[8,27,28] the American Academy of Pediatrics (AAP),[11] and the Association for Professionals in Infection Control and Epidemiology (APIC).[10] The most recent ACIP recommendations, which are summarized yearly, should always be consulted.[28] It is recommended that all HCP be immune to mumps, measles, rubella, varicella, pertussis, and influenza.[2,8,10,27,28] Depending on the vaccine-preventable disease, immunity may be assured by several different measures (**Table 1**). HCP who are not immune should receive appropriate immunization(s) (**Table 2**). Even if HCP are considered immune to a vaccine-preventable disease transmitted by the droplet (pertussis, invasive meningococcal infection, mumps, or rubella) or airborne route (varicella), they should wear a mask (don prior to entering the room) while providing care to a patient with one of these disease because immunization is not 100% effective in preventing infection.

All HCP with potential exposure to blood or body fluids should be immune to hepatitis B. Influenza vaccine should be offered to all HCP yearly. In the past few years, editorials and commentaries have recommended that yearly influenza immunization (unless contraindicated) should be a condition of employment for HCP.[29–31] In February 2012, the National Vaccine Advisory Committee issued a statement that provided recommendations on how to achieve the Healthy People 2020 annual influenza vaccine coverage goal (90%) for HCP; for facilities that have implemented the recommended initial strategies but have "not consistently achieved the Healthy People goal

**Box 2**
**Components of an occupational health service for health care personnel**

*At initial of employment or patient care*

- Evaluation for ability to perform job functions

- Screen for illicit drugs

- Medical evaluation of selected HCP
  - Department of transportation (required for use of certain motor vehicles)
  - Flight physical (required of pilots)
  - Police/security for use of weapons

- Review of immunity to vaccine-preventable diseases (see **Tables 1** and **2**)

- Evaluation for tuberculosis
  - Symptom review for active tuberculosis
  - Testing for latent tuberculosis (TST or IGRA)

- Allergy screening for common health care–associated products
  - Latex/natural rubber, germicides (antiseptics and disinfectants)

- Counseling for pregnant or immunocompromised personnel (voluntary)

- Education
  - Fire and electrical safety
  - Prevention of sharps injury
  - Appropriate hand hygiene and proper use of personal protective equipment
  - Workplace violence
  - Disaster planning: weather, bomb threats, biothreats, chemical spills
  - Reporting infectious disease exposures, injuries, illnesses
  - OHSA required (if applicable): blood-borne pathogens, tuberculosis/respiratory protection

*Annual*

- Evaluation for tuberculosis

- Review of immunity to vaccine-preventable diseases
  - Influenza immunization

- Miscellaneous
  - Hearing evaluation if part of OSHA-required hearing conservation program
  - Test for color blindness if performing high level disinfection

- Education
  - OHSA required (if applicable): blood-borne pathogens, tuberculosis/respiratory protection
  - Others as recommended/required by health care facility

*When needed*

- Evaluation for possible communicable disease
  - Consideration for treatment and job restriction/furlough if disease poses threat to patients or other HCP

- Evaluation for PEP
  - Consideration for treatment and job restriction/furlough if disease poses threat to patients or other HCP

- Evaluation of injured personnel (eg, strains, sprains, and lacerations)
  - Provide first aid
  - Refer to emergency department or specialize clinic for severe injuries
  - Provide long-term care
  - Communicate with workers' compensation department

- Return to work evaluation for non–work-related injuries/illnesses

- Fit for duty examination (may include drug and alcohol testing)

*Abbreviations:* IGRA, interferon gamma release assay; TST, tuberculin skin test.

**Table 1**
**Methods of demonstrating proof of immunity of health care personnel**

| Vaccine | Birth Before 1957 | Physician Diagnosis | Positive Serology | Self-Report | Documented Appropriate Vaccine Series[a] |
|---|---|---|---|---|---|
| Mumps (MMR) | Yes[b] | Yes[d] | Yes | No | Yes |
| Measles (MMR) | Yes[b] | Yes[c] | Yes | No | Yes |
| Rubella (MMR) | Yes[b,c] | No | Yes | No | Yes |
| Varicella | No | Yes | Yes | Yes[e] | Yes |
| Hepatitis B | No | — | $\geq$10 mIU/mL[f] | No | Yes |
| Pertussis (Tdap) | No | No | No | No | Yes |
| Influenza | No | No | No | No | Yes |

Yes in any column is acceptable evidence of immunity. Greater than 96% of HCP born before 1957 were demonstrated to be immune to measles, mumps or and rubella (2006–2008).[118]
  [a] Written documentation (ie, signed by a health care provider).
  [b] Consider immunization of HCP born before 1957; recommend during an outbreak.
  [c] All HCP of childbearing potential should be immunized.
  [d] Requires laboratory confirmation of infection.
  [e] Based on published literature: greater than 97% of HCP born before 1980 were demonstrated to be immune to varicella in 2014.[119]
  [f] Obtain anti-HBs titer, 1 to 2 months post last vaccine dose; if immunization remote and anti-HBs titer not available, see text for management.
*Adapted from* Weber DJ, Rutala WA, Schaffner W. Immunization for vaccine-preventable diseases: why aren't we protecting our students? Infect Contr Hosp Epidemiology 2011;32:912–4.

for vaccination coverage of HCP in an efficient and timely manner," it was recommended that they should "strongly consider an employer requirement for influenza immunization."[32] HCP should be provided vaccines that are recommended for adults,[28] such as human papillomavirus, herpes zoster (HZ), and pneumococcal vaccines, or referred to their local medical provider. In special circumstances, HCP and laboratory personnel and researchers should be offered immunization with other vaccines, including polio, rabies, hepatitis A, vaccinia (smallpox), and anthrax (**Box 3**). In addition, HCP who are traveling outside the United States for work-related activities should be evaluated and provided CDC recommended immunizations, such as typhoid, cholera, and Japanese encephalitis.[33,34]

Immunocompromised HCP require special consideration in the provision of immunizations.[8,27,28,35] First, live, attenuated virus vaccines (eg, measles-mumps-rubella [MMR] vaccine; varicella vaccine; and live, attenuated influenza vaccine [LAIV]) may be contraindicated. Second, vaccines not routinely recommended may be indicated (eg, pneumococcal, meningococcal, *Haemophilus influenzae* type b). Third, higher antigen doses (eg, hepatitis B vaccine in people with end-stage renal disease), additional doses of vaccine (eg, rabies vaccine in immunocompromised persons), or postimmunization serologic evaluation may be indicated (eg, antibody to hepatitis B surface antigen [anti-HBs] titer after hepatitis B vaccine or antibody response to rabies vaccine) because immunization of immunocompromised people may elicit a lower antibody response. Finally, such personnel should be individually evaluated for reassignment (with the consent of the employee) depending on their job duties. Caring for an immunocompromised patient is not a contraindication to receipt of a live, attenuated vaccine, although HCP receiving LAIV should not work in a protected environment (eg, stem cell transplant unit) for 7 days postimmunization.[28,36]

**Table 2**
**Immunizations recommended for nonimmune health care personnel**

| Vaccine | Health Care Personnel | Comments |
|---|---|---|
| Mumps | All (2 doses) | Provide as MMR |
| Measles | All (2 doses) | Provide as MMR |
| Rubella | All (1 dose) | Provide as MMR |
| Varicella | All (2 doses) | — |
| Hepatitis B | HCP with potential exposure to blood or contaminated body fluids (3 doses) | — |
| Meningococcal (serogroups A, C, Y, W) | Clinical microbiologists (1 dose; booster every 5 y) | Use conjugate vaccine for HCP 18–54 y of age and polysaccharide vaccine for HCP ≥55 y of age |
| Meningococcal (serogroup B) | Clinical microbiologists (2 doses) | — |
| Tdap | All (1 dose; no boosters recommended) | Especially important for HCP who have contact with children |
| Influenza | All (1 dose each year) | HCP who care for severely immunocompromised persons who require care in a protected environment should receive IIV or RIV; HCP who receive LAIV should avoid providing care for severely immunocompromised persons (ie, persons receiving care in "protected" hospital unit, such as BMTU) for 7 d after immunization. |

*Abbreviations:* BMTU, bone marrow transplant unit; IIV, inactivated influenza vaccine; RIV, recombinant influenza vaccine.

Pregnant HCP also require special consideration in the provision of immunizations. The risks from immunization during pregnancy are largely theoretic.[27] The benefit of immunization among pregnant women usually outweighs the potential risks for adverse reactions, especially when the risk for disease exposure is high, infection would pose a special risk to the mother or fetus, and the vaccine is unlikely to cause harm.[27,28,37–40] Furthermore, newer information continues to confirm the safety of vaccines given inadvertently during pregnancy. Ideally, women of childbearing age, including HCP, should have been immunized against measles, mumps, rubella, varicella, tetanus, diphtheria, pertussis, meningococcus, polio, hepatitis A, and hepatitis B as children or adolescents before becoming pregnant. Because this may not have occurred, however, it is especially important that all HCP be screened for immunity to vaccine-preventable diseases. Nevertheless, live, attenuated vaccines should be provided only to nonpregnant HCP and deferred for pregnant women. The ACIP has recommended that "healthcare personnel should administer [tetanus toxoid, reduced diphtheria toxoid, and acellular pertussis] Tdap during all pregnancies, preferably during the third or late second trimester (after 20 weeks' gestation)." If not administered during pregnancy, Tdap should be administered immediately postpartum. Women who are pregnant during respiratory virus season should receive inactivated influenza immunization.[28] There is no convincing evidence of risk from immunizing pregnant women with other inactivated virus or bacterial vaccines, or toxoids. Susceptible pregnant women at high risk for specific infections should receive, as indicated, the

---

**Box 3**
**Special use vaccines**

- Anthrax: PEP, research, biothreat attack
- Diphtheria (Tdap): Outbreak
- Hepatitis A: PEP, outbreak, travel
- Hepatitis B: PEP, travel
- Measles (MMR): PEP, outbreak
- Meningococcal serotypes A, C, W, Y: outbreak, travel
- Meningococcal serotype B: outbreak
- Mumps (MMR): outbreak
- Pertussis (Tdap): outbreak
- Poliomyelitis: research, outbreak
- Rabies: PEP, research, travel
- Rubella (MMR): outbreak
- Smallpox (Vaccinia): PEP, research, biothreat attack
- Tetanus (Tdap or Td): PEP
- Varicella: PEP, outbreak
- Vaccinia (smallpox): PEP, research, biothreat attack

Additional vaccines may be recommended for researchers or travel, such as yellow fever, Japanese encephalitis, cholera, and so forth.
*Abbreviation:* PEP, postexposure prophylaxis.

---

following vaccines: hepatitis A, hepatitis B, pneumococcal polysaccharide, meningococcal, rabies, and poliovirus (inactivated) (see **Box 3**).[27] The indications for use of immunoglobulin preparations are the same in pregnant and nonpregnant women. Breastfeeding does not adversely affect the response to immunization and is not a contraindication for any of the currently routinely recommended vaccines.

Before the administration of any vaccine, HCP should be evaluated for the presence of condition(s) that are listed as a vaccine contraindication or precaution.[27] If such a condition is present, the risks and benefits of vaccination need to be carefully weighed by the health care provider and the patient. The most common contraindication is a history of an anaphylactic reaction to a previous dose of the vaccine or to a vaccine component. Factors that are not contraindications to immunization include the following: household contact with a pregnant woman; breastfeeding; reaction to a previous vaccination, consisting only of mild to moderate local tenderness, swelling, or both, or fever less than 40.5°C; mild acute illness with or without low-grade fever; current antimicrobial therapy (except for oral typhoid vaccine) or convalescence from a recent illness; personal history of allergies except a history of an anaphylactic reaction to a vaccine component; and family history of allergies, serious adverse reactions to vaccination, or seizures.[27]

## POSTEXPOSURE PROPHYLAXIS

General guidelines on PEP are available from the CDC,[2] ACIP,[8] AAP,[41] APIC,[7] and the American Public Health Association (APHA).[42] All HCP should be educated at their initiation of employment or providing service when and how to report an infectious disease exposure. In general, HCP should complete an incident form, have it signed by their supervisor, and then report to the occupational health clinic. Occupational health evaluation should be available 24/7 for exposed HCP. The incident form should be reviewed by occupational health and communicated to the workers' compensation department. HCP with serious or life-threating injuries or exposures should be referred to an emergency department or specialty clinic as appropriate. If patient or visitor exposures also occurred, the infection control department should be notified.

A well-defined protocol should be in place that details the steps in evaluation of an HCP potentially exposed to an infectious agent (**Box 4**). Proper counseling of the exposed HCP is critical (**Box 5**). Appropriate first aid should be provided, including proper care of any sharp injury or mucosal membrane exposure (eg, copious rinsing of eyes in the case of splash to eyes). A proper evaluation of the source case should also be conducted to confirm the report by the exposed HCP that the source patient does have a communicable disease. Appropriate laboratory tests should be obtained from the source patient to determine if the source patient can transmit HIV, HBV, or HCV.

PEP is available for many diseases, including but not limited to, diphtheria, hepatitis A and B, HIV, influenza, measles, invasive meningococcal infection, pertussis, rabies, syphilis, tuberculosis, and varicella-zoster. PEP is also available for some exposures, including animal bites (eg, dogs, cats, rodents, and primates) and human bites. Unfortunately, PEP is not available for exposure to arboviruses, hepatitis C, mumps, parvovirus B-19, rubella, and Middle East respiratory syndrome–coronavirus. PEP may consist of antivirals, antibiotics, immunoglobulin preparations and/or vaccines (see **Box 3**). Immunoglobulin preparations may be indicated as part of PEP for exposure to hepatitis A (immune globulin [IG]), hepatitis B IG (HBIG), measles (IG), rabies IG, tetanus (tetanus IG), varicella (varicella-zoster IG), and vaccinia (vaccinia IG). More than 1 modality may be recommended. Pre-exposure prophylaxis with recommended immunization is not considered sufficient protection after an exposure to the following diseases, and postexposure antimicrobial prophylaxis is still recommended: pertussis, invasive meningococcal infection, and diphtheria (discussed later).

---

**Box 4**
**Management of an infectious disease exposure**

- Obtain name, medical record number, and location of source case
- Determine if source case has an infection and is infectious (ie, capable of transmitting infection)
- Determine if transmission possible (ie, appropriate exposure without appropriate personal protection)
- Determine if health care provider is susceptible (may require laboratory tests)
- Determine if PEP is available and indicated
- Consider alternative prophylaxis (if available) if health care provider has a contraindication to the prophylaxis of first choice
- Administer prophylaxis with informed consent (HCP may choose not to accept prophylaxis)
- Arrange follow-up
- Document all of the above in the medical record

---

**Box 5**
**Postexposure prophylaxis counseling of the exposed health care provider**

- Information to be provided to health care providers who are exposed to an infectious agent
  - Risk (if known) of acquiring the infectious disease
  - Risk (if known) of transmitting any infection that is acquired to patients, other HCP, and contacts (eg, household members)
  - Methods of preventing transmission of infection to other persons
  - Need for work restrictions (if any)
  - Recommended follow-up
- Information to be provided to health care providers who are offered prophylaxis
  - Recommendations for prophylaxis
  - Alternative methods of prophylaxis if the primary method is contraindicated
  - Degree of protection provided by the therapy
  - Potential side effects of the therapy
  - Safety laboratory tests (if recommended)
  - Risks (if known) of infection if PEP is refused

---

*Sharp Injuries*

Occupational blood and body fluid exposures to blood-borne pathogens remain a serious public health concern.[43] The CDC estimates that 5.6 million workers in the health care industry and related occupations are at risk of occupational exposure to blood-borne pathogens. More than 30 different pathogens have caused documented occupational infection after exposure to blood or body fluids in HCP or hospital laboratory personnel.[44] The most important blood-borne pathogens are HIV, HBV, and HCV.[44,45] The key features for assessing the risk of transmission of HBV, HCV, and HIV are for each agent their seroprevalence in the general population, their environmental survival, and transmissibility via percutaneous, mucous membrane or nonintact skin exposure. The seroprevalence of these viruses in the general population is HBV approximately 0.4%, HCV approximately 1.3%, and HIV approximately 0.31%.[46] HBV has been demonstrated to survive and remain infectious greater than 7 days on environmental surfaces.[47] The data on HCV environmental survival are varied, with articles reporting survival of 16 hours,[48] 5 days,[49] and up to 6 weeks.[50] For HIV, the half-life has been reported as 28 hours,[51] with a maximum of several days.[52] The risk of transmission of HBV depends on the route of exposure, whether the exposed person is immune (via immunization or natural infection), and serologic status of the source patient. Rates of clinical hepatitis/serologic evidence of HBV infection in susceptible exposed HCP after a percutaneous exposure have been reported as 22% to 31%/37% to 62% if the source is hepatitis B surface antigen (HBsAg) positive and but hepatitis B e antigen (HBeAg) positive; rates of transmission have been reported as 1% to 6%/23% to 37% if the source is HBsAg positive but HBeAg negative.[53] The risk of transmission of HCV after percutaneous exposure has been reported as 1.8% to 1.9% (range, 0%–7%).[46,54] The risk of transmission of HIV after percutaneous exposure has been reported as 0.3% (95% CI, 0.2%–0.5%).[46]

In addition to percutaneous transmission, the blood-borne viruses HBV, HCV, and HIV can be transmitted via blood or contaminated fluid exposure of mucous membranes, nonintact skin, or human bites. The risk of transmission by these routes has not been quantitated for HBV and HCV. The risk of transmission by the mucosal route for HIV has been reported to be 0.09% (95% CI, 0.01%–0.5%).[46] The risk of transmission of HIV via exposure of nonintact skin is likely less than 0.1% but has not been completely quantified. The risk from a human bite has also not been quantified. Transmission of HBV,[55] HCV,[56] and HIV[57] by human bites, however, has been reported. Human bites that penetrate the skin, however, should be considered as possible 2-way exposure (from patient-to-HCP and HCP-to-patient).

The CDC has estimated that approximately 385,000 percutaneous injuries occurred annually among HCP in the United States in the time period of 1997 to 1998.[43] Although the incidence of needlestick injuries has been reduced by advances in education, needle disposal, engineering changes, and personnel protection, institutions and HCP must continue to assume responsibility in further lowering the risk. Several methods of reducing exposure to blood and other potential infectious body fluids have been described (**Box 6**).

All occupational exposures to blood and other potentially infectious material place HCP at risk for infection with a blood-borne pathogen. OSHA defines blood to mean human blood, blood components, and products made from human blood.[24] Other potentially infectious material includes body fluids, such as semen, vaginal secretions, cerebrospinal fluid, synovial fluid, pericardial fluid, pleural fluid, peritoneal fluid, human milk, amniotic fluid, saliva associated with dental procedures, and body fluid that is visibly contaminated with blood. All body fluids should be considered infectious in situations where it is difficult or impossible to differentiate between bloody fluids. Any unfixed tissues or organs (other than intact skin) from a human (living or dead) are also considered potentially infectious material. For laboratory personnel, other potentially infectious material includes HIV-containing cell or tissue cultures, organ cultures, and HIV or hepatitis virus-containing culture medium or other solutions, as well as blood, organs, or tissues from experimental animals infected with HIV, HBV, or HCV.

Care for HCP who have been exposed to blood or potentially contaminated fluids has been reviewed.[46,53,54,58–62] Exposed HCP should immediately be provided with

---

**Box 6**
**Methods of reducing percutaneous, mucous membrane, or nonintact skin exposure to blood or potentially infectious body fluids**

- Strict adherence to standard precautions including appropriate hand hygiene and use of personal protective equipment (eg, gloves, gowns, masks, and eye shields)
- Use of safety engineered devices (needles, syringes, scalpels, etc.)
- Use of double-gloves during surgical procedures with an increased risk of glove puncture
- Use of blunted surgical needles, when possible
- Work practice controls to reduce risk of injuries, such as elimination of capping needles, using a tray to pass sharp devices, and immediately and appropriately discard used sharp instruments
- Puncture resistant sharp disposal units
- Precautions should be taken to prevent sharps injuries during procedures and during cleaning/disinfection of instruments
- Mouthpieces, resuscitation bags, or other ventilation devices should be available whenever their need can be anticipated
- Health care personnel who have exudative lesions or weeping dermatitis on exposed body areas (hands/wrist and face/neck) must be excused from providing direct patient care or working patient equipment (OSHA regulation)
- Enhanced education on the proper use of safety engineered device

first aid. Exposed mucous membranes should be flushed with water. Wounds and skin sites that have been in contact with blood or body fluids should be washed with soap and water. Antiseptics, such as chlorhexidine, have not been shown to reduce the risk of HBV transmission. There is no contraindication, however, to their use as long as they are not injected into the wound. It is not recommended to squeeze the wound to express fluid or using potentially harmful agents, such as bleach. The following exposures do not require PEP: (1) contact of intact skin with blood or body fluids; (2) skin was not breached by a sharp; (3) contact with saliva (nondental), urine, vomit, or feces that was not visibly contaminated with blood; and, (4) a sharp that was used before the injury.

The source patient for blood and body fluid exposures should be tested for HIV using a 4th-generation test (combined antibody and antigen test), HBsAg, hepatitis C antibody, and other tests as indicated by the source patient's medical history (eg, malaria, syphilis, or HTVL). If a source patient's HCV test is positive, an HCV polymerase chain reaction (PCR) should be obtained.

## Hepatitis B

The risk of HBV acquisition by HCP has declined dramatically over the years. The number of HBV infections among HCP declined by approximately 98% from an estimated 17,000 infections in 1983 to 263 acute HBV infections in 2010.[53] This decline was likely due to decreased exposure from improved work practice controls (see **Box 6**) and HBV immunization of HCP. The risk of HBV transmission from patient-to-HCP provider remains, however, because there are an estimated 800,000 to 1.4 million persons in the United States living with chronic HBV infection.[53]

The key method of preventing health care–associated HBV infection among HCP is HBV immunization prior to beginning direct patient care of all HCP with potential blood or body fluid exposure. Furthermore, all HCP should know their immune response to vaccination. For HCP immunized in training or at initiation of patient contact, an anti-HBs quantitative titer should be drawn 1 to 2 months after the last dose of vaccine. HCP with greater than or equal to 10 mIU/mL anti-HBs are considered immune for life. HCP who do not respond adequately should be reimmunized with 3 additional doses of vaccine and tested for immunity 1 to 2 months after the last (6th dose). HCP who have not responded adequately ($\geq$10 mIU/mL anti-HBs) should be tests for HBsAg. Nonresponders to 6 doses of vaccine should be counseled to return to report any exposures to blood or body fluids because they may be prophylaxed with HBIG (**Table 3**). HCP, especially trainees, with a remote history of hepatitis B vaccine should have their immunity to HBV assessed using the algorithm recommended by the CDC.[53]

HCP exposed to an HBsAg-positive patient should be evaluated for prophylaxis per the recommended CDC algorithm (see **Table 3**). HCP with known to have responded to vaccine ($\geq$10 mIU/mL anti-HBs) do not need any prophylaxis; unimmunized HCP or HCP with an unknown response should be managed per the CDC algorithm, which may entail the use of hepatitis B vaccine and/or HBIG. PEP should be provided as soon as possible but always within 7 days of exposure.[53] HBIG and hepatitis B vaccine can be administered simultaneously at separate injection sites.

## Human Immunodeficiency Virus

The number of persons living with HIV infection has increased over the years in the United States due to the success of antiviral medications. The CDC has estimated that there are approximately 1.2 million people in the United States living with HIV at the end of 2012, of whom approximately 12.8% did not know they were infected.[63]

**Table 3**
Postexposure management to prevent hepatitis B infection of health care personnel after occupational percutaneous and mucosal exposure to blood and body fluids

| HCP Status | Postexposure Testing | | Postexposure Prophylaxis | | Postvaccination Serologic Testing[b] |
|---|---|---|---|---|---|
| | Source Patient (HBsAg) | HCP Testing (Anti-HBs) | HBIG[a] | Vaccination | |
| Documented responder[c] after complete series (≥3 doses) | No action needed | | | | |
| Documented nonresponder[d] after 6 doses | Positive/unknown | —[e] | HBIG × 2 separated by 1 mo | — | No |
| | Negative | | No action needed | | |
| Response unknown after 3 doses | Positive/unknown | <10 mIU/mL[e] | HBIG × 1 | Initial revaccination | Yes |
| | Negative | <10 mIU/mL | None | — | — |
| | Any | ≥10 mIU/mL | No action needed | | |
| Unvaccinated/incompletely vaccinated or vaccine refusers | Positive/unknown | —[e] | HBIG × 1 | Complete vaccination | Yes |
| | Negative | — | None | Complete vaccination | Yes |

[a] HBIG should be administered intramuscularly as soon as possible after exposure when indicated. The effectiveness of HBIG when administered greater than 7 days after percutaneous, mucosal, or nonintact skin exposures is unknown. HBIG dosage is 0.06 mL/kg.

[b] Should be performed 1 to 2 months after the last dose of the HepB vaccine series (and 4–6 months after administration of HBIG to avoid detection of passively administered anti-HBs) using a quantitative method that allows detection of the protective concentration of anti-HBs (≥10 mIU/mL).

[c] A responder is defined as a person with anti-HBs ≥10 mIU/mL after ≥3 doses of HepB vaccine.

[d] A nonresponder is defined as a person with anti-HBs less than 10 mIU/mL after ≥6 doses of HepB vaccine.

[e] HCP who have anti-HBs less than 10 mIU/mL, or who are unvaccinated or incompletely vaccinated, and sustain an exposure to a source patient who is HBsAg-positive or has unknown HBsAg status, should undergo baseline testing for HBV infection as soon as possible after exposure, and follow-up testing approximately 6 months later. Initial baseline tests consist of total anti-HBc; testing at approximately 6 months consists of HBsAg and total anti-HBc.

*From* Schillie S, Murphy TV, Sawyer M, et al; Centers for Disease Control and Prevention. CDC guidance for evaluating health-care personnel for hepatitis B virus protection and for administering postexposure management. MMWR Recomm Rep 2013;62(RR-10):1–19.

In the United States, 58 confirmed and 150 possible cases of occupationally acquired HIV infection were reported to the CDC between 1985 and 2013.[64] Since 1999, only 1 confirmed case (a laboratory technician who sustained a needle puncture while working with a live HIV culture in 2008) has been reported.[64]

The management of HCP exposed to blood or body fluids from HIV-infected persons is well described in the literature.[45,46,59–61,65,66] OSHA requires that all US health care facilities provide postexposure management of HIV exposures consistent with the most recent US Public Health Service guideline.[60] This guideline delineates the situations for which expert consultation for HIV PEP is recommended as well as the recommended follow-up for HCP exposed to known or suspected HIV-positive sources.[60] The preferred HIV PEP regimen is Truvada (tenofovir disoproxil fumarate/TDF [Viread], 300 mg, plus emtricitabine/FTC [Emtrival] 200 mg), 1 tablet orally once daily, plus raltegravir/RAL (Isentress), 400 mg orally, twice daily (**Table 4**).[60] The authors' retrovirologists prefer raltegravir to dolutegravir because dolutegravir has more drug interactions and is substantially more expensive. The following antiretroviral agents should be used for PEP only with expert consultation: abacavir/ABC (Ziagen), efavirenz/EFV (Sustiva), enfuvirtide/T-20 (Fuzeon), fosamprenavir/FOSAPV (Lexiva), maraviroc/MVC (Selzentry), saquinavir/SQV (Invirase), and stavudine/d4t (Zerit). The following agents are generally not recommended for PEP: didanosine/ddI (Videx EC), nelfinavir/NFV (Viracept), and tipranavir/TPV (Aptivus). Neverapine/NVP (Viramune) is contraindicated at PEP.

**Table 4**
**Alternative regimens for HIV postexposure prophylaxis**

| Column A | Column B |
| --- | --- |
| Raltegravir/RAL (Isentress) | Tenofovir disoproxil fumarate/TDF (Viread) + emtricitabine/FTC (Emtriva); available as Truvada |
| Darunavir/DRV (Prezista) + ritonavir/RTV (Norvir) | |
| Etravirine/ETR (Intelence) | Tenofovir disoproxil fumarate/TDF (Viread) + lamivudine (Epivir; 3TC) |
| Rilpivirine/RPV (Edurant) | |
| Atazanavir/ATV (Reyataz) + ritonavir/RTV (Norvir) | Zidovudine/ZDV/AZT (Retrovir) + lamivudine (Epivir; 3TC); available as Combivir |
| Lopinavir/ritonavir LPV/RTV (Kaletra) | Zidovudine/ZDV/AZT (Retrovir) + emtricitabine/FTC (Emtriva) |

Should combine 1 drug or drug pair from the left column with 1 pair of nucleoside/nucleotide reverse-transcriptase inhibitors from the right column; prescribers unfamiliar with these agents/regimens should consult physicians familiar with the agents and their toxicities).

The following alternative is a complete fixed-dose combination regimen, and no additional antiretrovirals are needed: Stribild (elvitegravir, cobicistat, tenofovir DF, emtricitabine).

*Adapted from* Kuhar DT, Henderson DK, Struble KA, et al. Updated US Public Health Service guidelines for the management of occupational exposures to human immunodeficiency virus and recommendations for postexposure prophylaxis. Infect Control Hosp Epidemiol 2013;34:875–92.

## Invasive Meningococcal Infections

*Neisseria meningitidis*, a Gram-negative diplococcus and causative agent of invasive meningococcal disease, has at least 13 serogroups based on capsular typing. Five serogroups (A, B, C, W, and Y) cause most disease worldwide; 3 of these serogroups (B, C, and Y) cause most of the illness in the United States.[67,68] The incidence of invasive meningococcal disease varies over time and by age and location.[69,70] In recent years, the incidence of invasive disease has declined in the United States.[8] Based on reported cases in 2014, the CDC estimated that there were 450 cases (0.14/100,000) and 65 deaths (0.02/100,000) in the United States.[68]

N meningitidis is transmitted person-to-person via respiratory and throat secretions (saliva or spit) during close (eg, coughing or kissing) or lengthy contact (eg, living in the same household).[67] The carriage frequency of N meningitidis in children and young adults is approximately 10% in children and among young adults is approximately 10%.[71] Outbreaks most often occur in communities, schools, colleges, prisons, and other closed populations.[67] HCP have acquired invasive meningococcal infection as a result of providing direct care (eg, assisting in endotracheal intubation and airway suctioning) to infected patients.[72] It has been estimated that clinical microbiologists have an attack rate greater than 50 times high than the background rate of invasive meningococcal disease.[73] For this reason, the CDC/ACIP recommend that clinical and research microbiologist who might be routinely exposed to isolates of N meningitidis receive both the quadrivalent meningococcal vaccine (Men4ACWY) and the meningococcal serogroup B vaccine (MenB).[8,28] Fatal meningitis in a microbiologist due to N meningitidis serotype B was recently reported.[74] Such HCP should receive a booster dose of MenACWY every 5 years if they remain at increased risk.

Chemoprophylaxis of household members of an index case of invasive meningococcal disease is recommended.[41,42,75] Chemoprophylaxis of exposed HCP is advised for all persons who have had intensive, unprotected contact (eg, without wearing a mask) with infected patients (eg, via mouth-to-mouth resuscitation, endotracheal intubation, or endotracheal tube management). Chemoprophylaxis for HCP should be recommended even if the HCP has been vaccinated with either the conjugate or polysaccharide vaccine.[8] Because the rate of secondary disease for close contacts is highest immediately after onset of disease in the index patient, antimicrobial chemoprophylaxis should be administered as soon as possible (ideally less than 24 hours after identification of the index patient). Conversely, chemoprophylaxis administered greater than 14 days after exposure to the index patient is probably of limited or no value. Oropharyngeal or nasopharyngeal cultures are not helpful in determining the need for chemoprophylaxis and might delay institution of this preventive measure unnecessarily.

There is strong evidence that several antibiotics (ie, rifampin, ciprofloxacin, and ceftriaxone) and moderate evidence that other antibiotics (ie, azithromycin and cefixime) are highly effective in eradication of meningococcal carriage (90%–95%).[76–78] The preferred drugs for exposed HCP are rifampin (600 mg orally every 12 hours for 2 days) or ciprofloxacin (500 mg orally × 1 dose). The preferred agent in pregnant women is ceftriaxone (250 mg intramuscularly × 1 dose, diluted with 1% lidocaine to decrease pain at the injection site).[41] Although sporadic resistance to rifampin and ciprofloxacin have been reported worldwide, meningococcal resistance to chemoprophylaxis antibiotics remains rare in the United States.[78] This was recently reaffirmed in a recent population-based surveillance of antimicrobial resistance in N meningitis strains from the United States.[79] All strains tested were susceptible to ceftriaxone and azithromycin; 99% of strains were susceptible to ciprofloxacin and rifampin.

## Varicella

Prior to the introduction of the varicella vaccine in 1995, varicella was a common disease; an average of 4 million people got chickenpox; 10,500 to 13,000 were hospitalized (range, 8000–18,000) and 100 to 150 died each year.[80] Since the introduction of the varicella vaccine, there has been a dramatic decrease in the number of cases of varicella, hospitalizations and deaths.[80] Because varicella may be acquired from exposure to varicella or zoster, however, exposure in health care settings will continue to occur. Multiple nosocomial outbreaks of varicella-zoster virus (VZV) have been reported.[8] Nosocomial transmission has been attributed to delays in the diagnosis or reporting of varicella or HZ and in failures to implement control measures promptly. In hospitals and other health care settings, airborne transmission of VZV from patients with either varicella or HZ has resulted in varicella in HCP and patients who had no direct contact with the index case patient.[80] Although all susceptible patients in health care settings are at risk for severe varicella disease with complications, certain patients without evidence of immunity are at increased risk: pregnant women, premature infants born to susceptible mothers, infants born at less than 28 weeks' gestation or who weigh less than or equal to 1000 g regardless of maternal immune status, and immunocompromised persons of all ages (including persons who are undergoing immunosuppressive therapy, have malignant disease, or are immunodeficient).[80]

Guidelines for postexposure management of HCP exposed to varicella or zoster have been published by the CDC,[8] AAP,[41] and APHA.[42] Exposure to VZV is defined as close contact with an infectious person, such as close indoor contact (eg, in the same room) or face-to-face contact. Experts differ regarding the duration of contact; some suggest 5 minutes, and others up to 1 hour; all agree that it does not include transitory contact.[41] PEP with vaccination or varicella-zoster IG depends on immune status of the exposed HCP. HCP who have received 2 doses of vaccine and who are exposed to VZV (varicella, disseminated HZ, and uncovered lesions of a localized HZ) should be monitored daily during days 8 to 21 after exposure for fever, skin lesions, and systemic symptoms suggestive of varicella. HCP can be monitored directly by occupational health program or infection-control practitioners or instructed to report fever, headache, or other constitutional symptoms and any atypical skin lesions immediately. HCP should be excluded from a work facility immediately if symptoms occur.[8] HCP who have received 1 dose of vaccine and who are exposed to VZV should receive the second dose within 3 to 5 days after exposure to rash (provided 4 weeks have elapsed after the first dose). After vaccination, management is similar to that of 2-dose vaccine recipients. Those who did not receive a second dose or who received the second dose greater than 5 days after exposure should be excluded from work for 8 to 21 days after exposure (see work restrictions discussed later).

For HCP at risk for severe disease for whom varicella vaccination is contraindicated (eg, pregnant or immunocompromised HCP without evidence of immunity), varicella-zoster IG after exposure is recommended. The varicella-zoster IG product currently used in the United States is VariZIG (Cangene Corporation, Winnipeg, Canada).[81] VariZIG, if indicated, should be administered as soon as possible after VZV exposure, ideally within 96 hours for greatest effectiveness but always within 10 days.[81] VariZIG is supplied in 125-IU vials and should be administered intramuscularly; the recommended dose is 125 IU/10 kg of body weight, up to a maximum of 625 IU (5 vials). If VariZIG is indicated but not available or greater than 10 days have elapsed since the exposure, PEP can be provided with oral acyclovir (20 mg/kg per dose administered 4 times per day, maximum daily dose 3200 mg) or oral valacyclovir (20 mg/kg per dose administered 3 times per day, maximum daily dose 3000 mg) beginning on day 8 postexposure and continuing for 7 to 14 days.

## Pertussis

In the United States, the highest recorded annual incidence of pertussis occurred in 1934, when greater than 260,000 cases were reported.[82] After the introduction of diphtheria, tetanus, and whole-cell pertussis vaccine, the incidence dramatically declined. In recent years, however, there has been a resurgence of pertussis. Possible explanations for this increase in disease include (1) genetic changes in *Bordetella pertussis*, making the vaccine less effective; (2) waning immunity among children, adolescents, and adults vaccinated during childhood especially those who received acellular pertussis vaccines; (3) lessened effectiveness of acellular pertussis vaccines compared with whole-cell vaccines; (4) greater awareness of pertussis and hence more diagnostic testing; and (5) the general availability of better laboratory tests.[83]

At the University of North Carolina Hospitals, pertussis is now the most common source of infectious disease exposure evaluations (David Weber, unpublished data, 1994–2015). Multiple nosocomial outbreaks of pertussis have been reported, including outbreaks in which an infected HCP was the source.[84] Nosocomial outbreaks have occurred for several reasons: (1) failure to immunize all HCP with Tdap; (2) failure to recognize and appropriately isolate infected patients, (3) failure to provide antibiotic prophylaxis to exposed staff, and (4) failure to furlough symptomatic staff.[85,86] Seroprevalence studies of HCP who did not receive pertussis vaccine since childhood have revealed that 6.4%[87] and 15%[88] had evidence of recent infection.

Prevention of pertussis transmission in health care settings involves diagnosis and early treatment of clinical cases, droplet isolation of infectious patients, exclusion from work of HCP who are infectious, and PEP.[8] Guidelines for postexposure management of HCP exposed to pertussis have been published by the CDC,[8] AAP,[41] and APHA.[42] Data on the need for PEP in Tdap-vaccinated HCP are inconclusive.[89] Tdap might not preclude the need for PEP. Postexposure antimicrobial prophylaxis is recommended for all HCP who have unprotected exposure to pertussis and are likely to expose a patient at risk for severe pertussis (eg, hospitalized neonates and pregnant women). Other HCP should either receive postexposure antimicrobial prophylaxis or be monitored daily for 21 days after pertussis exposure and treated at the onset of signs and symptoms of pertussis.

*B pertussis* is highly susceptible in vitro to erythromycin[90,91] and the newer macrolides, azithromycin and clarithromycin.[92] It is also susceptible to trimethoprim-sulfamethoxazole.[91–95] Azithromycin has been demonstrated to be effective in the prophylaxis and treatment of pertussis.[96] It is now the preferred agent because, compared with erythromycin, it requires a short period of PEP or therapy (5 vs 7–14 days) and reduced dosing frequency (1 vs 4 times per day) and is less likely to result in gastrointestinal distress.[96] Trimethoprim-sulfamethoxazole is the recommended alternative for treatment and for chemoprophylaxis of individuals intolerant to a macrolide, although its efficacy as a chemoprophylactic agent has not been evaluated.

### Postexposure Prophylaxis: Others

#### Tetanus
Tetanus is an uncommon disease in the United States, with an average of 29 reported cases per year from 1996 through 2009.[97] Nearly all cases of tetanus are among people who have never received tetanus vaccine or adults did not stay current with their 10-year booster shots. HCP are not at greater risk for tetanus than the general population but like other adults may acquire tetanus if they are insufficiently immunized and they have puncture wounds, contaminate open wounds, burns, or crush injuries.[8] HCP with injuries that could lead to tetanus should be evaluated provided appropriate PEP based on the nature of the wound (clean, minor wound vs higher risk wounds) and their history of receipt of tetanus toxoid per recommendations of the CDC[98,99] and AAP.[41] If a tetanus toxoid and diphtheria toxoid (Td) booster is indicated, Tdap can be substituted if the HCP has not already received a Tdap.

## Diphtheria

Although diphtheria was a widespread disease in the United States prior to the use vaccines, it is now a rare disease. Between 2004 and 2015, only 2 cases were reported in the United States, although the disease continues to cause illness globally.[100] The case-fatality rate is still 5% to 10%. HCP are not at greater risk for diphtheria than the general population.[8] For HCP exposed to nasopharyngeal secretions of a patient known or suspected to have diphtheria, the following postexposure measures should be taken regardless of their immunization status: (1) surveillance for 7 days for evidence of disease; (2) culture for *Corynebacterium diphtheria*, and (3) antimicrobial prophylaxis with erythromycin (1 g orally for 7–10 days) or a single injection of penicillin G benzathine (1.2 million U intramuscularly $\times$ 1). Asymptomatic exposed HCP should also receive a booster dose of Td, if they have not received a booster dose of a diphtheria toxoid-containing vaccine within 5 years (Tdap is preferred if the HCP has not received a dose of Tdap previously).[41] Exposed HCP should not receive equine diphtheria antitoxin because there is no evidence that antitoxin provides additional benefits for contacts who have received antimicrobial prophylaxis.

## Measles

The incidence of measles has decreased dramatically since the widespread use MMR vaccine. Since 2000, when measles was declared eliminated from the United States, the annual number of cases has ranged from a low of 37 in 2004 to a high of 667 in 2014.[101] Measles cases in the United States occur as a result of importations by people who were infected while in other countries and from transmission that may occur from those importations. Nosocomial measles is well documented in the literature and may aid in the propagation of community outbreaks.[8,84,102–104] Investigations of individual outbreaks have reported that 17% to 59% of cases were acquired in a medical setting. Measles represents an important health hazard for HCP because of the following: (1) it is highly infectious; (2) transmission via the airborne route; (3) persons become infectious 4 days before the onset of the characteristic rash; and (4) transmission in the outpatient setting has occurred even though the index cases had left the waiting or examination room up to 75 minutes earlier. Because of the greater opportunity for exposure, HCP are at higher risk than the general population for becoming infected with measles.

If measles exposures occur in a health care facility, all nonprotected HCP should be evaluated immediately for presumptive evidence of measles immunity.[8] HCP without evidence of immunity should be offered the first dose of MMR vaccine and excluded from work from day 5 to 21 after exposure.[8] Available data suggest that live virus measles vaccine, if administered within 72 hours of measles exposure, prevents or modifies disease. HCP without evidence of immunity who are not vaccinated after exposure should be removed from all patient contact and excluded from the facility from day 5 after their first exposure through day 21 after the last exposure, even if they have received postexposure intramuscular IG of 0.50 mL/kg; (maximal dose by volume, 15 mL). Those with documentation of 1 vaccine dose may remain at work and should receive the second dose. Immunoglobulin PEP is especially recommended for serosusceptible pregnant women and immunocompromised persons intravenous (400 mg/kg). If IG is administered to an exposed person, observations should continue for signs and symptoms of measles for 28 days after exposure because IG might prolong the incubation period.

## Hepatitis A

Occasional outbreaks of hepatitis A virus (HAV) have been reported in hospitals.[105] Risk factors for HAV transmission to personnel have included activities that increase the risk of fecal-oral contamination, including caring for a person with unrecognized hepatitis A infection; sharing food, beverages, or cigarettes with patients, their families, or the staff; nail biting; handling bile without proper precautions; and not washing hands or wearing gloves when providing care to an infected patients.[105] Routine immunization of HCP with hepatitis A vaccine, however, is not recommended because seroprevalence studies have not demonstrated that HCP are at increased risk for HAV infection because of occupational exposure.[8,105] Maintenance workers may be exposed to sewage are also not at increased risk for acquisition of hepatitis A and do not need to be vaccinated.

Hepatitis A vaccine may be used for PEP and control of nosocomial outbreaks for persons 18 to 40 years of age.[41] In these cases, only monovalent hepatitis A vaccine should be used and should be administered within 14 days of exposure. For persons 41 years old and older, IG (0.02 mL/kg intramuscularly) can be used, although hepatitis A vaccine can be used if IG is not available.[41] The efficacy of hepatitis A vaccine and IG for PEP when administered more than 2 weeks after exposure has not been established.

### Human bites

HCP may occasionally suffer from a human bite, especially when caring for psychiatric patients. After a human bite, a semicircular or oval area of erythema or bruising is usually visible; the skin itself may or may not be intact. Wound care of a human bite is similar to that of an animal bite.[106] The bite area should be managed as follows: (1) clean the wound with an antiseptic; (2) trim any superficial devitalized tissue; (3) remove any foreign bodies or gross wound contaminants; and (4) assess the injury for tendon damage, vascular damage, or penetration into bone or joint. Most human bites should be left open to heal by secondary intention. If the wound may lead to a poor cosmetic result (eg, facial bites), however, the clinician may choose to close the wound. Human bites frequently develop infection. In general, all HCP with a human bite should receive antimicrobial prophylaxis with the first dose provided as soon as possible after the injury.[107] An initial parenteral dose of antibiotics is often provided to rapidly obtain an effective tissue level followed by 3 to 5 days of oral antibiotics.[107] Recommendations for specific antimicrobial therapy have been published.[107]

All HCP suffering bite should be assessed as to whether tetanus prophylaxis should be provided. As discussed previously, human bites may lead to patient-to-HCP and HCP-to-patient transmission of blood-borne pathogens (HIV, HBV, and HCV). Thus the HCP is both an exposed person as well as a potential source for transmission; hence, the same blood work ordered on the source patient should be obtained from the HCP.

### Rabies

Rabies is primarily a disease of animals.[108] The epidemiology of human rabies is a reflection of both the distribution of the disease in animals and the degree of contact with these animals. Rabies is most commonly acquired via a bite or scratch from a rabid animal or from contact between nonintact skin and infective saliva. Saliva and nerve tissue are highly infectious. Generally, contact with other body fluids does not constitute exposure. Uncommon routes of infection include contamination of mucous membranes, corneal transplantation, exposure to aerosols from spelunking or laboratory activities, and iatrogenic infection through improperly inactivated vaccines. Human-to-human transmission has been rarely reported.[108] Human rabies cases in the United States are rare, with only 1 to 3 cases reported annually.[109]

Rabies prophylaxis may occasionally need to be provided to HCP who work out-of-doors (eg, maintenance workers and personnel who care for grounds) and suffer a bite from a wild animal that could potentially transmit rabies (fox, raccoon, and so forth) or who have bat exposure. Concern about rabies transmission is frequent among HCP who have cared for human patients with rabies, especially because fluids from the upper and lower respiratory tracts of humans frequently test positive for rabies virus. One review article reported that approximately 30% of HCP who provided direct care for a patient with rabies were provided PEP.[110] The CDC recommends that patients with possible or known rabies be cared for using standard precautions.[15] Given HCP concerns and the rare possible risk of rabies transmission, however, the authors believe that HCP should use PPE to prevent contact with a patient's saliva and respiratory secretions (ie, gown, gloves, and face shield or mask with eye protection). HCP with mucous membrane or percutaneous skin exposure to a potentially rabid animal or human should receive postexposure rabies vaccine and rabies IG as recommended by the CDC.[111]

## Ectoparasites
Exposure of HCP to ectoparasites (eg, scabies or pediculosis) is likely common. Such exposed personnel should be evaluated for signs and symptoms of an infestation and provided appropriate therapy for confirmed or suspected scabies.[2] Prophylactic treatment should not be provided to personnel, however, who have had skin-to-skin contact with patients or other persons with ectoparasites (eg, scabies).[2]

## Syphilis
HCP are at risk for acquired syphilis via unprotected contact with syphilitic skin lesions, such as chancres (primary stage) and rashes or sores (secondary stage). It can also be acquired via contact with secretions of children with congenital syphilis.[112] Prior to the standard practice of using gloves by HCP to examine patients with skin lesions, there were reports of extragenital syphilitic lesions on HCP. Therefore, HCP who have had unprotected contact with a patient with early congenital syphilis before identification of the disease or during the first 24 hours of therapy should be examined clinically for the presence of lesions 2 to 3 week after contact.[41] Serologic testing should be performed and repeated 3 months after contact or sooner if symptoms occur. HCP with unprotected contact of skin lesions of a patient with primary or secondary state disease should be similarly managed. If the degree of exposure is considered substantial, immediate treatment should be considered.[41] The most current CDC sexually transmitted disease treatment guidelines should be used to guide postexposure therapy.[113]

## Influenza
As discussed previously, all HCP should be immunized annually against influenza. The CDC, however, has provided detailed recommendations on PEP for HCP exposed to influenza as well as the use of antivirals in outbreak situations.[114,115] Unvaccinated HCP who have occupational exposures and who did not use adequate personal protective equipment at the time of exposure are potential candidates for chemoprophylaxis. Decisions on whether to administer antivirals for chemoprophylaxis should take into account an exposed person's risk for influenza complications, the type and duration of contact, recommendations from local or public health authorities, and clinical judgment. Chemoprophylaxis with antiviral medications is not a substitute for influenza vaccination when influenza vaccine is available. HCP receiving PEP should be informed that chemoprophylaxis lowers but does not eliminate the risk for influenza, that susceptibility to influenza returns once the antiviral medication is stopped, and that influenza vaccination is recommended if available. Either oseltamivir or zanamivir is recommended for antiviral chemoprophylaxis of influenza A (2009 H1N1), influenza

**Table 5**
Recommended work restrictions for health care personnel colonized/exposed or infected with selected infectious agents

| Infection or Infectious Agent | Exposed or Colonized | Infected (Duration of Restrictions) |
|---|---|---|
| Conjunctivitis (adenovirus) | Exposed; no restriction unless illness develops | Restrict from patient contact and contact with the patient's environment (until discharge ceases) |
| Cytomegalovirus | No restriction | No restriction |
| Diarrheal diseases | No restriction unless illness develops | Acute disease: exclude from duty (until >48–72 h after symptoms resolve) Convalescent stage (Salmonella spp): restrict from care of high-risk patients and food handling (until symptoms resolve; consult local and state authorities for HCP/food handlers with Salmonella typhi) |
| Diphtheria | Exposed: no restriction unless illness develops | Exclude from duty (until antimicrobial therapy completed and 2 cultures obtained ≥24 h apart are negative) |
| Hepatitis A | Exposed: no restriction unless illness develops | Restrict from patient contact, contact with patient's environment, and food handling (until 7 d after onset of jaundice) |
| Hepatitis B (chronic) | — | Restrictions based on review of only HCP who perform exposure-prone procedures by expert panel (see text) |
| Hepatitis C | — | Restrictions based on review of HCP who perform exposure-prone procedures by expert panel (see text) |
| Herpes simplex (genital) | — | No restriction |
| Herpes simplex (hands; herpetic whitlow) | — | Restrict from patient contact and contact with the patient's environment (until lesions heal) |
| Herpes simplex (orofacial) | — | Evaluate for need to restrict from care of high-risk patients |
| HIV | — | Restrictions based on review of HCP who perform exposure-prone procedures by expert panel (see text) |
| Measles | Exposed (susceptible HCP): exclude from duty (From the 5th day after 1st exposure through 21st day after last exposure and/or after rash appears) | Exclude from duty (until 7 d after the rash appears) |
| Meningococcal infections | Exposed: no restriction unless illness develops Colonized (unrelated to invasive case): no restriction | Exclude from duty (until 24 h after start of effective therapy) |

| | | |
|---|---|---|
| Methicillin-resistant *Staphylococcus aureus* | Colonized: no restrictions unless or ill or epidemiologically/molecular test linked to patient infections | Allow to work provided lesions can be contained under a bandage and clothes; if lesions on exposed area (eg, hand/wrists, face/neck), exclude from duty (until lesions healed) |
| Mumps | Exposed (susceptible HCP): exclude from duty (from the 12th day after 1st exposure through 26th day after last exposure or after onset of parotitis) | Exclude from duty (until 9 d after onset of parotitis) |
| Pertussis | Exposure (asymptomatic): no restriction unless develops illness (PEP recommended) Exposed (symptomatic): per active disease | Exclude from duty (from beginning of catarrhal stage through 3rd week after onset of paroxysms or until 5 d after start of effective antimicrobial therapy) |
| Rubella | Exposed (susceptible HCP): exclude from duty (from 7th day after 1st exposure through 21st day after last exposure) | Exclude from duty (until 5 d after rash appears) |
| Group A streptococcus | Colonized: no restrictions unless or ill or epidemiologically/molecular test linked to patient infections | Restrict from patient care, contact with patient's environment, or food handling (until 24 h after adequate treatment started) |
| Tuberculosis | Latent tuberculous infection: no restrictions | Active pulmonary tuberculosis; exclude from duty (until proved noninfectious) |
| Varicella | Exposed (susceptible): exclude from duty (from 10th day after 1st exposure through 21st day [27th day if varicella IG provided] after last exposure) | Exclude from duty (until all lesions dried and crusted) |
| Zoster | Exposed (susceptible): same as varicella | Localized, in healthy HCP: Allow to work provided lesions can be contained under a bandage and clothes; if lesions on exposed area (eg, hand/wrists, face/neck), exclude from duty (until lesions dried and crusted) Generalized or localized in immunosuppressed HCP: exclude from duty (until all lesions dried and crusted) |
| Viral respiratory tract infections (acute) | No restrictions unless illness develops[a] | Febrile: exclude from duty (until afebrile for >24 h) Afebrile: exclude from care immunocompromised patients (ie, patients cared for in a protected environment) (until afebrile for >24 h or 7 d since onset of symptoms, whichever is longer) – HCP should wear a mask providing care until symptom-free |

[a] Consider restrictions if HCP exposed to high-contagious disease transmitted by the respiratory route or close contact (Middle East respiratory syndrome–coronavirus, Ebola virus, etc.).

*Adapted from* Boylard EA, Tablan OC, Williams WW, et al. Guideline for infection control in health care personnel. 1998. Available at: http://www.cdc.gov/hicpac/pubs.html; and Advisory Committee on Immunization Practices, Centers for Disease Control and Prevention. Immunization of Health-Care Personnel Recommendations of the Advisory Committee on Immunization Practices (ACIP). MMWR Recomm Rep 2011;60(RR-7):1–45.

A (H3N2), or influenza B influenza virus infection. An emphasis on early treatment is an alternative to chemoprophylaxis in managing HCP who have had a suspected exposure to influenza virus. Postexposure chemoprophylaxis is typically administered for a total of not more than 10 days after the most recent known exposure to a close contact known to have influenza.

Chemoprophylaxis can also be used as a control measure in outbreaks in health care facilities, especially if they house patients at higher risk for influenza complications.[114,115] In addition to antiviral medications, other outbreak-control measures include instituting droplet and contact precautions and establishing cohorts of patients with confirmed or suspected influenza, reoffering influenza vaccination (if available) to unvaccinated staff and patients, restricting staff movement between wards or buildings, and restricting contact between ill staff or visitors and patients. Chemoprophylaxis should be considered for all employees, regardless of their influenza vaccination status, if indications exist that the outbreak is caused by a strain of influenza virus that is not well matched by the vaccine. Such indications might include multiple documented breakthrough influenza virus infections among vaccinated persons who otherwise would be expected to respond to vaccination, studies indicating low vaccine effectiveness, or circulation in the surrounding community of suspected index case(s) of strains not contained in the vaccine. Specific antiviral dosing recommendations (drug, dose, route, and duration) are available from the CDC.

### EVALUATION OF ILL HEALTH CARE PERSONNEL

HCP exposed to a communicable disease for which they are susceptible should be considered for work restrictions or furlough (**Table 5**). Similarly, HCP ill with a communicable disease susceptible should be considered for work restrictions or furlough (see **Table 5**). Importantly, infectious HCP have been the source for patient infection and the index case for outbreaks.[84,102] HCP-to-patient transmission has been well documented for HIV, HBV, and HCV but has most commonly been reported with HBV. For this reason, infected HCP who perform invasive procedures should be evaluated by a special panel for the need for education, additional engineering controls, and/or work restrictions per current guidelines from the Society for Healthcare Epidemiology of America[116] and CDC.[117] The differences between these guidelines has been described.[120]

### REFERENCES

1. Centers for Disease Control and Prevention. Workplace safety & health topics. Healthcare workers. Available at: http://www.cdc.gov/niosh/topics/healthcare/. Accessed December 26, 2015.
2. Bolyard EA, Tablan OC, Williams WW, et al. Guideline for infection control in health care personnel. Am J Infect Control 1998;26:289–354.
3. Chong CY, Goldmann DA, Huskins WC. Prevention of occupationally acquired infections among health-care workers. Pediatr Rev 1998;19:219–31.
4. Health Canada. Prevention and control of occupational infections in health care. An infection control guideline. Can Commun Dis Rep 2002;28(Suppl 1):1–264.
5. Sepkowitz KA, Eisenberg L. Occupational deaths among healthcare workers. Emerg Infect Dis 2005;11:1003–8.
6. Weber DJ, Rutala WA, Schaffner W. Lessons learned: protection of healthcare workers from infectious disease risks. Crit Care Med 2010;38(Suppl):S306–14.

7. Sebazco S. Occupational health. In: Grota P, editor. APIC text of infection control and epidemiology. 4th edition. Washington, DC: Association for Professionals in Infection Control and Epidemiology; 2014. p. 100.1–100.16.

8. Centers for Disease Control and Prevention. Immunization of health-care personnel: recommendations of the advisory committee on immunization practices (ACIP). MMWR Recomm Rep 2011;60(RR–7):1–45.

9. Talbot TR. Update on immunizations for healthcare personnel in the United States. Vaccine 2014;32:4869–75.

10. Sparks V. Immunization of healthcare personnel. In: Grota P, editor. APIC text of infection control and epidemiology. 4th edition. Washington, DC: Association for Professionals in Infection Control and Epidemiology; 2014. p. 103.1–103.36.

11. American Academy of Pediatrics. Immunization in health care personnel. In: Kimberlin DW, Brady MT, Jackson MS, et al, editors. Red Book: 2015 report of communicable diseases. 30th edition. Elk Grove Village (IL): American Academy of Pediatrics; 2015. p. 95–8.

12. Tolle MA, Schwarzwald HL. Postexposure prophylaxis against human immunodeficiency virus [review]. Am Fam Physician 2010;82(2):161–6.

13. Grant RM. Antiretroviral agents used by HIV-uninfected persons for prevention: pre- and postexposure prophylaxis. Clin Infect Dis 2010;50(Suppl 3):S96–101.

14. Bader MS, McKinsey DS. Postexposure prophylaxis for common infectious diseases. Am Fam Physician 2013;88:25–32.

15. Seigel JD, Rhinehart E, Jackson M, et al. The Healthcare Infection Control Practices Advisory Committee. 2007 guideline for isolation precautions: preventing transmission of infectious agents in healthcare settings. Available at: www.cdc.gov/hicpac/pdf/isolation/Isolation2007.pdf. Accessed December 24, 2015.

16. Boyce JM, Pittet D. Guideline for hand hygiene in health-care settings. Am J Infect Control 2002;30:1–46.

17. World Health Organization. WHO guidelines on hand hygiene in health care. Available at: http://whqlibdoc.who.int/publications/2009/9789241597906_eng.pd. Accessed December 24, 2015.

18. Boyce JM. Update on hand hygiene. Am J Infect Control 2013;41(Suppl 5):S94–6.

19. Seigel JD, Rhinehart E, Jackson M, et al. The healthcare infection control practices advisory committee. Management of multidrug-resistant organisms in healthcare settings. 2006. Available at: www.cdc.gov/hicpac/pdf/guidelines/MDROGuideline2006.pdf. Accessed December 24, 2015.

20. Centers for Disease Control and Prevention. Guidance for control of infections with carbapenem-resistant or carbapenemase-producing Enterobacteriaceae in acute care facilities. MMWR Morb Mortal Wkly Rep 2009;58:256–60.

21. MacIntyre CR, Chughtai AA. Facemasks for the prevention of infection in health-care and community settings. BMJ 2015;350:h694.

22. Wagar E. Bioterrorism and the role of the clinical microbiology laboratory. Clin Microbiol Rev 2016;29:175–89.

23. Centers for Disease Control and Prevention. Biosafety in microbiological and biomedical laboratories (BMBL). 5th edition. Available at: http://www.cdc.gov/biosafety/publications/bmbl5/. Accessed March 10, 2016.

24. U.S. Occupational Safety and Health Administration. Bloodborne pathogens (1910.1030). Available at: https://www.osha.gov/pls/oshaweb/owadisp.show_document?p_table=STANDARDS&p_id=10051. Accessed January 29, 2016.

25. U.S. Occupational Safety and Health Administration. Respiratory Protection (1910.134). Available at: https://www.osha.gov/pls/oshaweb/owadisp.show_document?p_id=12716&p_table=standards. Accessed March 5, 2016.

26. Kanamori H, Weber DJ, DiBiase LM, et al. Impact of safety-engineered devices on the incidence of occupational blood and body fluid exposures among healthcare personnel in an academic facility, 2000-2014. Infect Control Hosp Epidemiol 2016;37(5):497–504.

27. Centers for Disease Control and Prevention. General recommendations on immunization: Recommendations of the Advisory Committee on Immunization Practices (ACIP). MMWR Recomm Rep 2011;60(2):1–61.

28. Centers for Disease Control and Prevention. Advisory committee on immunization practices recommended immunization schedule for adults aged 19 years or older — United States, 2016. MMWR Morb Mortal Wkly Rep 2016;64:88–90.

29. Talbot TR, Babcock H, Caplan AL, et al. Revised SHEA position paper: influenza vaccination of healthcare personnel. Infect Control Hosp Epidemiol 2010;31: 987–95.

30. Lee LM. Adding justice to the clinical and public health ethics arguments for mandatory seasonal influenza immunization for healthcare workers. J Med Ethics 2015;41:682–6.

31. Poland GA. Mandating influenza vaccination for health care workers: Putting patients and professional ethics over personal preference. Vaccine 2010;28: 5757–9.

32. National Vaccine Advisory Committee. Recommendations on strategies to achieve the Healthy People 2020 annual vaccine coverage goal for health care personnel. Available at: nvac_adult_immunization_work_group.pdf. Accessed March 10, 2016.

33. Centers for Disease Control and Prevention. CDC information for international travel 2016. Available at: http://wwwnc.cdc.gov/travel/page/yellowbook-home-2014. Accessed March 10, 2016.

34. Centers for Disease Control and Prevention. Epidemiology and prevention of vaccine-preventable diseases. Available at: http://www.cdc.gov/vaccines/pubs/pinkbook/index.html. Accessed March 10, 2016.

35. Rubin LG, Levin MJ, Ljungman P, et al. 2013 IDSA clinical practice guideline for vaccination of the immunocompromised host. Clin Infect Dis 2014;58:309–18.

36. Talbot TR, Babcock H, Cotton D, et al. The use of live attenuated influenza vaccine (LAIV) in healthcare personnel (HCP): guidance from the Society for Healthcare Epidemiology of America (SHEA). Infect Control Hosp Epidemiol 2012;33:981–3.

37. Bazan JA, Mangino JE. Infection control and postexposure prophylaxis for the pregnant healthcare worker. Clin Obstet Gynecol 2012;55:571–88.

38. Rasmussen SA, Watson AK, Kennedy ED, et al. Vaccines and pregnancy: past, present, and future. Semin Fetal Neonatal Med 2014;19:161–9.

39. Chu HY, Englund JA. Maternal immunization. Clin Infect Dis 2014;59:560–8.

40. Swamy GK, Beigi RH. Maternal benefits of immunization during pregnancy. Vaccine 2015;33:6436–40.

41. American Academy of Pediatrics. Section 3: summaries of infectious diseases. In: Kimberlin DW, Brady MT, Jackson MS, et al, editors. Red Book: 2015 report of communicable diseases. 30th edition. Elk Grove Village (IL): American Academy of Pediatrics; 2015. p. 225–870.

42. American Association of Public Health. Control of communicable diseases. In: Heymann DL, editor. Control of Communicable Diseases Manual. 20th edition. Washington, DC: APHA Press; 2015. p. 1–692.

43. Centers for Disease Control and Prevention. Sharps safety for healthcare settings. Available at: http://www.cdc.gov/sharpssafety/index.html. Accessed March 11, 2016.
44. Tarantola A, Abiteboul D, Rachline A. Infection risks following accidental exposure to blood or body fluids in health care workers: a review of pathogens transmitted in published cases. Am J Infect Control 2006;34:367–75.
45. Deuffic-Burban S, Delarocque-Astagneau E, Abiteboul D, et al. Blood-borne viruses in health care workers: prevention and management. J Clin Virol 2011;52: 4–10.
46. Centers for Disease Control and Prevention. Recommendations for postexposure interventions to prevent infection with hepatitis B virus, hepatitis C virus, or human immunodeficiency virus, and tetanus in persons wounded during bombings and other mass-casualty event, US, 2008. MMWR Recomm Rep 2008;57(RR06):1–19. Available at: http://www.cdc.gov/mmwr/preview/mmwrhtml/rr5706a1.htm. Accessed March 10, 2016.
47. Bond WW, Favero MS, Petersen NJ, et al. Survival of hepatitis B virus after drying and storage for one week. Lancet 1981;1(8219):550–1.
48. Kamili S, Krawczynski K, McCaustland K, et al. Infectivity of hepatitis C virus in plasma after drying and storing at room temperature. Infect Control Hosp Epidemiol 2007;28:519–24.
49. Doerrbecker J, Friesland M, Ciesek S, et al. Inactivation and survival of hepatitis C virus on inanimate surfaces. J Infect Dis 2011;204:1830–8.
50. Paintsil E, Binka M, Patel A, et al. Hepatitis C virus maintains infectivity for weeks after drying on inanimate surfaces at room temperature: implications for risks of transmission. Infect Dis 2014;209:1205–11.
51. Tjøtta E, Hungnes O, Grinde B. Survival of HIV-1 activity after disinfection, temperature and pH changes, or drying. J Med Virol 1991;35:223–7.
52. van Bueren J, Simpson RA, Jacobs P, et al. Survival of human immunodeficiency virus in suspension and dried onto surfaces. J Clin Microbiol 1994;32:571–4.
53. Centers for Disease Control and Prevention. CDC guidance for evaluating health-care personnel for hepatitis B virus protection and for administering postexposure management. MMWR Recomm Rep 2013;62(RR–10):1–19.
54. Henderson D. Managing occupational risks for hepatitis C transmission in the healthcare setting. Clin Microbiol Rev 2003;16:546–68.
55. Gane E, Calder L. Transmission of HBV from patient to healthcare worker. N Z Med J 2008;121:87–8.
56. Akhtar S, Moatter T, Azam SI, et al. Prevalence and risk factors for intrafamilial transmission of hepatitis C virus in Karachi, Pakistan. J Viral Hepat 2002;9: 309–14.
57. Richman KM, Rickman LS. The potential for transmission of human immunodeficiency virus through human bites. J Acquir Immnune Defic Syndr 1993;6: 402–6.
58. Michelin A, Henderson DK. Infection control guidelines for prevention of health care-associated transmission of hepatitis B and C viruses. Clin Liver Dis 2010; 14:119–36.
59. Henderson DK. Management of needlestick injuries: a house officer who has a needlestick. JAMA 2012;307:75–84.
60. Kuhar DT, Henderson DK, Struble KA, et al. US Public Health Service Working Group. Updated US Public Health Service guidelines for the management of occupational exposures to human immunodeficiency virus and

recommendations for postexposure prophylaxis. Infect Control Hosp Epidemiol 2013;34:875–92.

61. Beekmann SE, Henderson DK. Prevention of human immunodeficiency virus and AIDS: postexposure prophylaxis (including health care workers). Infect Dis Clin North Am 2014;28:601–13.

62. Riddell A, Kennedy I, Tong CY. Management of sharps injuries in the healthcare setting. BMJ 2015;351:h3733.

63. Centers for Disease Control and Prevention. HIV/AIDS: Basic statistics. Available at: http://www.cdc.gov/hiv/basics/statistics.html. Accessed March 10, 2016.

64. Joyce MP, Kuhar D, Brooks JT. Notes from the field: occupationally acquired HIV infection among health care workers - United States, 1985-2013. MMWR Morb Mortal Wkly Rep 2015;63:1245–6.

65. Grant RM, Smith DK. Integrating antiretroviral strategies for human immunodeficiency virus prevention: post- and pre-exposure prophylaxis and early treatment. Open Forum Infect Dis 2015;2(4):ofv126.

66. Ford N, Shubber Z, Calmy A, et al. Choice of antiretroviral drugs for postexposure prophylaxis for adults and adolescents: a systematic review. Clin Infect Dis 2015;60(Suppl 3):S170–6.

67. Centers for Disease Control and Prevention. Meningococcal disease. Available at: http://www.cdc.gov/meningococcal/index.html. Accessed March 10, 2016.

68. Centers for Disease Control and Prevention. ABCs Report: Neisseria meningitidis, provisional-2014. Available at: http://www.cdc.gov/abcs/reports-findings/survreports/mening14.html. Accessed March 10, 2016.

69. Halperin SA, Bettinger JA, Greenwood B, et al. The changing and dynamic epidemiology of meningococcal disease. Vaccine 2012;30(Suppl 2):B26–36.

70. Dwilow R, Fanella S. Invasive meningococcal disease in the 21st century—an update for the clinician. Curr Neurol Neurosci Rep 2015;15:2.

71. Abio A, Neal KR, Beck CR. An epidemiological review of changes in meningococcal biology during the last 100 years. Pathog Glob Health 2013;107:373–80.

72. Centers for Disease Control and Prevention. Occupational transmission of Neisseria meningitidis - California, 2009. MMWR Morb Mortal Wkly Rep 2010;59:1480–3.

73. Sejvar JJ, Johnson D, Popovic T, et al. Assessing the risk of laboratory-acquired meningococcal disease. J Clin Microbiol 2005;43:4811–4.

74. Sheets CD, Harriman K, Zipprich J, et al. Fatal meningococcal disease in a laboratory worker–California, 2012. MMWR Morb Mortal Wkly Rep 2014;63:770–2.

75. Telisinghe L, Waite TD, Gobin M. Chemoprophylaxis and vaccination in preventing subsequent cases of meningococcal disease in household contacts of a case of meningococcal disease: a systematic review. Epidemiol Infect 2015;143:2259–68.

76. Hanquet G, Stefanoff P, Hellenbrand W, et al. Strong public health recommendations from weak evidence? Lessons learned in developing guidance on the public health management of meningococcal disease. Biomed Res Int 2015;2015:569235.

77. Zalmanovici Trestioreanu A, Fraser A, Gafter-Gvili A, et al. Antibiotics for preventing meningococcal infections. Cochrane Database Syst Rev 2013;(10):CD004785.

78. Centers for Disease Control and Prevention. Prevention and control of meningococcal disease: recommendations of the advisory committee on immunization practices (ACIP). MMWR Recomm Rep 2013;62(2):1–28.

79. Harcourt BH, Anderson RD, Wu HM, et al. Population-based surveillance of Neisseria meningitidis antimicrobial resistance in the United States. Open Forum Infect Dis 2015;2(3):ofv117.
80. Centers for Disease Control and Prevention. Monitoring the impact of varicella immunization. Available at: http://www.cdc.gov/chickenpox/hcp/monitoring-varicella.html. Accessed March 10, 2016.
81. Centers for Disease Control and Prevention. Updated recommendations for use of VariZIG — United States, 2013. MMWR Morb Mortal Wkly Rep 2013;62: 574–6.
82. Centers for Disease Control and Prevention. Pertussis: surveillance and reporting. Available at: http://www.cdc.gov/pertussis/surv-reporting.html. Accessed March 10, 2016.
83. Cherry JD. Pertussis: challenges today and for the future. PLoS Pathog 2013; 9(7):e1003418.
84. Sydnor E, Perl TM. Healthcare providers as sources of vaccine-preventable diseases. Vaccine 2014;32:4814–22.
85. Weber DJ, Rutala WA. Pertussis: an underappreciated risk for nosocomial outbreaks. Infect Control Hosp Epidemiol 1998;19:825–8.
86. Weber DJ, Rutala WA. Pertussis: a continuing hazard for healthcare facilities. Infect Control Hosp Epidemiol 2001;22:736–40.
87. Cunegundes KS, de Moraes-Pinto MI, Takahashi TN, et al. Bordetella pertussis infection in paediatric healthcare workers. J Hosp Infect 2015;90:163–6.
88. Urbiztondo L, Broner S, Costa J, et al. Seroprevalence study of B. pertussis infection in health care workers in Catalonia, Spain. Hum Vaccin Immunother 2015;11:293–7.
89. Goins WP, Edwards KM, Vnencak-Jones CL, et al. A comparison of 2 strategies to prevent infection following pertussis exposure in vaccinated healthcare personnel. Clin Infect Dis 2012;54:938–45.
90. Zackrisson G, Brorson J-E, Krantz I, et al. In-vitro sensitivity of Bordetella pertussis. J Antimicrob Chemother 1983;11:407–11.
91. Kurzynski T, Boehm DM, Rott-Petri JA, et al. Antimicrobial susceptibilities of Bordetella species isolated in a multicenter pertussis surveillance project. Antimicrob Agents Chemother 1988;32:137–40.
92. Hoppe JE, Eichhorn A. Activity of new macrolides against Bordetella pertussis and Bordetella parapertussis. Eur J Clin Microbiol Infect Dis 1989;8:653–4.
93. Granstrom G, Sterner G, Nord CE, et al. Use of erythromycin to prevent pertussis in newborns of mothers with pertussis. J Infect Dis 1987;155:1210–4.
94. Sprauer MA, Cochi SL, Zell ER, et al. Prevention of secondary transmission of pertussis in households with early use of erythromycin. Am J Dis Child 1992; 146:177–81.
95. De Serres G, Boulianne N, Duval B. Field effectiveness of erythromycin prophylaxis to prevent pertussis within families. Pediatr Infect Dis J 1995;4:969–75.
96. Altunaiji S, Kukuruzovic R, Curtis N, et al. Antibiotics for whooping cough (pertussis). Cochrane Database Syst Rev 2007;(3):CD004404.
97. Centers for Disease Control and Prevention. About tetanus. Available at: http://www.cdc.gov/tetanus/about/index.html. Accessed March 8, 2016.
98. Centers Disease Control and Prevention. Tetanus: epidemiology and prevention of vaccine-preventable disease. In: Hamborsky J, Kroger A, Wolfe CS, editors. The pink book. 13th edition. Atlanta (GA): Centers for Disease Control and Prevention; 2015. p. 341–52. Available at: http://www.cdc.gov/vaccines/pubs/pinkbook/tetanus.html. Accessed March 10, 2016.

99. Centers Disease Control and Prevention. Preventing tetanus, diphtheria, and pertussis among adults: use of tetanus toxoid, reduced diphtheria toxoid and acellular pertussis vaccine. recommendations of the advisory committee on immunization practices (ACIP) and Recommendation of ACIP, supported by the healthcare infection control practices advisory committee (HICPAC), for use of Tdap among health-care personnel. MMWR Recomm Rep 2006;55(RR17):1–33.
100. Centers for Disease Control and Prevention. Diphtheria. Available at: http://www.cdc.gov/diphtheria/clinicians.html. Accessed March 8, 2016.
101. Centers for Disease Control and Prevention. Measles: Clinical features. Available at: http://www.cdc.gov/measles/hcp/index.html. Accessed March 20, 2016.
102. Huttunen R, Syrjänen J. Healthcare workers as vectors of infectious diseases. Eur J Clin Microbiol Infect Dis 2014;33:1477–88.
103. Maltezou HC, Wicker S. Measles in health-care settings. Am J Infect Control 2013;41:661–3.
104. Botelho-Nevers E, Gautreta P, Biellke R, et al. Nosocomial transmission of measles: an updated review. Vaccine 2012;30:3996–4001.
105. Weber DJ, Rutala WA, Weigle K. Selection and use of vaccines for healthcare workers. Infect Control Hosp Epidemiol 1997;18:682.
106. Weber DJ, Hansen AR. Infections resulting from animal bites. Infect Dis Clin North Am 1991;5:663–80.
107. Endom EE. Initial management of animal and human bites. UpToDate 2016.
108. Weber DJ, Rutala WA. Risks and prevention of nosocomial transmission of rare zoonotic diseases. Clin Infect Dis 2001;32:446–56.
109. Centers for Disease Control and Prevention. Rabies: human rabies. Available at: http://www.cdc.gov/rabies/location/usa/surveillance/human_rabies.html. Accessed March 10, 2016.
110. Helmick CG, Tauxe RV, Vernon AA. Is there a risk to contacts of patients with rabies? Rev Infect Dis 1987;9:511–8.
111. Centers for Disease Control and Prevention. Use of a reduced (4-dose) vaccine schedule for postexposure prophylaxis to prevent human rabies: recommendations of the advisory committee on immunization practices. MMWR Recomm Rep 2010;59(RR02):1–9.
112. Stoltey JE, Cohen SE. Syphilis transmission: a review of the current evidence. Sex Health 2015. http://dx.doi.org/10.1071/SH14174.
113. Workowski K, Bolan GA. Sexually transmitted diseases treatment guidelines, 2015. MMWR Morb Mortal Wkly Rep 2015;64(3):1–144.
114. Centers for Disease Control and Prevention. Influenza: use of antiviral. http://www.cdc.gov/flu/professionals/antivirals/antiviral-use-influenza.htm. Available at: Accessed March 10, 2016.
115. Fiore AE, Fry A, Shay D, et al. Antiviral agents for the treatment and chemoprophylaxis of influenza: recommendations of the advisory committee on immunization practices (ACIP). MMWR Recomm Rep 2011;60(RR01):1–24.
116. Henderson DK, Dembry L, Fishman NO, et al. SHEA guideline for management of healthcare workers who are infected with hepatitis B virus, hepatitis C virus, and/or human immunodeficiency virus. Infect Control Hosp Epidemiol 2010;31:203–32.
117. Centers for Disease Control and Prevention. Updated CDC recommendations for the management of hepatitis B virus-infected health-care providers and students. MMWR Recomm Rep 2012;61(RR–3):1–12.

118. Weber DJH, Consoli S, Sickbert-Bennett E, et al. Susceptibility to measles, mumps, and rubella in newly hired (2006-2008) healthcare workers born before 1957. Infect Contr Hosp Epidemiology 2010;31:655–7.

119. Troioni L, Hill JJ 3rd, Consoli S, et al. Varicella-Zoster Immunity in US Healthcare Personnel With Self-Reported History of Disease. Infect Contr Hosp Epidemiol 2015;36:1467–8.

120. Henderson DK. Changing times, changing landscapes: comparing the Society for Healthcare Epidemiology of America's infected provider guidelines with the Centers for Disease Control and Prevention's Guidelines for managing providers INFECTED with hepatitis B virus. Infect Control Hosp Epidemiol 2012;33: 1152–5.

# Informatics in Infection Control

Michael Y. Lin, MD, MPH[a],*, William E. Trick, MD[a,b]

## KEYWORDS

- Infection control • Informatics • Surveillance • Prevention • Public health

## KEY POINTS

- In the age of digitized medical data, informatics tools are integral to routine infection control activities.
- Computer software can partially or fully automate infection surveillance, improving efficiency and reliability.
- Informatics are used for infection prevention, primarily through clinical decision support.
- Informatics link clinical and public health activities through electronic laboratory reporting, syndromic surveillance, and enhanced interfacility communication, which improves the timeliness of disease reporting, and outbreak detection and intervention.

The term "informatics" describes the use of computer information systems to answer questions, solve problems, and make decisions[1]; for the purpose of this paper, it refers to the use of computer information systems to control and prevent infection. As medical information becomes digitized, computer applications are an important part of everyday infection control practice. Informatics has the potential to improve infection control outcomes in three major domains: (1) surveillance, (2) prevention, and (3) connections with public health (**Box 1**). Furthermore, informatics can connect individual facility infection control programs with each other in a way that is similar to what the Internet did for stand-alone desktop computers; such connectedness improves regional control of antibiotic resistance by enhancing interfacility communication and facilitating outbreak detection across multiple facilities. This article reviews the current and emerging use of informatics for infection control.

## BACKGROUND

The adoption of electronic medical record systems in the United States has skyrocketed; the percentage of hospitals with at least a basic electronic medical record

Disclosure Statement: The authors have nothing to disclose.
[a] Department of Medicine, Rush University Medical Center, 600 South Paulina Street, Suite 143, Chicago, IL 60612, USA; [b] Department of Medicine, Cook County Health and Hospitals System, 1900 West Polk Street, Suite 1600, Chicago, IL 60612, USA
* Corresponding author.
E-mail address: Michael_Lin@rush.edu

---

**Box 1**
**Uses of informatics in infection control**

*Surveillance*

- Fully or semiautomated surveillance of infections
- Fully automated device counting (denominator)
- Outbreak detection, single institution or ward

*Prevention*

- Awareness of multidrug-resistant organism carriage on admission
- Enhanced interfacility communication
- Identifying inappropriate infection precautions
- Reducing device use
- Antimicrobial stewardship

*Public health*

- Electronic communicable disease reporting
- Syndromic surveillance
- Regional outbreak detection

---

increased from approximately 10% in 2008 to 75% in 2014.[2] Patient information relevant to the infection control department (including microbiology and laboratory test results, patient location, presence of invasive devices, and infection precautions status) is stored electronically, enabling computers to automate processes that were previously performed by hand.

The automation of infection control has improved efficiency, allowing a single infection preventionist to perform more surveillance than previously possible. Historically, surveillance of hospital-acquired bloodstream infections focused on the intensive care unit in part because of feasibility; now, with the use of automated surveillance, bloodstream infection surveillance is performed across the entire hospital. Whether the adoption of informatics results in a net savings of time is unclear; the trade-off of surveillance efficiency is the generation of more data to review, which competes with time spent on the hospital floor interacting with hospital staff. Ultimately, the critical question is whether the implementation of informatics improves patient safety.

## INFECTION SURVEILLANCE

Surveillance is a cornerstone of infection prevention. Hospitals use surveillance data to identify trends within wards (eg, is infection increasing in the particular intensive care unit); public health officials, payors, and consumers use surveillance data to compare performance among hospitals (eg, does Hospital A have a higher infection rate than Hospital B). The objectives of surveillance definitions are clearly different from that of clinical diagnostic criteria, which are used to help providers treat patients. Thus, although clinical diagnostic criteria relies heavily on human judgement to determine whether or not a patient has a disease, surveillance definitions work best when the definitions are as objective as possible, to reduce subjectivity and increase reliability between infection preventionists.[3]

An example of subjective versus objective surveillance definition is *Clostridium difficile* surveillance. The National Healthcare Safety Network (NHSN) endorses two options for tracking *C difficile*: the Infection Surveillance definition (subjective) and the laboratory-identified (LabID) event (objective).[4] Although the infection surveillance definition requires that the infection preventionist determine onset of diarrheal symptoms via review of chart documentation (which requires interpretation of nonspecific stool description, such as "loose"), the LabID event ignores symptoms and is only concerned with the collection date of the first positive *C difficile* test and whether that falls within the first 3 calendar days of admission (community onset) or later (hospital onset). Although clinicians and some reviewers are frustrated with not being able to interpret nuanced information, laboratory-based surveillance events are computable and theoretically do not need human effort, improving reliability and reducing burden on infection preventionists.

Surveillance metrics typically comprise numerator counts (how many events occurred) and denominator counts (how many patient days at risk). Ideally, infection control software assists infection preventionists with determining both types of counts.

### Fully Automated Versus Semiautomated Surveillance

In general, computer surveillance of health care–associated infections can be fully automated or semiautomated.[5,6] Fully automated surveillance can occur when the surveillance definition is completely computable (eg, *C difficile* LabID event). Alternatively, semiautomated surveillance occurs when the computer performs part of the surveillance (eg, case-finding using specified criteria) and a human performs the rest. For example, a computer may identify a candidate central line–associated bloodstream infection (CLABSI), based on a positive blood culture and the presence of a central line; the infection preventionist then reviews the chart to judge whether the bloodstream pathogen originated from a central line versus an extravascular source (eg, a urinary tract infection).

### Common Data Sources Needed for Surveillance Informatics

All computer software programs for infection control (whether provided by a commercial vendor or home grown) require access to specific types of data. For all types of infection surveillance, software systems need microbiology and laboratory results to determine positive cultures and diagnostic tests. To determine where the patient is at the time of infection, software programs also need access to the admission/discharge/transfer dataset. Other metric-specific data requirements are outlined next and in **Table 1**.

### Examples of Surveillance Metrics Enhanced by Informatics

#### Central line–associated bloodstream infections
The NHSN definition of CLABSI requires judgement on the part of infection preventionists, who must decide whether an organism recovered from a positive blood culture originated from a central line versus an extravascular source. Thus, agreement between infection preventionists is imperfect, even when reviewing an identical case,[7] hampering the ability to compare hospitals based on CLABSI rates.[8] In response, NHSN has made the CLABSI definition more objective over time (eg, making the definition of a secondary bacteremia stricter). Because some subjective elements require human judgment, most surveillance software programs offer a semiautomated approach to bloodstream infection surveillance: candidate positive blood cultures that occur in the presence of a central line are presented by the software to the infection preventionist for review. Semiautomated approaches work best when the computer algorithm has a high negative predictive value for infection,[9] thereby sparing

**Table 1**
**Key data elements necessary for electronic surveillance of health care–associated infections**

| NHSN Surveillance Metric | Key Electronic Data Elements | Barriers to Fully Automated Electronic Surveillance |
|---|---|---|
| Central line–associated line infection | Microbiology cultures (blood and nonblood sites), ADT, central venous catheter presence | Current definition requires judgment regarding the origin of the blood pathogen |
| Catheter-associated urinary tract infection | Microbiology cultures (urine only), urinalysis, ADT, vital signs (fever), urinary catheter presence | Current definition requires assessment of patient symptoms |
| Surgical site infection | Microbiology cultures (superficial or deep wound cultures), procedure billing codes (eg, CPT codes), hospital billing codes (eg, ICD-9), ADT (to detect readmissions), antibiotic administration (optional) | Current definition requires judgment as to whether infection occurred, because not all infections have a positive culture; designation of depth of infection is often nuanced |
| Ventilator-associated event (VAC, IVAC) | Ventilator settings (PEEP, Fio$_2$), presence of endotracheal intubation device, ADT, antimicrobial use, vital signs (temperature), laboratory (white blood cell count), microbiology culture results | None |
| MDRO module (LabID) | Microbiology cultures, ADT | None |
| *Clostridium difficile* module (LabID) | Microbiology (*C difficile*), ADT | None |

*Abbreviations:* ADT, admission/discharge/transfer system; CPT, current procedural therapy; Fio$_2$, fraction inspired oxygen; ICD-9, International Classification of Diseases, 9th revision; IVAC, infection-related ventilator-associated complication; MDRO, multidrug-resistant organism; PEEP, positive expiratory-end pressure; VAC, ventilator-associated condition.
*Adapted from* Woeltje KF, Lin MY, Klompas M, et al. Data requirements for electronic surveillance of healthcare-associated infections. Infect Control Hosp Epidemiol 2014;35(9):1088; with permission.

the infection preventionist from having to review positive blood cultures that are unlikely to be true CLABSIs. To perform CLABSI surveillance, basic database sources are needed: microbiology; admission/discharge/transfer; and ideally, patient-specific central line data.

Some investigators have implemented fully automated CLABSI surveillance, as an alternative to traditional surveillance.[8–10] Such approaches are useful in performing surveillance in hospital units where there may not be enough resources to perform traditional surveillance (eg, non–intensive care unit areas of the hospital).[11] Additionally, completely automated approaches are likely more reliable when performing inter-facility comparisons, compared with traditional surveillance.[12] However, because fully automated CLABSI measurements result in infection rates that are higher than those derived from traditional methods, hospitals reporting automated CLABSI rates would need to be compared with other hospitals using the same automated surveillance definition.

*Surgical site infections*

Surgical site infections (SSI) surveillance requires some human judgment, because the depth of infection (superficial vs deep vs organ/space) must be determined, and not all SSIs involve a positive microbiologic culture. Thus, SSI surveillance is typically semi-automated, with software used to identify candidate surgical cases and to count the denominator of qualified procedures in a given time. SSI rates are typically risk adjusted by the American Society of Anesthesiologists score, wound class, and duration of surgery; these elements are usually available electronically through the surgical information system, but the accuracy of these data sources must be validated at each hospital before use.

Case finding of SSIs is extremely valuable, reducing the amount of chart review needed. Because not all SSIs result in a positive culture, surveillance systems that rely solely on positive cultures likely undercount infections. Ideally, case-finding algorithms would use a combination of culture results, diagnosis codes, hospital readmission, and antibiotic use; different algorithms have been developed for a variety of SSIs.[13–17] For example, a multicenter study of SSI surveillance focusing on coronary artery bypass graft, caesarian section, and breast surgeries showed that enhanced surveillance (that identified postoperative patients with inpatient antimicrobial exposure of various thresholds of duration) had sensitivity of 88% to 91% sensitivity, compared with 38% to 64% for routine surveillance, and surveillance for cesarean section infection was further enhanced with the addition of infection diagnosis codes.[13]

*Ventilator-associated pneumonia/ventilator-associated events*

In 2013, NHSN released new surveillance definitions for ventilator-associated events (VAE); these definitions were designed to rely only on objective criteria (eg, changes in ventilator settings). The VAE definition marked a departure from older definitions that relied heavily on subjective criteria (eg, interpretation of clinical signs/symptoms and radiographic signs). In the process, the VAE definition shifted the focus of prevention from pneumonia alone to general complications of mechanical ventilation.

VAE surveillance starts by identifying patients with "ventilator-associated conditions," defined as a sustained increase in ventilator settings after a period of stable or improving ventilator settings.[18] Additional criteria (white blood cell count, temperature, antibiotic receipt) define a subgroup of ventilator-associated conditions as "infection-related ventilator-associated conditions"; further subgroups of "possible pneumonia" and "probable pneumonia" are defined by sputum purulence and respiratory culture results. VAE surveillance can be fully automated in hospitals that can electronically access all required data elements: daily minimum positive expiratory end pressure, daily minimum fraction inspired oxygen, daily minimum and maximum temperature, daily minimum and maximum white blood cell count, and antibiotic start/stop dates. To assess possible and probable ventilator-associated pneumonia, Gram stain neutrophil and epithelial cell counts and respiratory culture results are needed. Hospitals that cannot access all required data elements may perform the surveillance in a semiautomated manner, which may include manual data entry or manual review of some data elements.

*Catheter-associated urinary tract infection*

The current NHSN definition for catheter-associated urinary tract infection (CAUTI) relies on determining whether bacteria in the urine (bacteriuria) is associated with symptoms of infection (eg, fever, urgency, frequency, dysuria, suprapubic tenderness, and costovertebral angle pain or tenderness) and whether a urinary catheter is present.

Symptoms, as documented in clinical notes, are difficult for software to extract from the medical record; thus, CAUTI surveillance usually is semiautomated with a human making a final determination based on chart review. The presence or absence of an indwelling urinary catheter is the starting point for determining whether a CAUTI has occurred and also for counting denominator data (urinary catheter days). Furthermore, surveillance software must be able to interpret a urine culture result based on NHSN criteria, by counting the number of species in the urine culture (no more than two species allowed, with at least one species at a concentration of $\geq 10^5$ colony-forming units).

### Multidrug-resistant organism module

The NHSN multidrug-resistant organism (MDRO) module contains the LabID surveillance option, which relies on completely objective and computable metrics (microbiology culture results and patient location data). Candidate MDROs include methicillin-resistant *Staphylococcus aureus* (MRSA), vancomycin-resistant *Enterococcus*, cephalosporin-resistant *Klebsiella*, carbapenem-resistant Enterobacteriaceae, multidrug-resistant *Acinetobacter* spp, and *C difficile*. These surveillance metrics allow for determination of community-onset versus hospital-onset infection, and unit-specific surveillance. The LabID surveillance definitions are an example of the future of infection surveillance, where metrics are calculated completely by computers without human effort.

### Outbreak Detection

Infection preventionists typically perform outbreak detection of hospital-acquired infections using simple rules, such as three or more new cases of a single pathogen within 2 weeks in a single ward. Such approaches do not account for the natural variation of pathogen prevalence over time, and can miss outbreaks spanning multiple hospital units. Surveillance software offers the opportunity to perform automated cluster detection using statistical principles. For example, in one study, investigators used a space-time permutation scan statistic (WHONET-SaTScan) approach to identify clusters of pathogens that were of same species and antibiotic susceptibility profiles.[19] Over 5 years, such an approach identified 59 clusters, 95% of which were deemed by the hospital epidemiologists to merit consideration or warrant active investigation/intervention; importantly, 72 of 73 previously designated MRSA clusters and 87 of 87 vancomycin-resistant *Enterococcus* clusters were found to have likely occurred by chance alone (ie, not significant), potentially saving infection preventionist resources. Statistical surveillance systems use baseline prevalence data to automate evaluation of whether a statistically significant increase in infections or organisms has occurred.

## INFECTION PREVENTION

Although infection control software is used predominantly to improve data collection and surveillance, there are many opportunities for software to actively prevent infections and improve patient care. Such approaches often use "clinical decision support" tools that present information to the end user (infection preventionist or hospital staff) to prompt immediate action.[20]

### Increasing the Recognition of Multidrug-Resistant Organism Carriage on Admission

The Centers for Disease Control and Prevention encourages hospitals to identify patients who are colonized with MDROs at the time of admission, to place them in appropriate contact precautions.[21] Infection control software, or the health system's electronic medical record, can flag patients with MDROs so that on hospital readmission, health care workers know to put the patient in isolation precautions.[22] For example, a computer alerting system allowed a hospital to increase staff awareness of patient MRSA colonization from 15% at baseline to 90%, with a similar increase in appropriate contact precautions.[23] Other investigational systems allow hospitals to identify those patients who are at higher risk of MDRO carriage, to then prompt further culture testing at the time of admission (ie, active surveillance).[24]

Health care facilities find it difficult to ascertain patients' MDRO status at the time of admission if the MDRO test information resides at another health care facility. Such awareness requires a regional health informatics system (sometimes called a health information exchange) to share MDRO information among facilities. MDRO information sharing is being developed in certain regions of the United States.[25] One example is the Illinois XDRO registry, which facilitates or automates sharing of carbapenem-resistant Enterobacteriaceae (CRE) information among all facilities in Illinois.[26] Infection preventionists are mandated to report CRE patients to the Illinois Department of Public Health, and thereafter, any hospital can query the registry to determine whether a given patient has ever been reported to the registry. Such CRE alerts can be automated, which is important for large health care facilities with high admission rates.

### Identifying Inappropriate Infection Precautions

During a patient's hospitalization, infection preventionists spend considerable time ensuring that appropriate isolation precautions are placed for patients with relevant pathogens. For example, a patient with a positive AFB smear may need to be placed in airborne precautions because of tuberculosis transmission risk. If a given patient's infection control precautions can be captured electronically in real time, then infection control software can identify patients with specific pathogens (eg, MDROs, C difficile, varicella zoster virus, Mycobacterium tuberculosis) and identify patients with inappropriate isolation precautions for further infection preventionist review.[27,28]

### Reducing Device Use

Clinical decision support can reduce device use, leading to fewer device-related infections. For example, a multihospital academic system instituted measures to reduce the use of indwelling urinary catheters, including alerts to providers to reassess the need for the urinary catheter if not removed within the recommended time. Urinary catheter use declined during the study period, as did CAUTIs.[29] Similar interventions for urinary catheters have been described elsewhere.[30]

### Antibiotic Stewardship

Antimicrobial stewardship is a complementary component of infection control, because antimicrobial use affects C difficile infection rates and increases risk for antimicrobial resistance. Many software programs are available for pharmacists and antimicrobial stewards.[31] Various stewardship strategies are augmented by informatics. Prospective audit and feedback strategy is enhanced by electronically identifying patients on target antimicrobials for review (eg, all patients on broad-spectrum antimicrobials) or for patients treated with antimicrobials that have redundant spectra.[32] Formulary restriction and preauthorization uses clinical decision support at the time of antimicrobial prescribing to alter prescribing behavior (eg, avoiding certain antimicrobial drug classes, or prompting the ordering provider to obtain approval from the infectious diseases department). Guideline-based treatment recommendations are provided to physicians by the computer software at the time of antibiotic decision-making. Lastly, software can encourage appropriate antimicrobial use by identifying new clinical information (eg, a positive blood culture result) that should prompt modification of antimicrobial therapy.

Numerous examples of computer-assisted antimicrobial stewardship are available,[33–35] including a randomized-control trial that demonstrated a clinical decision support system could increase appropriate antimicrobial therapy and decrease antimicrobial expenditures.[36] This topic is discussed in further detail in elsewhere in this issue (see Nagel JL, Kaye KS, LaPlante KL, et al: Antimicrobial stewardship for the infection control practitioner, in this issue on antimicrobial stewardship).

## INFORMATICS AND PUBLIC HEALTH

Informatics systems have strengthened and expanded the interface between infection preventionists and public health agencies. Incentives, such as the Centers for Medicare and Medicaid's Meaningful Use Program, have encouraged hospitals to adopt such technologies as electronic laboratory reporting and syndromic surveillance, although uptake has been inconsistent and hampered by the complexity of microbiology data.[37] Such connections facilitate opportunities for infection prevention activities to be integrated across regions, which is essential for control of MDROs.[38]

### Electronic Communicable Disease Reporting

Most public health reporting of communicable diseases has now moved to the Internet, with users reporting via a World Wide Web interface. A World Wide Web interface allows the infection preventionist to input complete report information, including microbiology results and patient demographic/epidemiologic information. Electronic laboratory reporting automates some of the reporting, allowing the microbiology laboratory information to be automatically sent to the public health department using reporting rules. Electronic laboratory reporting has been shown to increase the completeness and timeliness of communicable disease reporting,[39] although a major limitation is that certain patient data, such as demographic and epidemiologic data, still require manual infection preventionist entry.[40]

### Syndromic Surveillance and Outbreak Detection

Syndromic surveillance is preferred over traditional case reporting for monitoring common conditions, such as influenza, or for rapid identification of outbreaks and bioterrorism events.[37] Personal identifiers do not need to be sent to the public health department because such reports do not require patient-specific public health response. To track influenza, public health officials monitor for influenza-like illness by looking for trends in specific chief complaints from emergency departments and some ambulatory care settings. Reports typically contain basic demographic information, but lack clinical, vaccination, or laboratory information. Future iterations of syndromic surveillance would be enhanced by sharing patient identifiers through an encrypted master patient identifier. Such an enhancement would allow public health agencies to deduplicate events across systems and communicate public health alerts across facilities.

## GENERAL CONSIDERATIONS FOR IMPLEMENTING INFORMATICS SOFTWARE

Infection preventionists and hospital epidemiologists need to work closely with their information technology and laboratory specialists to implement and maintain informatics software, whether home-grown or commercial. Here, we discuss some of the general considerations in working with informatics software and strategies to maintain quality of data through internal/external validation.

## Challenges of Microbiology Data

Microbiology data are inherently complex. Although some tests have a single result value (eg, human immunodeficiency virus antibody test is positive/negative), other tests, such as cultures can have results that include multiple organisms, each with its own antibiotic susceptibility profile. Furthermore, the bacterial taxonomy can change based on genetic analysis; for example, in 1995 *Bacteroides gracilis* was renamed *Campylobacter gracilis*.[41] Thus, informatics software must map each organism to standardized terminology (eg, Systemized Nomenclature of Medicine, College of American Pathologists), and determine when new data are coming from the microbiology laboratory that are unrecognized because of naming or format changes. Furthermore, any changes in the underlying information systems that supply data to infection control software require a complete reassessment of data integrity at the time of change.

## Challenges of Device Data

Information from routine nurse charting can allow software to detect the presence of invasive devices, such as central lines, indwelling urinary catheters, and mechanical ventilation.[42] Based on our experience, insertion/discontinuation orders for devices are contributory, but less reliable than daily nursing assessments for determining whether a device is present. For example, a patient can be discharged from the hospital without a device discontinuation order, and then it is unclear on readmission whether the device is still present.

When working with electronic device data, infection control personnel are responsible for mapping local device names to device types. For example, the NHSN CAUTI definition surveys complications of indwelling urethral catheters, so suprapubic catheters (which are outside the urethra) should not count as qualifying catheters. If local device names cannot discriminate between qualifying versus nonqualifying devices, infection control personnel need to work with the informatics team to modify the device name list.

## Validation of Data

Surveillance of health care–associated infections has high stakes implications; besides the direct role of surveillance in monitoring patient safety, hospital infections rates are publicly reported and affect hospital reimbursement in pay-for-performance models.[43,44] Validation is the process that ensures high quality of infection control data. In the context of informatics, it means that the products of electronic surveillance are compared with a reference standard (usually, manual review). Validation can be divided into two activities: internal validation, which is refers to self-assessment by the reporting facility; and external validation, which is performed by an agency outside the reporting facility (usually the health department). Validation is an iterative process that should be performed on a scheduled basis (eg, yearly). Both numerator and denominator data need validation, because poor quality in either domain can adversely affect infection rates.

NHSN recommends each facility's infection control program use the following steps for internal validation. (1) Ensure and document current training in NHSN surveillance competency. (2) Ensure that risk adjustment variables are accurate and reliable (eg, for CLABSI/CAUTI, this involves verifying location mapping, bed size, and teaching hospital type). (3) Ensure numerator quality by maintaining a decision record of all positive culture investigation results (blood cultures and urine cultures for CLABSI and CAUTI, respectively), and request a summary line listing of all positive cultures from the laboratory to compare with the list of previously investigated cultures. (4) Verify that denominator collection is accurate; if performed electronically, facilities are required to document that electronic data counts are within 5% of manual data counts for 3 months. Validation steps specific for infection type can be found on NHSN's data validation Web site (http://www.cdc.gov/nhsn/validation/).

## SUMMARY

Infection control personnel benefit most from computer technology when they recognize the strengths and limitations of software systems in carrying out everyday infection control tasks. Computer programs excel in applying surveillance rules when little or no judgement is needed. However, computers are only as valid as the data fed into the programs, and thus periodic validation of data inputs is required. As surveillance becomes more efficient, the challenge for infection preventionists is in translating the knowledge gained from electronic surveillance systems into action. The ability of informatics tools to motivate behavior change by hospital personnel to prevent infections is a key determinant in how well informatics can ultimately improve patient safety.

## REFERENCES

1. Kulikowski CA, Shortliffe EH, Currie LM, et al. AMIA Board white paper: definition of biomedical informatics and specification of core competencies for graduate education in the discipline. J Am Med Inform Assoc 2012;19(6):931–8.
2. Adler-Milstein J, DesRoches CM, Kralovec P, et al. Electronic health record adoption in US hospitals: progress continues, but challenges persist. Health Aff (Millwood) 2015;34(12):2174–80.
3. Rubin MA, Mayer J, Greene T, et al. An agent-based model for evaluating surveillance methods for catheter-related bloodstream infection. AMIA Annu Symp Proc 2008;6:631–5.
4. CDC. Multidrug-resistant organism (MDRO) & Clostridium difficile infection (MDRO/CDI) module. 2016. Available at: http://www.cdc.gov/nhsn/PDFs/pscManual/12pscMDRO_CDADcurrent.pdf. Accessed February 4, 2016.
5. Woeltje KF, Lin MY, Klompas M, et al. Data requirements for electronic surveillance of healthcare-associated infections. Infect Control Hosp Epidemiol 2014; 35(09):1083–91.
6. Klompas M, Yokoe DS, Weinstein RA. Automated surveillance of health care-associated infections. Clin Infect Dis 2009;48(9):1268–75.
7. Mayer J, Greene T, Howell J, et al. Agreement in classifying bloodstream infections among multiple reviewers conducting surveillance. Clin Infect Dis 2012; 55(3):364–70.
8. Lin MY, Hota B, Khan YM, et al. Quality of traditional surveillance for public reporting of nosocomial bloodstream infection rates. JAMA 2010;304(18):2035–41.
9. Woeltje KF, Butler AM, Goris AJ, et al. Automated surveillance for central line-associated bloodstream infection in intensive care units. Infect Control Hosp Epidemiol 2008;29(9):842–6.
10. Trick WE, Zagorski BM, Tokars JI, et al. Computer algorithms to detect bloodstream infections. Emerg Infect Dis 2004;10(9):1612–20.
11. Woeltje KF, McMullen KM, Butler AM, et al. Electronic surveillance for healthcare-associated central line-associated bloodstream infections outside the intensive care unit. Infect Control Hosp Epidemiol 2011;32(11):1086–90.

12. Lin MY, Woeltje KF, Khan YM, et al. Multicenter evaluation of computer automated versus traditional surveillance of hospital-acquired bloodstream infections. Infect Control Hosp Epidemiol 2014;35(12):1483–90.

13. Yokoe DS, Noskin GA, Cunnigham SM, et al. Enhanced identification of postoperative infections among inpatients. Emerg Infect Dis 2004;10(11):1924–30.

14. Yokoe DS, Khan Y, Olsen MA, et al. Enhanced surgical site infection surveillance following hysterectomy, vascular, and colorectal surgery. Infect Control Hosp Epidemiol 2012;33(8):768–73.

15. Calderwood MS, Ma A, Khan YM, et al. Use of Medicare diagnosis and procedure codes to improve detection of surgical site infections following hip arthroplasty, knee arthroplasty, and vascular surgery. Infect Control Hosp Epidemiol 2012;33(1):40–9.

16. Olsen MA, Fraser VJ. Use of diagnosis codes and/or wound culture results for surveillance of surgical site infection after mastectomy and breast reconstruction. Infect Control Hosp Epidemiol 2010;31(5):544–7.

17. Bolon MK, Hooper D, Stevenson KB, et al. Improved surveillance for surgical site infections after orthopedic implantation procedures: extending applications for automated data. Clin Infect Dis 2009;48(9):1223–9.

18. Magill SS, Klompas M, Balk R, et al. Developing a new, national approach to surveillance for ventilator-associated events: executive summary. Clin Infect Dis 2013;57(12):1742–6.

19. Huang SS, Yokoe DS, Stelling J, et al. Automated detection of infectious disease outbreaks in hospitals: a retrospective cohort study. PLoS Med 2010;7(2): e1000238.

20. Wright MO, Robicsek A. Clinical decision support systems and infection prevention: to know is not enough. Am J Infect Control 2015;43(6):554–8.

21. CDC. Facility guidance for control of carbapenem-resistant enterobacteriaceae (CRE). 2015. Available at: http://www.cdc.gov/hai/pdfs/cre/CRE-guidance-508. pdf. Accessed February 4, 2016.

22. Kho AN, Dexter PR, Warvel JS, et al. An effective computerized reminder for contact isolation of patients colonized or infected with resistant organisms. Int J Med Inform 2008;77(3):194–8.

23. Kac G, Grohs P, Durieux P, et al. Impact of electronic alerts on isolation precautions for patients with multidrug-resistant bacteria. Arch Intern Med 2007;167(19): 2086–90.

24. Robicsek A, Beaumont JL, Wright MO, et al. Electronic prediction rules for methicillin-resistant *Staphylococcus aureus* colonization. Infect Control Hosp Epidemiol 2011;32(1):9–19.

25. Kho AN, Lemmon L, Commiskey M, et al. Use of a regional health information exchange to detect crossover of patients with MRSA between urban hospitals. J Am Med Inform Assoc 2008;15(2):212–6.

26. Trick WE, Lin MY, Cheng-Leidig R, et al. Electronic public health registry of extensively drug-resistant organisms, Illinois, USA. Emerg Infect Dis 2015;21(10): 1725–32.

27. Ross B, Marine M, Chou M, et al. Measuring compliance with transmission-based isolation precautions: comparison of paper-based and electronic data collection. Am J Infect Control 2011;39(10):839–43.

28. Chen ES, Wajngurt D, Qureshi K, et al. Automated real-time detection and notification of positive infection cases. AMIA Annu Symp Proc 2006;883.

29. Baillie CA, Epps M, Hanish A, et al. Usability and impact of a computerized clinical decision support intervention designed to reduce urinary catheter utilization

and catheter-associated urinary tract infections. Infect Control Hosp Epidemiol 2014;35(9):1147–55.

30. Meddings J, Rogers MA, Macy M, et al. Systematic review and meta-analysis: reminder systems to reduce catheter-associated urinary tract infections and urinary catheter use in hospitalized patients. Clin Infect Dis 2010;51(5):550–60.

31. Forrest GN, Van Schooneveld TC, Kullar R, et al. Use of electronic health records and clinical decision support systems for antimicrobial stewardship. Clin Infect Dis 2014;59(Suppl 3):S122–33.

32. Glowacki RC, Schwartz DN, Itokazu GS, et al. Antibiotic combinations with redundant antimicrobial spectra: clinical epidemiology and pilot intervention of computer-assisted surveillance. Clin Infect Dis 2003;37(1):59–64.

33. Pestotnik SL, Classen DC, Evans RS, et al. Implementing antibiotic practice guidelines through computer-assisted decision support: clinical and financial outcomes. Ann Intern Med 1996;124(10):884–90.

34. Evans RS, Pestotnik SL, Classen DC, et al. A computer-assisted management program for antibiotics and other antiinfective agents. N Engl J Med 1998;338(4):232–8.

35. Samore MH, Bateman K, Alder SC, et al. Clinical decision support and appropriateness of antimicrobial prescribing: a randomized trial. JAMA 2005;294(18):2305–14.

36. McGregor JC, Weekes E, Forrest GN, et al. Impact of a computerized clinical decision support system on reducing inappropriate antimicrobial use: a randomized controlled trial. J Am Med Inform Assoc 2006;13(4):378–84.

37. Birkhead GS, Klompas M, Shah NR. Uses of electronic health records for public health surveillance to advance public health. Annu Rev Public Health 2015;36:345–59.

38. Slayton RB, Toth D, Lee BY, et al. Vital signs: estimated effects of a coordinated approach for action to reduce antibiotic-resistant infections in health care facilities—United States. MMWR Morb Mortal Wkly Rep 2015;64(30):826.

39. Effler P, Ching-Lee M, Bogard A, et al. Statewide system of electronic notifiable disease reporting from clinical laboratories: comparing automated reporting with conventional methods. JAMA 1999;282(19):1845–50.

40. Dixon BE, Siegel JA, Oemige TV, et al. Electronic health information quality challenges and interventions to improve public health surveillance data and practice. Public Health Rep 2013;128:546–53.

41. Somer HJ, Summanen P. Recent taxonomic changes and terminology update of clinically significant anaerobic gram-negative bacteria (excluding spirochetes). Clin Infect Dis 2002;35(Suppl 1):S17–21.

42. Wright MO, Fisher A, John M, et al. The electronic medical record as a tool for infection surveillance: successful automation of device-days. Am J Infect Control 2009;37(5):364–70.

43. Totten AM, Wagner J, Tiwari A, et al. Closing the quality gap: revisiting the state of the science (vol. 5: public reporting as a quality improvement strategy). Evid Rep Technol Assess (Full Rep) 2012;(208.5):1–645.

44. Kahn CN, Ault T, Potetz L, et al. Assessing Medicare's hospital pay-for-performance programs and whether they are achieving their goals. Health Aff (Millwood) 2015;34(8):1281–8.

# Antimicrobial Stewardship for the Infection Control Practitioner

Jerod L. Nagel, PharmD[a], Keith S. Kaye, MD, MPH[b],
Kerry L. LaPlante, PharmD[c,d,e], Jason M. Pogue, PharmD[f],*

## KEYWORDS

- Antimicrobial stewardship • Antibiotic management
- Antibiotic resistance infection control • Education • Multidrug resistance

## KEY POINTS

- Antibiotic misuse is a serious patient safety concern and a national public health priority.
- Years of indiscriminant antibiotic use have led to selection of antibiotic-resistant bacteria and *Clostridium difficile* infection, which ultimately led to poor patient outcomes.
- Antimicrobial stewardship programs are designed to promote judicious use of antimicrobials by optimizing antimicrobial selection, dose, route, and duration.
- Infection preventionists can enhance stewardship efforts through patient identification, prevention of device-related infections, and through input in the development of drug and disease state bundles.

## CONSEQUENCES OF ANTIMICROBIAL RESISTANCE: IMPACT ON PUBLIC HEALTH AND SAFETY

One of the greatest achievements in science and medicine of the last century was the discovery and the subsequent development of antibiotics for human use. Antibiotics have enabled many of the achievements in modern medicine including transplantation, invasive forms of surgery, chemotherapy, and successful management of the critically ill.[1] Unfortunately, this situation has become compromised due to the introduction and vast expansion of antimicrobial resistance. The impact that antimicrobial resistance has on the international community is well recognized by governing bodies. The World Health Organization has identified antimicrobial resistance as 1 of the 3 greatest

[a] Department of Pharmacy Services, University of Michigan Health System, Ann Arbor, MI 48109, USA; [b] Department of Medicine, Detroit Medical Center, Wayne State University, Detroit, MI 48201, USA; [c] College of Pharmacy, University of Rhode Island, Kingston, RI 08221, USA; [d] Alpert Medical School, Brown University, Providence, RI 02912, USA; [e] Department of Pharmacy Services, Providence Veterans Medical Center, Providence, RI 02908, USA; [f] Department of Pharmacy Services, Sinai-Grace Hospital, Detroit Medical Center, Wayne State University School of Medicine, Detroit, MI 48235, USA
* Corresponding author.
*E-mail address:* jpogue@dmc.org

Infect Dis Clin N Am 30 (2016) 771–784
http://dx.doi.org/10.1016/j.idc.2016.04.012
0891-5520/16/$ – see front matter © 2016 Elsevier Inc. All rights reserved.

threats to human health,[2] placing it in the same category as climate change and widespread poverty. In 2004, the Infectious Diseases Society of America (IDSA) raised the alert level in the United States with their Bad Bugs, No Drugs campaign introducing the cleverly titled ESKAPE pathogens,[3] which can escape the effects of the antimicrobial armamentarium and to which vulnerable patients cannot escape the devastating outcomes due to infections with these organisms. The ESKAPE pathogens include the Gram-positive pathogens methicillin-resistant *Staphylococcus aureus* (MRSA) and vancomycin-resistant *Enterococcus* (VRE), as well as the Gram-negative pathogens *Klebsiella pneumoniae, Pseudomonas aeruginosa, Acinetobacter baumannii,* and Enterobacter species.[3] The Centers for Disease Control (CDC) built on this awareness and call for action in their 2013 Antibiotic Resistance Threats Report, in which they detailed the unfathomable impact that resistant organisms have on patient outcomes. In this report, the CDC estimates that each year in the United States at least 2 million people become infected with bacteria that are resistant to antibiotics and at least 23,000 people die each year as a direct result of these infections, with even more perishing from conditions that were complicated by these infections.[4]

## THE IMPACT OF ANTIMICROBIAL USE, MISUSE, AND OVERUSE

The overuse and misuse of antimicrobial agents have detrimental effects to the individual patient, the health care system, and society as a whole. Among other negative consequences, inappropriate antimicrobial use has contributed to the rising costs of health care, the emergence of multidrug-resistant organisms (MDROs) and superinfections (most notably *Clostridium difficile* infections), and unnecessary adverse drug reactions. It is estimated that up to 50% of antimicrobial use is inappropriate in acute care settings[5] and up to 75% of antibiotic use in inappropriate in long-term care facilities.[6] These staggering numbers add considerable costs to patient care. According to the Office of Technology Assessment, antibiotics are the second most commonly prescribed class of drugs in the United States.[7] Upwards of 40% of all hospitalized patients receive antibiotics annually.

   Although it is intuitive that use of a particular antimicrobial, through the process of selective pressure, will lead to the development of resistance to that agent or class of agents in an organism present in a patient; it is actually a much more complex process. Cross-resistance to structurally unrelated antimicrobials can also occur with alarming frequency. This can occur by 1 of 2 main methods. First is the presence of shared resistance pathways (eg, multidrug-resistant efflux pumps that pump structurally unrelated drugs out of the bacterial cell). Second is the presence of resistance islands within the genetic material of certain pathogens that carry diverse resistance mechanisms to structurally different antimicrobials. In this second scenario, receipt of antibiotic A can select for the strain of bacteria with resistance to that antibiotic. However, because that resistance determinant exists in combination with other resistance determinants for other antimicrobials, the strain selected actually displays multidrug resistance. Therefore, scrutiny of every antimicrobial exposure is warranted to prevent the emergence of MDROs. For example, the impact of each antimicrobial exposure on the development and subsequent isolation of carbapenem-resistant Enterobacteriaceae (CRE), an organism the CDC has given the highest threat level, is well described. In addition to data showing carbapenem exposure as a risk factor for isolation of CRE,[8] there are equally convincing data showing that any antimicrobial exposure,[9] each additional antimicrobial exposure,[10] and each additional day of antimicrobial exposure[11] are all associated with an increased risk of CRE isolation. Furthermore, a recent meta-analysis showed an independent association with virtually every class of antimicrobial agents and the development of *C difficile* infection.[12] Encouragingly, however, a separate meta-analysis investigating the impact stewardship programs can have on *C difficile* rates reported that a variety of stewardship strategies can be used to decrease rates by more than 50%.[13] In addition to the association between antibiotic use and antibiotic resistance and *C difficile*, data show that a prolonged duration of antimicrobial exposure can increase the chance of potentially serious adverse events. For these reasons, it is essential that health care professionals are continually assessing all patients on antimicrobials to determine whether or not there is a continued need for antimicrobial therapy.

## NATIONAL INITIATIVES CALLING FOR IMPROVED ANTIMICROBIAL USAGE

Due to the large degree of inappropriate antimicrobial use, the impact that all usage has on resistance, superinfections, and safety, and the negative impact of infections due to resistant pathogens and *C difficile* on patient outcomes, national initiatives have been implemented to optimize antimicrobial usage. In September of 2014, President Barack Obama signed an executive order titled Combating Antibiotic-Resistant Bacteria, furthering the previous efforts of the CDC and continuing to move forward the call for enhanced antimicrobial stewardship to combat this natural security priority. This executive order led to the development of a task force that has since developed an action plan recommending enhanced antimicrobial stewardship to decrease inappropriate antimicrobial use by at least 20%.[14] This action plan is not limited to inpatient settings but applies to enhancing stewardship efforts across the continuum of care, including the community, as well as long-term care facilities where up to 75% of antimicrobial use is inappropriate.[6] These types of activities will soon be mandatory for participation, reimbursement, or recognition with The Centers for Medicare and Medicaid Services (CMS), The Joint Commission, and The Leapfrog Group. These agencies are finalizing minimum stewardship requirements that an institution must perform as a condition of participation. It is hoped that these initiatives will lead to enhanced resources allocated for development and expansion of stewardship programs over the next 5 years, and infection control practitioners will be called on for assistance.

## WHAT IS ANTIMICROBIAL STEWARDSHIP AND WHAT ARE THE GOALS?

Antimicrobial stewardship is globally defined as any activity to optimize the drug selection, dose, duration, or route of an antimicrobial.[15,16] Antimicrobial stewardship programs implement, direct, and monitor appropriate antimicrobial use at a health care institution. Antimicrobial stewardship programs provide a standard, evidence-based approach to judicious antimicrobial use. The most effective antimicrobial stewardship programs incorporate multiple strategies after collaborating with the various specialties within a given health care facility, although interventions on a smaller scale to improve antimicrobial use are also valuable in some settings.

There are multiple goals of antimicrobial stewardship programs and, although many of the initiatives described previously have been driven by the alarming rise in antimicrobial resistance, it must be understood that the primary function of stewardship programs is to optimize the outcome of a given patient with an infectious disease.[16] This is done by optimizing the 4 components of antimicrobial therapy for a patient: agent selection, dose, route, and duration. Antimicrobial selection encompasses the narrowest spectrum of therapy to treat the suspected organism that also penetrates the site of infection. Appropriate selection includes empiric therapy, which takes into account likely pathogens, local susceptibility data, and patient-specific factors, such as allergies, severity of illness, and comorbidities. Once a causative pathogen is identified therapy should be de-escalated or streamlined to the narrowest spectrum therapy that covers that pathogen. Dose optimization includes strategies for optimizing likelihood of achieving pharmacokinetic or pharmacodynamic targets (eg, extended infusion of beta-lactams) or dose reduction in the presence of renal insufficiency to ensure that patients do not have elevated concentrations of the antimicrobial, which can be associated with increased toxicity. Appropriate route includes transitioning patients to oral therapy once indicated and optimal duration based on the clinical course of the infection, in combination with evidence-based guidelines.

In optimizing these 4 facets of antimicrobial exposures, clinicians can minimize the unintended consequences of antimicrobial usage. Most notably, from a public health standpoint, reduction of emergence of antimicrobial resistance and preservation of existing and future antimicrobial agents are priorities. Although there are numerous examples of stewardship approaches in the literature that have led to decreases in unnecessary antimicrobial use, there are fewer that have demonstrated short-term reductions in antimicrobial resistance, and even fewer, if any, that have demonstrated long-term reductions. The lack of evidence is likely related to difficulties in measuring these outcomes rather than suggestive that stewardship programs are ineffective in meeting this goal. As described previously, there are clear data describing the impact of stewardship programs on the reduction of *C difficile*.[13]

Nevertheless, it is useful to consider benefits other than reduction in resistance when justifying the existence of a program. Improvements in patient safety, reducing inappropriate exposure, and optimizing outcomes in the area of antimicrobial prescribing are easier to demonstrate and may be more palatable for individual providers as reasons to endorse stewardship. An additional goal of antimicrobial stewardship, and of particular interest to administrators, is to reduce health care costs without compromising the quality of medical care. Antimicrobials account for up to 20% of hospital pharmacy budgets.[16] It is estimated that up to 50% of antimicrobial use is inappropriate,[5] adding considerable costs to patient care. As previously discussed, antibiotics are the second most commonly prescribed class of drugs in the United States and upwards of 40% of all hospitalized patients receive antibiotics in the United States annually.[7] Antimicrobial stewardship programs have demonstrated significant annual savings in both large academic hospitals as well as smaller community hospitals in the range of $200,000 to $900,000, while not sacrificing the quality of clinical care.[17–23]

## KEY MEMBERS AND DEPARTMENTS REPRESENTED ON THE ANTIMICROBIAL STEWARDSHIP TEAM

Antimicrobial stewardship programs must harness the talents of all members of the health care team to effectively develop and maintain a program with optimal patient outcomes. The following section discusses the members of the antimicrobial stewardship team and provides a brief overview of their roles.[16]

### Infectious Diseases Physician

Essential to a successful antimicrobial stewardship program is the presence of at least 1 infectious disease-trained physician who dedicates a portion of his or her time to the design, implementation, and/or evaluation of the program. Having a stewardship team led by an infectious diseases physician may increase acceptance and compliance of the program by other physicians. This may also reduce the perception that a stewardship program is a pharmacy-driven cost-savings scheme. Even if the infectious diseases physician does not perform many of the daily activities of the program, it is essential to have someone trained in infectious diseases is available to provide clinical guidance to support those administering the program.

### Clinical Pharmacist

One or more clinical pharmacists with specialized training in infectious diseases is highly recommended for establishing and maintaining a stewardship program. Infectious diseases pharmacists can perform most day-to-day activities of a stewardship program, including antimicrobial education, before and after prescription review, and guideline development. Because many institutions do not currently have access to infectious diseases-trained clinical pharmacists, it is important to note that pharmacists without training in infectious diseases can play an important part in antimicrobial stewardship. Their roles should be tailored based on the structure of the stewardship program. Multiple stewardship training programs are available in the United States to further their development.

### Infection Preventionist and Health Care Epidemiologist

Expertise in infection control and prevention, and health care epidemiology plays a pivotal role in the development, justification, and impact measurement of an antimicrobial stewardship program.[24] Health care professionals with this expertise can assist with early identification of organisms and infected patients to further the mission of stewardship programs (see later discussion of opportunities for collaboration). Additionally, these individuals are a standing presence within the health care institution and can promote compliance with standard and transmission-based precautions, bundle-care practices, vaccination efforts, and hand hygiene to help limit the development and spread of MDROs and C difficile. They also provide experience in educating staff, patients, and visitors.

### Microbiology Laboratory

The clinical microbiology laboratory plays a critical role in antimicrobial stewardship by providing patient-specific culture and susceptibility data to optimize individual therapy. A stewardship program and the microbiology laboratory should work collaboratively on the institution's antibiogram. Local antibiograms with microbe-specific susceptibility data updated at least annually can assist with developing treatment guidelines for certain infections within an institution. In addition, because the stewardship program directly observes how providers use and interpret microbiology data, it can provide important feedback to the laboratory regarding optimal mechanisms for communication of laboratory tests and testing modalities that should be considered to enhance patient care. Furthermore, stewardship programs can work with the microbiology laboratory to select for which agents susceptibility results are visible to clinicians on in the medical record. Selective reporting of antimicrobial susceptibilities can help improve compliance with institutional recommendations for pathogen-specific therapy (eg, if a program wants to limit fluoroquinolone use they can work with the microbiology laboratory to hide susceptibility information for fluoroquinolones.)

### Information Technology

Access to experts in information technology is critical while developing and managing a stewardship program. These individuals can assist with the harnessing of data on microbiology and antimicrobial use from existing electronic sources, can facilitate the detection of patients warranting daily intervention by stewardship personnel, and assist with measuring the impact of the program.

### Hospital Administration

It is unlikely that an antimicrobial stewardship program will be successfully implemented without at least passive endorsement by the hospital administration. Commitment to implementation of antimicrobial stewardship programs must come from upper levels of hospital administration that are willing to invest resources in program development; otherwise funding for initiating and sustaining a stewardship program may be inadequate. If support from hospital leadership is lacking, some physicians may be less likely to comply with antimicrobial recommendations.

### Pharmacy and Therapeutics Committee

The pharmacy and therapeutics (P & T) committee determines which drugs, including antibiotics, should be placed on an institution's formulary. Antimicrobials are chosen based on efficacy, costs, safety profiles, and pathogen-resistance profiles. An effective committee limits the number of agents that have a similar antimicrobial spectrum to simplify therapeutic options, reduce the impact of pharmaceutical detailing on antimicrobial selection by physicians, and reduce antimicrobial costs through contract negotiation. Members of the stewardship team should be involved in the P & T committee to assist in antimicrobial formulary selection.

### INFECTION CONTROL AND ANTIBIOTIC STEWARDSHIP

Although all of the aforementioned team members are essential to stewardship efforts, the role of infection control practitioners should not be understated. The following section discusses how infection control practitioners can work with stewardship programs to help further optimize patient therapy.

### Drug-Based Antimicrobial Stewardship

The cornerstone of antimicrobial stewardship is promoting appropriate antimicrobial use, which includes initiating the correct antimicrobial at the optimal time and at the appropriate dose, route, frequency, and duration.[16] Additionally, antibiotic de-escalation to narrow-spectrum therapy should occur once diagnostic data, laboratory results, or clinical improvements are obtained. There are many passive and active methods to help guide appropriate antimicrobial therapy. Examples of passive antimicrobial stewardship include the development of guidelines, pathways, or protocols; educational presentations or posting of educational materials on Intranet or Internet; and automatic computer-generated hard or soft discontinuation of antibiotic therapy after a predetermined duration. Prospective audit with feedback on a case-by-case basis, or utilization of well-designed computerized decision support alerts based on patient-specific information are examples of active stewardship methods. Although, all passive and active stewardship methods are intended to promote appropriate use, without question, the most effective method is prospective audit and feedback on a case-by-case basis.[16,25] To perform drug-based prospective audit and feedback, an institution must first determine which antimicrobials will be targeted for active review and intervention and a priori decide what criteria are appropriate and inappropriate for each targeted antimicrobial. Using prospective audit and feedback, antimicrobial stewardship programs have consistently demonstrated a reduction of excessive antimicrobial therapy and decreased costs.[25]

Although the responsibilities of antimicrobial stewardship programs and infection control departments are different, collaboration between these groups is essential in promoting optimal outcomes, providing cost-effective care, reducing the development of resistance, and preventing the spread of infection. Antibiotic exposure is a main driver for the development or acquisition of infection due to an MDRO. This finding is consistent among most publications evaluating risk factors for the development of bacterial resistance, regardless of which organisms or infection is analyzed.[26] Thus, infection control departments must rely on stewardship programs to help minimize excessive antibiotic exposure, which ultimately decreases the level of risk that patients face with regard to acquiring infections due to multidrug-resistant organisms. Antimicrobial stewardship programs rely on good infection-control practices, in a complementary fashion, to minimize the patient-to-patient spread of multidrug-resistant bacteria. Poor infection control practices can lead to increasing number of patients with multidrug-resistant infections, which leads to a downward spiral of increased utilization of broad-spectrum antibiotics and the further development of resistance.

Additionally, the information gained through infection control screening for colonization by target organisms, such as VRE, CRE, MRSA, or extended spectrum beta-lactamase–producing Enterobacteriaceae, can be extremely valuable for antimicrobial stewardship programs in determining appropriate empiric antimicrobial therapy for individual patients. For example, publications have consistently demonstrated VRE colonization in high-risk populations as a risk factor for the development of VRE bacteremia.[27,28] Thus, communication between infection control and stewardship team members regarding which patients are colonized with VRE within an institution can improve prompt timely anti-VRE therapy, in certain clinical scenarios. The importance of this cannot be overstated because a recent analysis showed that in patients with enterococcal bloodstream infections delay of effective therapy of longer than 48 hours was associated with a 3-fold increase in 30-day mortality.[29] Additionally, the lack of colonization with VRE is associated with a strong negative predictive value for the development of VRE infection.[27,28] Therefore, informing stewardship personnel about which patients screen negative for VRE could help antimicrobial stewardship programs avoid or de-escalate unnecessary empiric anti-VRE therapy.

### Disease-Based Antimicrobial Stewardship and Multidisciplinary Bundles

As stated previously, the IDSA antimicrobial stewardship guidelines state that the primary goal of stewardship programs should be optimization of clinical outcomes while minimizing unintended consequences. These guidelines align with the shifting focus of health care towards increased emphasis on quality, safety, and patient outcome metrics linked to specific disease states.[30] Various organizations that track quality have demonstrated that process measures and associated outcomes may be suboptimal at given institutions, and the CMS started implementing reimbursement penalties in 2008 for institutions that are outliers among peer institutions with regard to process and management for a variety of disease states.[31] Antimicrobial stewardship programs that dedicate efforts to improving outcomes commonly focus on specific diseases. Additionally, antimicrobial stewardship programs and infection control practitioners are well positioned to identify and improve patient outcomes linked to a specific disease because they already target patients with specific infections, disease states, or patients receiving certain antimicrobials.

Implementation of guidelines has significantly improved appropriate antimicrobial therapy for a variety of disease states, including skin-and-soft tissue infections, intra-abdominal infections, bacteremia and candidemia, C difficile disease, and urinary tract infections.[32–39] Additionally, prospective audit and feedback pertaining to treatment of targeted disease states has improved antimicrobial prescribing and clinical outcomes. Traditionally, antimicrobial stewardship programs have used disease-based stewardship to focus on appropriate antibiotic prescribing. However, stewardship programs can facilitate improvement in other aspects of patient care and have used consult services and infection control as needed. For example, the IDSA guidelines identify 7 evidence-based quality performance measures that every patient with *S aureus* bacteremia should receive.[40] Historically, compliance with these quality performance measures is suboptimal and has ranged from 0% to 72.9%.[41,42] A study by Nguyen and colleagues[43] reported an antimicrobial stewardship-led interventional bundle significantly improved compliance with all quality performance measures compared with a conventional control group (84.1% vs 56.1%, P<.001), and this was associated with a reduction in hospital readmissions due to *S aureus* bacteremia. Notably, the stewardship team at this institution used a multidisciplinary approach for this *Staphylococcus* bacteremia initiative, which included representation and input from the microbiology, pharmacy, infectious diseases, and infection control departments to improve performance measures and outcomes.

Collaborations between infection control and antimicrobial stewardship programs are also well documented for the prevention or management of *C difficile* disease.[13,32] As previously described, a recent meta-analysis evaluated the impact of antimicrobial stewardship on the incidence of *C difficile* disease and demonstrated that focused interventions on reduction in antimicrobial prescribing reduced the risk of *C difficile* infection by 52% (pooled risk ratio of 0.48, 95% CI 0.38–0.62).[13] Most of the studies included in this analysis reported collaboration with infection control and acknowledged that a multifaceted intervention approach led to the improved *C difficile* infection rates. Improving clinical outcomes for diseases often requires multifaceted interventions and multidisciplinary collaboration. Infection control and antimicrobial stewardship programs can prospectively identify targeted organisms or diseases towards which they can implement an evidence-based approach to facilitate appropriate management and outcomes.

### Device-Associated Infection Prevention

Prevention of device-associated infections, such as central line-associated bloodstream infection (CLABSI) and catheter-associated urinary tract infection (CAUTI), present opportunities for collaboration between the infection control and stewardship teams. Obtaining cultures only when indicated using appropriate technique can improve the accuracy and impact of culture results from both infection control and stewardship perspectives. Obtaining cultures appropriately can lead to decreased likelihood of culture contamination (ie, of having a false-positive culture) and will reduce the possibility that a patient might be falsely categorized as having a CAUTI or CLABSI. In addition, fewer contaminated cultures will reduce the likelihood that a patient will receive unnecessary antimicrobial therapy.

### Barriers to Implementation and Maintenance of Stewardship Programs

Implementing a successful stewardship program is challenging and faces numerous potential barriers. Programs may struggle with pulling together a multidisciplinary team from pharmacy, infectious diseases, infection control, and informatics that has resources and adequate effort provided to accomplish stewardship goals. A recent survey suggested only 18% of infectious diseases physicians participating in antimicrobial stewardship programs are reimbursed for their services, despite guideline recommendations recommending compensation.[16,44] Additionally, multidisciplinary stewardship programs need to establish clear goals and expectations with hospital administration. Developing appropriate goals is a common barrier in defining the success of a stewardship program. Although stewardship programs agree that prescribing appropriate antibiotics on a case-by-case basis is a core goal, there is not a consistent definition of what appropriate antimicrobial prescribing entails.[45] Although most physicians recognize that the emergence of resistance as an important issue, they are primarily concerned with the acute needs of the individual patient who they are caring for rather than the public health consequences of excessive antimicrobial prescribing.[46] Thus, when developing a stewardship program, it is imperative to assemble a multidisciplinary team with well-defined goals and obtain the backing of hospital administration.

Practicing antimicrobial stewardship on a day-to-day basis with a properly established antimicrobial stewardship team also faces several barriers. One barrier relates to infectious diseases physicians sometimes accommodating antimicrobial requests to make their daily interactions with the requesting physicians more collegial. Forty-five percent of infectious diseases physicians believe that participation in antimicrobial stewardship programs leads to a loss of consultation requests.[44] Stewardship programs should facilitate educational sessions that promote communication and include infectious diseases physicians in the decision-making process. Antimicrobial stewardship programs should augment the activities of infectious diseases departments by encouraging primary physicians to request formal infectious diseases consultations in medically complex cases. Other barriers related to stewardship programs include developing a process to handle situations in which stewardship recommendations are not accepted, the need to continually educate incoming residents and interns, and continuing to identify areas of inappropriate prescribing in the face of ever-changing rates of antimicrobial resistance and publication of new literature.

### Making a Business Case for Antimicrobial Stewardship

Antimicrobial stewardship activities currently do not directly impact hospital reimbursement or generate revenue. Similar to most infection control activities, stewardship activities are mostly cost-avoiding in nature. Stewardship teams have consistently and successfully demonstrated a reduction in cost associated with decreased antimicrobial utilization. Additionally, some disease-based stewardship activities have demonstrated a reduction in length of stay and hospital readmissions, which improve profit margins in a fixed-reimbursement system. Finally, stewardship teams that reduce unnecessary antimicrobial utilization will likely reduce the risk for *C difficile* infection and the risk for development of multidrug-resistant pathogen colonization or infection, which impacts the cost of health care.

Building a business case for stewardship will depend on the activities of the stewardship program, and the current state of health care–associated infections and level of resistance at the institution. Hospitals with very high rates of hospital-acquired *C difficile* infection or high rates of multidrug-resistant infections could have an increase in the perceived value of the stewardship program.

### Measuring the Impact of the Program

There are no current standardized metrics to evaluate the performance of stewardship programs, and measuring the impact of a program remains a primary challenge of antimicrobial stewardship. Measuring the success of an antimicrobial stewardship program depends on the predefined goals. Although programs should be encouraged to evaluate antibiotic utilization and costs, the impact of interventions on the quality of care and patient outcomes are likely more important. The 3 most common metrics for antibiotic utilization include days of therapy (DOTs), defined daily dose, and mean duration of antimicrobial therapy. Evaluating utilization trends over time within the hospital can help identify areas of potential inappropriate antimicrobial overutilization. Furthermore, antimicrobial stewardship programs can compare utilization across similar hospitals. The National Healthcare Safety Network (NHSN) offers benchmarking of DOTs per 1000 patient days stratified by location type, which are identical to the location codes used by infection control when reporting health care–associated infections.[47] Additionally, the University Heath Consortium offers benchmarking capabilities for academic medical centers. Benchmarking of antimicrobial utilization is still in the early stages compared with the current reporting performed by infection control programs and is currently not required. However, as antimicrobial utilization benchmarking improves, facilities will have the capability to better understand the relationship between antimicrobial utilization, health care–associated infections, and patient outcomes. Additionally, improvements are needed to compare antibiotic utilization among different patient populations, which may not be linked to an NHSN unit classification, such as solid organ transplant patients, neurosurgical patients, or patients with diabetic foot infections. Polk and colleagues[48] evaluated utilization stratified by these types of patient populations using International Classification of Diseases-9 codes; however, current benchmarking at this level is not available to most hospitals.

Although, antimicrobial stewardship programs have consistently documented a reduction in antimicrobial costs following implementation, there is a plateau effect that is reached over time and it is important that this is portrayed to administration before implementation of a program. The focus of antimicrobial stewardship should not be continual reduction of cost year-over-year; however, evaluating costs can help programs identify areas for cost improvement. Antimicrobial stewardship programs can adjust the formulary, guidelines, and antimicrobial-restriction criteria to reduce the antimicrobial budget, without influencing overall utilization rates.

The primary goal of antimicrobial stewardship programs is to improve patient outcomes. The ideal way to improve and measure outcomes is through disease-based stewardship and/or multidisciplinary bundles. Individual hospitals will need to decide on which diseases to focus efforts, evaluate outcomes, and measure costs. One common area of focus is real-time stewardship team review and intervention in patients who have positive blood culture results (with or without implementation of rapid diagnostic testing). Numerous studies have demonstrated that stewardship review improves timeliness of appropriate antibiotic therapy, a reduction in antimicrobial costs, and improvements in clinical outcomes, including both mortality and length of hospitalization. Three studies have evaluated the impact of total hospital costs, instead of just antimicrobial costs, and demonstrated a total cost savings ranging from $19,583 to $26,298 per blood stream infection. This can lead to millions in cost savings over the course of a year.[49–51] Stewardship programs that implement blood culture review should clearly communicate the impact on outcomes and costs to hospital administration. In many situations, microbiology cost is increased with the implementation of new technology or modifying technician workflow to alert the stewardship program to positive results. There might not be major changes in antimicrobial expenses because antimicrobials are often started or modified, rather than discontinued. Therefore, a silo cost structure might not demonstrate any significant reduction in costs for the microbiology or pharmacy departments, despite there being a reduction in overall hospital costs due to the collaborative efforts of microbiology and pharmacy. Thus, it is important to communicate expectations and outcomes to garner the necessary resources to implement and maintain effective disease-based stewardship and quality improvement efforts.

## SUMMARY

The continued increase in the rates of antimicrobial-resistant organisms, the devastating impact of infections due to these pathogens on patient outcomes, and the lean antibiotic pipeline has created a health care industry in desperate need of enhanced antimicrobial stewardship strategies to both optimize outcomes in patients infected with these pathogens and to decrease their development and spread. These common goals lead to a natural alliance between antimicrobial stewardship clinicians and infection control practitioners.

Antimicrobial stewardship and infection control within an institution should convene and develop collaborative goals and strategies for decreasing the development and spread of problematic pathogens, as well as defining optimal evidence-based strategies for management of patients infected with these pathogens. These strategies could include targeting high-risk antimicrobials and enhanced hand hygiene and contact precaution compliance due to increased *C difficile* rates, and screening for problematic MDROs within an institution to ensure both rapid isolation of colonized patients as well as communication to stewardship personnel so that future empiric therapies can be tailored accordingly. Furthermore, infection control and stewardship teams can work together to tailor educational strategies throughout the institution using existing relationships to ensure that the message of each discipline reaches the widest possible audience.

Finally, stewardship and infection control personnel should determine the best metrics for measuring the success (or failures) of their combined efforts. These could include outcomes in patients infected with target pathogens (including time to appropriate or optimal antimicrobial therapy and time until a patient is placed in contact isolation), trends in *C difficile* rates within hospitalized patients, and/or antimicrobial use metrics. Ideally, institutions will develop a multifaceted dashboard of several such metrics to most appropriately measure the success of these complementary programs.

## ACKNOWLEDGMENTS

The authors would like to acknowledge Pranita Tamma and colleagues for their contributions to a previous version of this article.

## REFERENCES

1. Laxminarayan R, Duse A, Wattal C, et al. Antibiotic resistance-the need for global solutions. Lancet Infect Dis 2013;13(12):1057–98.
2. Infectious Diseases Society of America. The 10 x '20 Initiative: pursuing a global commitment to develop 10 new antibacterial drugs by 2020. Clin Infect Dis 2010; 50(8):1081–3.
3. Boucher HW, Talbot GH, Bradley JS, et al. Bad bugs, no drugs: no ESKAPE! An update from the Infectious Diseases Society of America. Clin Infect Dis 2009; 48(1):1–12.
4. Centers for Disease Control and Prevention. Antibiotic resistance threats in the United States, 2013. Atlanta (GA): US Department of Health and Human Services; Available at: http://www.cdc.gov/drugresistance/threat-report-2013/. Accessed April 6, 2016.
5. Reimann HA, D'Ambola J. The use and cost of antimicrobials in hospitals. Arch Environ Health 1966;13:631–6.
6. Morrill HJ, Caffrey AR, Jump RL, et al. Antimicrobial stewardship in long-term care facilities: a call to action. J Am Med Dir Assoc 2016;17(2): 183.e1–16.
7. Office of Technology Assessment USC. Impacts of antibiotic-resistant bacteria. OTA-H-629. Washington, DC: Government Printing Office; 1995.

8. McLaughlin M, Advincula MR, Malczynski M, et al. Correlations of antibiotic use and carbapenem resistance in Enterobacteriaceae. Antimicrob Agents Chemother 2013;57(10):5131–3.

9. Marchaim D, Chopra T, Bhargava A, et al. Recent exposure to antimicrobials and carbapenem-resistant Enterobacteriaceae: the role of antimicrobial stewardship. Infect Control Hosp Epidemiol 2012;33(8):817–30.

10. Patel N, Harrington S, Dihmess A, et al. Clinical epidemiology of carbapenem-intermediate or -resistant Enterobacteriaceae. J Antimicrob Chemother 2011; 66(7):1600–8.

11. Swaminathan M, Sharma S, Poliansky Blash S, et al. Prevalence and risk factors for acquisition of carbapenem-resistant Enterobacteriaceae in the setting of endemicity. Infect Control Hosp Epidemiol 2013;34(8):809–17.

12. Slimings C, Riley TV. Antibiotics and hospital-acquired *Clostridium difficile* infection: update of systematic review and meta-analysis. J Antimicrob Chemother 2014;69(4):881–91.

13. Feazel LM, Malhotra A, Perencevich EN, et al. Effect of antibiotic stewardship programmes on *Clostridium difficile* incidence: a systematic review and meta-analysis. J Antimicrob Chemother 2014;69(7):1748–54.

14. Morton JB, LaPlante KL. Impact of the presidential executive order on decreasing antimicrobial resistance. Am J Health Syst Pharm 2015;72(14):1171–2.

15. Centers for Disease Control and Prevention. The core elements of antibiotic stewardship for nursing homes. Atlanta (GA): US Department of Health and Human Services; CDC; 2015. Available at: http://www.cdc.gov/longtermcare/index.html. Accessed April 6, 2016.

16. Dellit TH, Owens RC, McGowan JE Jr, et al. Infectious Diseases Society of America and the Society for Healthcare Epidemiology of America guidelines for developing an institutional program to enhance antimicrobial stewardship. Clin Infect Dis 2007;44:159–77.

17. Schentag JJ, Ballow CH, Fritz AL, et al. Changes in antimicrobial agent usage resulting from interactions among clinical pharmacy, the infectious disease division, and the microbiology laboratory. Diagn Microbiol Infect Dis 1993;16:255–64.

18. Carling P, Fung T, Killion A, et al. Favorable impact of a multidisciplinary antibiotic management program conducted during 7 years. Infect Control Hosp Epidemiol 2003;24:699–706.

19. LaRocco A Jr. Concurrent antibiotic review programs- a role for infectious diseases specialists at small community hospitals. Clin Infect Dis 2003;37:742–3.

20. Ansari F, Gray K, Nathwani D, et al. Outcomes of an intervention to improve hospital antibiotic prescribing: interrupted time series with segmented regression analysis. J Antimicrob Chemother 2003;52:842–8.

21. Ruttimann S, Keck B, Hartmeier C, et al. Long-term antibiotic cost savings from a comprehensive intervention program in a medical department of a university-affiliated hospital. Clin Infect Dis 2004;38:348–56.

22. Lutters M, Harbarth S, Janssens J-P, et al. Effect of a comprehensive, multidisciplinary, educational program on the use of antibiotics in a geriatric university hospital. J Am Geriatr Soc 2004;52:112–6.

23. Scheckler WE, Bennett JV. Antibiotic usage in seven community hospitals. JAMA 1970;213(2):264–7.

24. Moody J, Cosgrove SE, Olmsted R, et al. Antimicrobial stewardship: a collaborative partnership between infection preventionists and healthcare epidemiologists. Infect Control Hosp Epidemiol 2012;33(4):328–30.

25. Wagner B, Filice GA, Drekonja D, et al. Antimicrobial stewardship programs in inpatient hospital settings: a systematic review. Infect Control Hosp Epidemiol 2014;35(10):1209–28.

26. Andersson DI. Improving predictions of the risk of resistance development against new and old antibiotics. Clin Microbiol Infect 2015;21(10):894–8.

27. Ziakas PD, Thapa R, Rice LB, et al. Trends and Significance of VRE Colonization in the ICU: a Meta-Analysis of Published Studies. PLoS One 2013;8(9):e75658.

28. Weinstock DM, Conlon M, Iovino C. Colonization, bloodstream infection, and mortality caused by vancomycin-resistant enterococcus early after allogeneic hematopoietic stem cell transplant. Biol Blood Marrow Transplant 2007;13:615–21.

29. Zasowski EJ, Claeys KC, Lagnf AM, et al. Time is of the essence: the impact of delayed antibiotic therapy on patient outcomes in hospital-onset enterococcal bloodstream infections. Clin Infect Dis 2016;62(10):1242–50.

30. Nagel JL, Stevenson JG, Eiland EH III, et al. Demonstrating the value of antimicrobial stewardship programs to hospital administrators. Clin Infect Dis 2014; 59(Suppl 3):S146–53.

31. CMS. Available at: https://www.cms.gov/Medicare/Medicare.html8. Accessed December 14, 2015.

32. Yeung SS, Yeung JK, Lau TT, et al. Evaluation of a Clostridium difficile infection management policy with clinical pharmacy and medical microbiology involvement at a major Canadian teaching hospital. J Clin Pharm Ther 2015;40(6): 655–60.

33. Bauer KA, Perez KK, Forrest GN, et al. Review of rapid diagnostic tests used by antimicrobial stewardship programs. Clin Infect Dis 2014;59(Suppl 3):S134–45.

34. Loeb M, Brazil K, Lohfeld L, et al. Effect of a multifaceted intervention on number of antimicrobial prescriptions for suspected urinary tract infections in residents of nursing homes: cluster randomised controlled trial. BMJ 2005;331(7518):669.

35. Skarda DE, Schall K, Rollins M, et al. Response-based therapy for ruptured appendicitis reduces resource utilization. J Pediatr Surg 2014;49(12):1726–9.

36. Antworth A, Collins CD, Kunapuli A, et al. Impact of an antimicrobial stewardship program comprehensive care bundle on management of candidemia. Pharmacotherapy 2013;33(2):137–43.

37. Pogue JM, Mynatt RP, Marchaim D, et al. Automated alerts coupled with antimicrobial stewardship intervention lead to decreases in length of stay in patients with gram-negative bacteremia. Infect Control Hosp Epidemiol 2014;35(2):132–8.

38. Jardin CG, Palmer HR, Shah DN, et al. Assessment of treatment patterns and patient outcomes before vs after implementation of a severity-based Clostridium difficile infection treatment policy. J Hosp Infect 2013;85(1):28–32.

39. Kelley D, Aaronson P, Poon E, et al. Evaluation of an antimicrobial stewardship approach to minimize overuse of antibiotics in patients with asymptomatic bacteriuria. Infect Control Hosp Epidemiol 2014;35(2):193–5.

40. Liu C, Bayer A, Cosgrove SE, et al. Clinical practice guidelines by the Infectious Diseases Society of America for the treatment of methicillin-resistant Staphylococcus aureus infections in adults and children: executive summary. Clin Infect Dis 2011;52(3):285–92.

41. Lopez-Cortes L, del Toro MD, Galvez-Acebal J, et al. Impact of an evidence-based bundle intervention in the quality-of-care management and outcome of Staphylococcus aureus bacteremia. Clin Infect Dis 2013;57:1225–33.

42. Borde JP, Nadide B, Rieg S, et al. Adherence to an antibiotic stewardship bundle targeting Staphylococcus aureus blood stream infections at a 200-bed community hospital. Infection 2014;42:713–9.

43. Nguyen CT, Gandhi T, Chenoweth C, et al. Impact of an antimicrobial stewardship-led intervention for *Staphylococcus aureus* bacteraemia: a quasi-experimental study. J Antimicrob Chemother 2015;70(12):3390–6.

44. Sunenshine RH, Kiedkte LA, Jernigan DB, et al. Role of infectious diseases consultants in management of antimicrobial use in hospitals. Clin Infect Dis 2004;38: 934–8.

45. DePestel DD, Eiland EH 3rd, Lusardi K. Assessing appropriateness of antimicrobial therapy: in the eye of the interpreter. Clin Infect Dis 2014;59(Suppl 3): S154–61.

46. Metlay JP, Shea JA, Crossette LB, et al. Tensions in antibiotic prescribing: pitting social concerns against interests of individual patients. J Gen Intern Med 2002; 17:87–94.

47. National Healthcare Safety Network; Antimicrobial Use and Resistance Options website. Available at: http://www.cdc.gov/nhsn/acute-care-hospital/aur/. Accessed December 15, 2015.

48. Polk RE, Hohmann SF, Medvedev S, et al. Benchmarking risk-adjusted adult antibacterial drug use in 70 US academic medical center hospitals. Clin Infect Dis 2011;53(11):1100–10.

49. Perez KK, Olsen RJ, Musick WL, et al. Integrating rapid diagnostics and antimicrobial stewardship improves outcomes in patients with antibiotic-resistant Gram-negative bacteremia. J Infect 2014;69(3):216–25.

50. Perez KK, Olsen RJ, Musick WL, et al. Integrating rapid pathogen identification and antimicrobial stewardship significantly decreases hospital costs. Arch Pathol Lab Med 2013;137(9):1247–54.

51. Wong JR, Bauer KA, Mangino JE, et al. Antimicrobial stewardship pharmacist interventions for coagulase-negative staphylococci positive blood cultures using rapid polymerase chain reaction. Ann Pharmacother 2012;46(11):1484–90.

# Infection Control in Alternative Health Care Settings: An Update

Elaine Flanagan, RN, BSN, MSA, CIC[a], Marco Cassone, MD, PhD[b],
Ana Montoya, MD[b], Lona Mody, MD, MSc[b,c,*]

## KEYWORDS

- Infection control • Health care delivery • Nursing homes • Hand hygiene

## KEY POINTS

- With changing health care delivery, patients receive care at various settings, including acute care hospitals, nursing homes, outpatient primary care and specialty clinics, as well as at home. Each of these settings exposes patients to pathogens.
- Each health care setting faces unique challenges, requiring individualized infection control programs.
- Infection control programs in nursing homes should address: surveillance for infections and antimicrobial resistance, outbreak investigation and control plan for epidemics, isolation precautions, hand hygiene, staff education, and employee and resident health programs.

## BACKGROUND

Health care delivery in the United States has evolved significantly over the latter part of the twentieth century. Health care delivery has moved from acute care facilities to rehabilitation units, nursing homes (NHs), assisted living facilities, home, and outpatient settings. Measures to reduce health care costs have led to a reduced number of hospitalizations and shorter lengths of stay, along with increased outpatient, home care, and NH stays for older adults.[1–3]

This article focuses on infection control issues in NHs and outpatient settings.

Portions of this article originally appeared in Volume 25, Issue 1 (March 2011) of *Infectious Disease Clinics of North America*.

[a] Quality and Patient Safety, Detroit Medical Center Healthcare System, 399 John R Street, Detroit, MI 48201, USA; [b] Division of Geriatric Medicine, University of Michigan Medical School, Ann Arbor, MI, USA; [c] Geriatrics Research Education and Clinical Center, Veterans Affairs Ann Arbor Healthcare System, 2215 Fuller Drive, Ann Arbor, MI 48105, USA
* Corresponding author. AAVAMC, 11-G GRECC, 2215 Fuller Drive, Ann Arbor, MI 48105.
*E-mail address:* lonamody@umich.edu

Infect Dis Clin N Am 30 (2016) 785–804
http://dx.doi.org/10.1016/j.idc.2016.05.001
0891-5520/16/$ – see front matter © 2016 Elsevier Inc. All rights reserved.

id.theclinics.com

## INFECTION PREVENTION PROGRAMS IN NURSING HOMES

NHs host approximately 1.5 million residents, which is more than in acute care hospitals and centers. About 3–15% of such residents acquire an infection in these facilities (1.8–13.5 infections per 1000 residents care days). Infections are among the top five causes of death[4,5] and rank even higher among preventable causes. It is no surprise then that NH residents are more likely to be prescribed antimicrobial therapy than any other drug class. Antimicrobial therapy accounts for 20% or more of all recorded adverse drug reactions.[6,7] Every year there are more than 2 million discharges, and these numbers will grow following shifts in the demographic curve.[2] The high volume of transfers from and to hospitals is a major determinant in shaping the epidemiology of infections in NHs.

Even with the evolution of health care delivery within the United States, NHs are institutions that provide health care to people who are unable to manage independently in the community in two different circumstances: (1) for chronic care management, and (2) for short-term rehabilitative services following an acute care hospital stay, to complete their medical treatment plan before returning to independent living. As NHs accept increasingly medically complex patients from acute care, infection prevention becomes crucial. Infection prevention research in the NH setting has made enormous strides in the last 2 decades.

However, NHs have unique characteristics that create special challenges in implementing an infection prevention program. First, effective infection control programs require human and capital investment. Initial access to funds and to personnel experienced in infection prevention can be a challenge. Second, NH residents are particularly susceptible to infections because of comorbidities, greater severity of illness, functional and cognitive impairment, incontinence, and indwelling device use such as urinary catheters and feeding tubes. These factors also make the diagnostic process more challenging, especially when cognitive deficit is present or when fever response is inadequate. Third, NH residents may also serve as host reservoirs for antimicrobial-resistant pathogens such as methicillin-resistant *Staphylococus aureus* (MRSA) and vancomycin-resistant *Enterococcus* (VRE). Indeed, a previous stay in a NH is considered to be a risk factor for colonization with multidrug-resistant organisms (MDROs). With reduction in the hospital length of stay, the severity of illness among post-acute care residents has increased, with resultant inherent transfers back to the hospital. Thus, residents serve as vectors, transmitting pathogens from one setting to another. Fourth, the diagnostic yield of specimens is often subpar because of sampling difficulties (eg, obtaining a sputum sample or clean-catch urine sample). Delays in access to technology such as chest radiographs, blood, and microbiology tests may postpone diagnosis and affect clinical evaluation. Communication with off-site clinical providers is an additional challenge, since indirect assessment of residents encourages risk-aversion practices such as overuse of long-term empirical antibiotic therapy. This starts the vicious cycle of selection of MDROs, leading in time to further overuse of empiric wide-spectrum antibiotics.

To help navigate through those challenges, specific criteria for the diagnosis of infection were developed. These criteria have been recently modified incorporating the larger body of evidence and improvements in diagnostic tools now available.[8] Loeb's minimum criteria should be used to help determine when it is appropriate to initiate antimicrobial therapy.[9] Unfortunately, adherence to these criteria is still suboptimal.[10,11]

## INFECTION PREVENTION PROGRAMS IN NURSING HOMES: FUNCTIONS, COMPONENTS, AND OVERSIGHT

Main functions for an infection prevention program include

- Obtaining and managing critical data, including surveillance information for endemic infections and outbreaks
- Developing and updating policies and procedures
- Developing individualized interventions to prevent infections and antimicrobial resistance
- Educating and training health care workers (HCWs), residents, visitors, and nonmedical caregivers[1]

An effective infection prevention program includes a method of surveillance for infections and antimicrobial-resistant pathogens, an outbreak control plan for epidemics, isolation and standard precautions, hand hygiene (HH), staff education, an employee health program, a resident health program, policy formation and periodic review with audits, and a policy to communicate reportable diseases to public health authorities.

An infection preventionist (IP) is the central figure among many indispensable individuals in developing and executing an infection prevention program. Due to the constant evolution and the adoption of best practices, the IP must be an engaged professional continually pursuing new knowledge and education.

In the last 10 years, successful infection prevention programs have increasingly utilized bundles, usually 3 to 5 interventions each with demonstrated efficacy, which are deployed together to greatly increase the power of the program and at the same time maximize effort and resources (**Box 1**). The advantages of intervention bundles are many and often reach beyond the stated goal of the specific program itself: Promoting cost-effective measures, engaging personnel at all levels, creation of a culture of safety and quality, promoting a chain of accountability, facilitating learning rather than blaming, and helping to establish ripe translational frameworks for further interventions, which is key in such an evolving and resource intensive setting. Bundles may also have disadvantages in certain cases (eg, the specific impact of each individual component of the intervention cannot be quantified). Also, in populations with unique characteristics, there may not be multiple proven interventions available for inclusion in the bundle.

Recent examples of successful protocols using bundles include

- A multimodal intervention including preemptive barrier precautions, active surveillance for MDROs and infections, and NH staff education, leading to a decrease in overall MDRO prevalence density, new MRSA acquisition, and catheter associated urinary tract infection (CAUTI)[12]
- A nationwide initiative in 133 Veterans Administration (VA) NHs, consisting of universal nasal surveillance for MRSA, contact precautions for patients colonized or infected with MRSA, HH, and direct accountability of everyone who had contact with patients, leading to a 36% decrease in MRSA health care-associated infections[13]
- An active protocol of decolonization with nasal mupirocin and chlorhexidine bathing, coupled with enhanced environmental cleaning, which reduced MRSA colonization from 16% to 10% in a high-risk population[14]
- A comprehensive protocol based on the World Health Organization (WHO) multimodal HH improvements strategy, including the use of alcohol-based handrub placed at point of care on dedicated racks; the use of pull reels; HH posters and reminders; an educational program; and performance feedback, which

---

**Box 1**
**Resources for infection preventionists**

1. SHEA and APIC both have long-term care committees that publish and approve NH infection guidelines and publish periodic position papers related to pertinent infection control issues. Their websites have several educational resources for staff education and in-services. In addition, APIC also publishes a quarterly long-term care newsletter.

2. Local professional infection prevention society chapters provide a network to socialize, discuss infection control challenges and practical solutions to overcome them, and provide access to educational resources and services. ICPs should become members of these professional societies at both the local and national level to remain up-to-date with practice guidelines, position statements, information technology resources, and changes in policies and regulations.

3. Hospital epidemiology and infection control, 3rd edition; C. Glen Mayhall Ed.: Lippincott Williams & Wilkins: Philadelphia, PA.

4. Selected internet websites:
   a. CDC: http://www.cdc.gov
   b. SHEA: http://www.shea-online.org/
   c. APIC: http://www.apic.org
   d. OSHA: http://www.osha.gov
   e. Joint Commission on Accreditation of Healthcare Organizations—Infection Control Initiatives: http://www.jcaho.org/accredited+organizations/patient+safety/infection+control/ic+index.htm
   f. AAMI Standards and Recommended Practices Sterilization in Health Care Facilities 2015 Edition: www.aami.org
   g. Guidelines for Perioperative Practice 2015 Edition: www.aorn.org
   h. CDC Guide to Infection Prevention for Outpatient Settings: Minimum Expectations for Safe Care Web site 2011: http://www.cdc.gov/hai/pdfs/guidelines/ambulatory-care-04-2011.pdf

---

resulted in both compliance improvement and reduction in respiratory outbreaks and MRSA infection requiring hospital admission[15]

- A multimodal protocol targeted at HCWs that reduced hand colonization and resolved longstanding issues of enteral feed contamination[16]

### Information Transfer During Care Transitions

Transitional care is defined as "a set of actions designed to ensure the coordination and continuity of health care as patients transfer between different locations or different levels of care in the same location".[17] For older adults, these locations can include acute care hospitals, NHs, skilled nursing facilities, rehabilitation units, assisted living facilities, inpatient hospice care, home care, and outpatient primary and specialty clinics. During these care transitions, older adults are particularly prone to fragmented care, which can lead to errors and omissions in health care delivery. These transitions also provide an opportunity for pathogens to be transferred from one setting to another. Risk factors at discharge, such as presence of central venous catheters or other invasive devices, and presence of chronic wounds, for example, are predictors of subsequent colonization with MRSA in transitioning residents.[18] It then becomes important for the NHs to request clinical information from the transferring facility regarding current culture reports of the resident's body sites that may be infected or colonized with pathogenic organisms, especially MDROs. This action will enable the physician providers and HCWs to determine the nursing care interventions necessary to meet the resident's needs and to prevent spread of pathogens in the facility. An important step would be to provide every transitioning resident a standardized form with key information about their specific risk factors for infections, history of MDRO colonization or infection, and antibiotic therapy, including specific agents and duration. This information should be readily accessible in a common and recognizable format. In a not so distant future, nationwide compatibility and communication in electronic records should make it possible to mandate effortless, automatic creation and update of such standardized forms.

### Hand Hygiene

HH remains the most effective and least expensive measure to prevent transmission of pathogenic organisms in health care settings. Despite calls from numerous local, national, and international organizations and infection prevention societies, compliance with HH remains dismal, averaging only 30% to 50%.[19-26] Reasons frequently reported for poor compliance with HH measures by HCWs include skin irritation from frequent washing, too little time due to a high workload, and simply forgetting.

The WHO launched its first Global Patient Safety Challenge, "Clean Care is Safer Care," in October 2005.[21] The objective of this initiative was to reduce health care–associated infections around the globe. The program's initial focus was the promotion of HH practices in diverse health care systems. WHO has also developed an innovative core theme, "My Five Moments of Hand Hygiene," which details appropriate situations for compliance with HH measures during health care delivery. This approach provides guidelines and specific recommendations to enhance HH compliance and is targeted at a broad audience of HCWs, hospital administrators, and health authorities. A systematic review of 56 studies suggested that HH helped decrease the infection risk in NHs, with major impacts on respiratory infections and influenza (80%) and gram-positive bacterial infections (76%), and a lower impact on gram-negative bacterial infections (44%).[2] In a recent survey, it was noted that although HH was an important focus of infection control programs, formal policies regarding monitoring of staff compliance were lacking.[23]

To improve HH bundles of simple and effective measures should be used. In a recent meta-analysis,[24] several strategies proved useful towards improving overall HH compliance:

- Ensure HH resources are accessible facility wide and at the point of care.
- Reinforce HH behavior and accountability.
- Provide regular reminders.
- Establish ongoing monitoring and feedback of HH compliance.
- Establish ongoing monitoring and feedback on infection rates.
- Establish administrative leadership and support.
- Establish a multidisciplinary design and response team.
- Provide ongoing education and training for staff, patients, families, and visitors.

The use of waterless, alcohol-based handrubs as an adjunct to resident washing hands with soap and water has become a routine practice by HCWs in acute care facilities.[25] Introduction of alcohol-based handrubs has been shown to significantly improve HH compliance among HCWs in acute care hospitals and to decrease overall nosocomial infection rates and transmission of MRSA infections. Alcohol-based handrubs have also been shown to enhance compliance with HH in NHs and should be used to complement educational initiatives.[27] Although the cost of introducing alcohol-based handrubs could be a concern for NHs, a study in acute care has shown that the total costs of a HH promotion campaign including alcohol-based handrub corresponded to less than 1% of costs that could be attributed to nosocomial infections.[28]

While introducing alcohol-based handrub in health care settings is a prudent, cost-effective measure, several issues need to be considered. Alcohol-based handrubs should not be used if hands are visibly soiled, in which case HH with antimicrobial soap and water is recommended. Alcohol-based handrubs can cause dry skin; however, recent data on rubs containing emollients have shown that handrubs cause significantly less skin irritation and dryness than soap and water.[26] NH staff should be aware that alcohols are flammable. NH staff should work with their local fire marshals to ensure that installation of alcohol-based handrub containers is consistent with local fire codes. More information on HH is available elsewhere in this issue (See Bolon MK: Hand Hygiene, in this issue).

Compliance in the use of gown and gloves still needs improvement and must be enforced. In addition, it is important to stress the importance of gown and glove changes when appropriate, to prevent contamination. In a recent study, dressing, transferring, providing hygiene, changing linens and toileting a resident were found to be high-risk care activities for the transmission of MRSA from colonized resident to HCW gown and gloves.[29]

### Multidrug-Resistant Organisms

Infection and colonization with antimicrobial-resistant pathogens are important concerns in NHs and develop primarily due to widespread use of empiric antibiotics, functional impairment, use of indwelling devices, limited adherence to HH programs among HCWs, and cross-transmission during group activities. In 2013, the US Centers for Disease Control and Prevention (CDC) identified 18 most important antibiotic resistant threats.[30] Of those 18, at least 11 are common in NH residents. The most important are MRSA, which in the United States accounts for more than half of all *S aureus* isolates, VRE, and multi-drug resistant gram-negative bacilli (MDR-GNB), defined as resistant to 3 or more antibiotic classes. Among MDR-GNB, the most common species are *Escherichia coli, Klebsiella pneumoniae, Proteus spp, Acinetobacter baumanii,* and *Pseudomonas aeruginosa.*[31] *Burkholderia cepacia* and *Stenotrophomonas maltophilia*, although isolated less often, are important, because they are commonly resistant to most broad-spectrum antibiotics.[32]

The most important risk factors for MDRO infection in NHs are use of indwelling devices, functional disability, presence of wounds,[33] prior antimicrobial use,[34] and prior hospitalization. Interestingly, some functional disability and comorbidity scoring systems, such as the Physical Self Maintenance Score (PSMS) and Charlson's Comorbidity Score, which have been established to aid in prognostic and effort/cost evaluations, might also prove useful in quantifying infection risk.[35] NHs can reduce infections and colonization with resistant pathogens by emphasizing HH, developing an antimicrobial utilization program, encouraging evidence-based clinical evaluation and management of infections, and ensuring that the facility has a well-established individualized infection prevention program. Guidelines and expert reviews to control MRSA and VRE provide a good base for developing facility-specific policies.[1,36–38]

There has been some debate on the role of active surveillance cultures and their impact on isolation policies in acute care hospitals. The Society for Healthcare Epidemiology of America (SHEA) guideline for preventing nosocomial transmission of MDROs advocates for use of active surveillance cultures,[39] whereas the recent draft of the CDC's Healthcare Infection Control and Prevention Advisory Committee (HICPAC) guidelines call for individual facilities to assess their own needs and conduct surveillance cultures as they deem necessary.[40] These guidelines refer to studies from acute care hospitals serving a sicker, shorter-stay population than those served by NHs. The role of active surveillance cultures in NHs has not been clearly defined. In a rural setting comprised of 1 hospital, 5 affiliated NHs, and 1 ambulatory center, active surveillance resulted in a dramatic decrease in MRSA colonization in NH residents and MRSA infections in hospital patients.[41] Although these results may not translate as well to highly populated areas with complex health care networks, they serve as proof that facilities should be familiar with guidelines and evidence, and monitor rates of MRSA and VRE, and any recent outbreaks.

## Isolation Precautions

HICPAC has proposed a 2-tiered structure for isolation precautions. The first tier is standard precautions, which apply to the care of all patients in health care settings regardless of their infectious status. Standard precautions constitute the primary strategy for preventing transmission of organisms between patients and health care workers. In the second tier are transmission-based precautions, which are used for the care of patients suspected of or known to be infected with epidemiologically important pathogens when the route of transmission (eg, physical contact, or airborne or droplet transmission) is not completely interrupted by standardized precautions.[42]

Standard precautions apply to blood, all body fluids, secretions and excretions regardless of whether they contain visible blood, nonintact skin, and/or mucous membrane material. Designed to reduce the risk of transmission of pathogens, both from apparent and ambiguous sources of infection, standard precautions include HH compliance, gowns, glove use, masks, eye protection or face shield, as well as avoiding injuries from sharps. Two new elements of standard precautions added in the HICPAC isolation precautions guidelines respiratory hygiene/cough etiquette and safe injection practices, also apply to NHs. The elements of respiratory hygiene/cough etiquette include

- Education of health care facility staff, residents, and visitors
- Use of language and education appropriate posters and signs
- Source control measures such as covering the mouth/nose with a tissue and prompt disposal of used tissues or sneezing into the elbow area rather than the hand if tissues are not available
- HH after contact with respiratory secretions and spatial separation of greater than 3 feet in common areas if possible

Safe injection practices include the use of single-use, sterile, disposable needle and syringe for each injection and prevention of contamination of any injection equipment and medication.[42] Injuries caused by needles and other sharps have been associated with the transmission of hepatitis B virus, hepatitis C virus, and human immune deficiency virus (HIV).

Transmission-based precautions are intended for use with patients who may be infected with highly transmissible or epidemiologically significant pathogens. There are three main types of transmission-based precautions: airborne precautions (eg, for tuberculosis), droplet precautions (eg, for influenza), and contact precautions (eg, for *Clostridium difficile*). Contact precautions are recommended for residents with MDROs who are ill, or whose secretions or drainage cannot be contained. Single rooms are preferred for these residents if available, as well as for residents with excessive coughing or widespread skin disease. Often NHs have high occupancy rates and a paucity of single-resident rooms. In such situations, residents should be cohorted or kept in a semiprivate room, preferably with a resident who is at low risk of developing an infection (such as one who is well nourished, ambulatory, can perform daily activities independently, and has no indwelling catheters/lines or open wounds). Spatial separation of at least 3 feet between beds is advised to reduce the opportunities for inadvertent sharing of items between the infected/colonized residents.[42] Although these guidelines were designed for acute care settings, several of them, especially standard precautions, apply to NHs also. These recommendations have to be adapted to the needs of the individual facility.

Residents colonized with a specific pathogen should participate in facility activities and be able to dine in the dining hall. Because there are both recognized and unrecognized pathogen carriers participating in these group activities, all residents should have wounds or invasive device sites cleansed and covered, and have hands washed before leaving their rooms.

### Surveillance for Infections and Antimicrobial Usage

Overuse of antibiotics or use of inappropriate regimens such as wide-spectrum antibiotics, is of concern in NHs and often leads to infections with antimicrobial-resistant organisms in residents who receive antibiotics as well as those in NHs who do not receive antibiotics.[34,43] NHs are often are major reservoirs of MDROs.[44–46] Furthermore, there are immense geographic variations, demanding locally relevant policies and practices. For example, in European NHs, empirical and prophylactic antibiotics account for 80% of all treatments. Specific regimens and indications vary greatly across countries, with conditions such as antibiotic overuse in residents with bacteriuria standing out as one area needing much improvement in every single region and making a case for structured, sustained surveillance practices.[47]

Infection surveillance in NHs involves collection of data on facility-acquired infections. Surveillance is defined as "ongoing, systematic collection, analysis, and interpretation of health data essential to the planning, implementation, and evaluation of public health practice, closely integrated with timely dissemination of these data to those who need to know."[48] Surveillance can be limited based on a particular objective, a particular ward, or an unusual organism or may be facility-wide.

For surveillance to be conducted correctly, utilization of standardized NH-appropriate definitions of infections is crucial.[49,50] Besides using valid surveillance definitions, a facility must have clear goals and aims for setting up a surveillance program. These goals, as with other elements of an infection control program, have to be reviewed periodically to reflect changes in the facility's population, pathogens of interest, and changing antimicrobial resistance patterns. Plans to analyze the data and use of these data to design and implement proven preventive measures must also be clearly delineated in advance. The analysis and reporting of infection rates in NHs are typically conducted monthly, quarterly, and annually to detect trends. Infection rates (preferably reported as infections per 1000 resident days) can be calculated by using as the denominator resident days or average resident census for the surveillance period.

These data can then be used to establish endemic baseline infection rates, and to recognize variations from the baseline that could represent an outbreak. This information should eventually lead to specific, targeted infection control initiatives and to evaluate the success of the changes. Additionally, a facility's surveillance system should include monitoring for appropriate antibiotic use. For example a positive culture in a person without clinical symptoms rarely requires treatment with antibiotics. Surveillance strategies may alternatively focus the effort on screening for MDROs in high-risk residents such as those with indwelling devices or functional disability.[51,52] Evidence on the optimal strategy to screen for MDROs is not yet clear. Screening in research settings has included screening for multiple anatomic sites, which greatly improves not just sensitivity, but also the quality of screening data and allows for the uncovering of important specific strain epidemiology.[53–55]

For high-risk groups, surveillance could be conducted using the PRECEDE (Predisposing, Reinforcing and Enabling Constructs in Educational Diagnosis and Evaluation) model, which follows 4 stages:

- The starting stage is defining predisposing factors, by assessing the local, current epidemiology of infection and colonization with MDROs, and the relevant attitude, practices, and knowledge in HCWs.
- The second stage focuses on enabling HCWs using education, involvement in leadership and promotion of prevention practices, HH campaigns, and by making related products and infrastructure available.
- Reinforcement is then provided to NH staff using simple, regular feedback on infection and colonization rate.
- The fourth stage, which is intended to feed back into the first, consists of outcome evaluation by knowledge and adherence reassessment and by determining how rates of infection and colonization have been impacted.[51]

### Outbreak Management

An illness in a community or region is considered an outbreak when the frequency of this illness clearly exceeds the normal rate of expectancy. The existence of an outbreak is thus always defined relative to the number of cases that are expected to occur in a specific population in a specific time period.

The main objectives of an outbreak investigation are discovery and elimination of the source and prevention of new cases. To prevent future outbreaks, research is carried out to gain additional knowledge about the infectious agent, its mode of transmission, and conditions that facilitate it. This new knowledge leads to re-evaluation of infection control programs and strategies for improvement are devised.

It is vital that the IP, in conjunction with physician support, has the skills to recognize an outbreak, conduct appropriate data collection methods, analyze and interpret the data using simple epidemiologic measures, conduct an initial outbreak investigation efficiently, and institute emergent, effective and appropriate outbreak control measures. Although local health departments are available for counseling, it may also be beneficial for the IP to have access to a hospital epidemiologist for consultation. More information about outbreak investigations is available elsewhere in this issue (See Sood G, Perl TM: Outbreaks in Healthcare Settings, in this issue).

### Rehabilitation Services

NHs also provide post-acute care rehabilitation, including physical therapy (PT), occupational therapy (OT), and wound care with or without hydrotherapy. These therapists, like other clinical staff such as nurses and nurses' aides, frequently come into contact with residents and thus have many opportunities to transmit pathogens. In a NH, PT and OT services can be provided either at the bedside or in a central therapy unit. For bedside therapy, therapists may move between rooms and units and do not routinely wear gloves and gowns. For care at a central therapy unit, residents are transported to an open unit, where handwashing sinks may not be readily available. Although therapists are seldom directly linked to hospital outbreaks,[56] hydrotherapy for wounds has been shown to facilitate outbreaks with resistant pathogens.[57]

A detailed infection control program for rehabilitation services should be prepared and focus on facility design to promote HH compliance including convenient and easy access to sinks and the use of alcohol-based handrubs. Patients who are infectious should not be treated at the central therapy unit. Facilities providing hydrotherapy should consider providing the service in a dedicated room with a separate resident entrance.

### Environmental Hygiene

Cleaning and disinfection of frequently touched surfaces reduce the risk of transmission of MDROs and *C difficile*. NH residents share common areas such as rehabilitation rooms, dining areas, common halls, and activity rooms, offering opportunities for pathogen exchange. Staff should be educated on the use of the chemicals, and annual competencies are recommended to be required for specific disinfection procedures in compliance with CDC guidelines.[58]

### Resident and Employee Health Program

The resident health program should focus on immunizations, tuberculin testing, and infection control policies to prevent specific infections. The program should include areas such as skin care, oral hygiene, prevention of aspiration, and catheter care to prevent urinary tract infections. Adults over the age of 65 should receive pneumococcal vaccination at least once and influenza vaccination every year. New pneumococcal vaccinations covering additional serotypes should be also considered in residents who received previous formulations. Standing orders for pneumococcal vaccination have improved vaccination rates in NHs.[59] Tetanus, diphtheria and pertussis (Tdap) vaccination is also recommended among older adults in NHs.

The employee health program mainly concerns employees with potentially communicable diseases, policies for sick leave, immunizations, and Occupational Safety and Health Administration (OSHA) regulations to protect them from blood-borne pathogens. It is a requirement that NHs bar employees with known communicable diseases or infected skin lesions from providing direct contact with the residents, and that employees with infected skin lesions or infectious diarrhea be prevented from having direct contact with residents' food. Moreover, when hiring new employees, an initial medical history must be obtained along with a physical examination and screening for tuberculosis. Immunization status should also be assessed.

Infection control policies and measures in NHs must be in place to address postexposure prophylaxis for infections such as HIV and hepatitis B. Varicella vaccine should be given to employees not immune to the virus. Employees are expected to be up-to-date with their tetanus boosters and to receive influenza vaccinations every year. Influenza vaccine has been associated with decreased absenteeism among HCWs and decreased influenza mortality in NH residents.[60] Annual influenza vaccination campaigns play a central role in deterring and preventing nosocomial transmission of the influenza virus and should be promoted by the IP and NH leadership. Employee immunization records should reflect immunity status for indicated vaccinations and those administered during employment, and should be accessible in the event of an outbreak situation.[61]

### Role of Infection Preventionist

An IP, usually a staff nurse, is assigned the responsibility of directing infection control activities in an NH. The IP is responsible for implementing, monitoring, and evaluating the infection control program. To maintain compliance with regulations, NHs have increased the rate of NH IP employment from 8.1% in 2003 to 44% in 2008.[62] However, often an IP has additional responsibilities such as employee health or staff education.[63] For an infection control program to succeed, the IP should be empowered with sufficient time and resources to carry out infection control activities. The IP should also be familiar with the federal, state, and local regulations regarding infection control. Collaborating with an infectious diseases epidemiologist should be encouraged. Such collaborations could also provide assistance with outbreak investigations, emergency preparedness in the event of bioterrorism and vaccine shortages, and the use of microbiologic and molecular methods for infection prevention.

### Environmental Rounds

The IP should conduct walking rounds on a regular basis to make observations regarding equipment decontamination and cleaning procedures, and adherence to infection control guidelines. Observations should be made regarding availability of soap and paper towels, handling of sharps and infectious waste, and storage of health care supplies, medications and food.

### Staff Education

The IP plays a vital role in meeting infection control requirements and in educating NH personnel on various infection control measures, particularly in view of rapid staff turnover common in NHs. A lack of understanding of key infection prevention concepts among NH staff has been reported.[64] A recent study on nursing assistants reported language, knowledge, part-time status, workload demands, and accountability as barriers to using infection control practices, and proposed translating in-services, hands-on training, on-spot training for part time staff, and increased staffing ratios and inclusion and empowerment as strategies to overcome those barriers.[65] Informal education during infection control and quality improvement meetings as well as during infection control walking rounds should be complemented with in-service education on HH, appropriate and early diagnosis of infections, indications for antibiotic usage and antimicrobial resistance, and isolation precautions and policies.

Ongoing staff education is important due to the new research and guidelines published every year, advancements in technology, and regulatory demands. The Joint Commission (TJC) expects new employee orientation to include the facility's infection prevention program, and the employee's individual responsibility is to prevent infections. In addition, OSHA requires training for blood-borne pathogens and tuberculosis on any employee expected to potentially come into contact with infectious agents.

### Oversight Committee

The Federal Nursing Home Reform Act from the Omnibus Budget Reconciliation Act of 1987 mandated the formation of a formal infection control committee to evaluate infection rates, implement infection control programs, and review policies and procedures. This mandate has been dropped by OBRA at the federal level. However, some states may still require them. A small subcommittee or a working group comprised of the medical director, administrator or nursing supervisor, and IP should evaluate the NH infection rates on a regular basis and present the data at quality control meetings, review policies and any relevant research, and make decisions regarding infection control changes. This subcommittee can review and analyze the surveillance data, assure that these data are presented to the nursing and physician staff, and approve targeted recommendations to reduce the incidence of infections. Records pertaining to these activities and infection data should be kept and filed for future reference. Given that infection control involves multiple disciplines, the participation of representatives from food services, maintenance, housekeeping, laundry services, clinical services, resident activities, and employee health should be considered. It is recommended that the infection control committee meet at least quarterly throughout the year and on an emergent basis as needed.

## AMBULATORY CARE CENTERS

Ambulatory care settings have the same infection prevention and control requirements as inpatient hospital settings, but the method of application to comply with the standards will vary depending on the type of care provided by that clinic to their population. The settings range from clinics that provide medical specialty expertise to clinics that provide invasive procedures such as hemodialysis, endoscopy, and surgical centers. There are many challenges in ambulatory care to reduce infection risk and improve patient safety. Infection control oversight and accountability are often lacking, especially if the clinics are not part of a hospital or system.

### Communicable Disease and Isolation Management

Patients may be exposed to infectious diseases in the ambulatory waiting rooms. HCWs need to use standard precautions in the care of all patients, but patients exhibiting communicable disease symptoms should be managed per CDC isolation precautions.[42] Because most ambulatory centers do not have adequate private rooms, a triage policy should be followed. The goal is to promptly identify and process patients with symptoms compatible with communicable disease in order to protect other patients and ambulatory care staff from exposure or infection. Symptoms of a communicable disease may include tuberculosis symptoms such as cough, bloody sputum production, night sweats, weight loss, anorexia, and fever. Symptoms of other communicable diseases might include rash of unknown origin or persistent cough. Patients with respiratory symptoms should wear a mask and should be promptly processed to a waiting area or examination room apart from other patients. If the ambulatory site has a negative pressure room for acid fast bacillus (AFB) and airborne isolation, patients with suspected tuberculosis and other communicable diseases transmitted by the airborne route should be triaged to these rooms as soon as possible.[66] When entering the room of a patient with suspected or confirmed tuberculosis, all ambulatory staff should wear a fit-tested particulate respirator. Cough-inducing procedures such as aerosol administration of medication, bronchoscopy, and sputum inductions on patients with a respiratory illness pose a high risk of aerosolization of organisms and infection of staff and other patients. Rooms in which these aerosol-producing procedures are performed must be modified to meet airborne isolation standards to protect ambulatory care staff and other patients. Ambulatory surgery centers must provide particulate respirators to staff caring for patients maintained in AFB and airborne isolation. Dental clinics should defer treatment on a patient with known or suspected active *Mycobacterium tuberculosis* or other potentially communicable airborne disease unless it is determined that the procedure is an emergency.

Respiratory hygiene/cough etiquette is an infection control component of standard precautions. The protocol is optimized by giving patients tissues and instructions to cover their mouth and nose when coughing or sneezing and disposing of tissues in the trash. Handwashing must be reinforced with accessible handwashing facilities or waterless alcohol-based handrub. Patients with a persistent cough are to be given a surgical mask while in a waiting room or other common areas and instructed to ask for a new mask if their old mask becomes soiled or moistened. Respiratory etiquette signage is a Joint Commission requirement for ambulatory centers within hospital institutions, but is encouraged to be used in all ambulatory centers, especially during the influenza season.

### Environmental Hygiene—Cleaning Disinfection and Sterilization

Cleaning and disinfection of frequently touched surfaces reduce the risk of transmission of MDROs and *C difficile*. Ambulatory settings need to standardize cleaning procedures, types of chemicals used, and establish a monitoring system to assure that the patient care equipment and environment are cleaned, disinfected and stored appropriately so that patient safety is optimized.[67–70] Staff should be educated on the use of the chemicals, and annual competencies are recommended for specific disinfection and sterilization procedures. All cleaning, disinfection, and sterilization processes should comply with CDC guidelines.[67]

High-level disinfection and sterilization of patient care equipment are important for infection control in many ambulatory settings and are discussed in the next section and in more detail elsewhere in this issue (See Rutala WA, Weber DJ: Disinfection and Sterilization in Health-Care Facilities: An Overview and Current Issues, in this issue).

### Ambulatory Surgical Centers

The same aseptic technique and environmental standards apply to all surgical settings. The National Patient Safety Goals (NPSG) for ambulatory and office-based surgery provide the elements of performance to achieve safe patient care.[71] One of the NPSG elements requires improvement in HH compliance. Another element requires evidence-based practices for preventing surgical site infections. The IP can provide guidance to implement the practices. Major components include: hair removal only with clippers and not shaving the surgical site, administration of antimicrobial agents for prophylaxis for a particular procedure or disease according to guidelines, and education regarding surgical site infection prevention provided to patients and families as well as staff and licensed independent practitioners involved in surgical procedures. Process and outcome measures need to be documented and reviewed as determined by the ambulatory site's risk assessment. These measures might include incidence of surgical site infection, compliance with antibiotic prophylaxis, time out practices by the operating team, preoperative chlorhexidine bath, surgical skin prep, use of wound protectors, supplemental oxygen, or compliance with hair removal methods. The IP can collaborate with the surgery team in identifying the high risk or most frequent surgical procedures performed, so that the surveillance program can be targeted to address key components of operative care. Currently there are no external benchmarks available for surgical site infection (SSI) or other process measures for surgery performed in ambulatory centers. It is recommended that internal benchmarks be used (ie, ambulatory centers track SSI and compliance rates at their institution over time and look for changes over time). Overall surgical infection rates and procedure-specific rates (for procedures primarily performed in hospitals), as published by the CDC, may be used.[72]

IPs and other HCWs who clean and process patient care equipment should be familiar with the basic principles for sterilization and disinfection outlined by Earle H. Spaulding, which classify patient care items and equipment into three categories based on the degree of risk of infection involved in the use of the items: critical, semicritical, and noncritical.[70] This classification provides guidance for determining the level of disinfection required and items requiring sterilization. Immediate use steam sterilization (IUSS) must be kept to a minimum and should not be used as a reason for shortage of instruments or back-to-back cases per Association for the Advancement of Medical Instrumentation (AAMI) guidelines.[68] Efforts should be made to purchase equipment and minimize the number of back-to-back cases to reduce the use of IUSS. Implants are not to be sterilized by IUSS, and biological monitoring is required before use. The Joint Commission Infection Control Standards have now placed a focus on immediate-use steam sterilization procedures in the operating room to assure optimal procedural compliance.[69] A major challenge to ambulatory surgical centers and the IP is to remain current with changes in sterilization technology and disinfectant products. New surgical equipment is becoming available, and manufacturer processing guidelines need to be followed to prevent damage to the instruments as well as adequate disinfection or sterilization. The Joint Commission and Centers for Medicare/Medicaid require documentation of staff competencies and knowledge of the manufacturer guidelines for management of surgical equipment in their surveys. Endoscopy centers must comply with AAMI standards for flexible and semirigid endoscope cleaning and disinfection processing to prevent cross-contamination between patients.[69]

### Safe Injection Practices

The CDC has implemented recommendations relating to safe injection practices as part of their standard precautions to provide safety to both the HCW and patient. Injuries due to needles and other sharps have been associated with the transmission of hepatitis B virus, hepatitis C virus, and HIV. The federal Needlestick Safety and Prevention Act signed into law in November 2000 authorized OSHA's revision of its Bloodborne Pathogens Standard to require the use of safety-engineered sharp devices.[73] Ambulatory services need to provide policies and infection control in-services to staff regarding aseptic technique and correct management of sharps during patient care.

Syringes, needles, insulin pens, and all sharps must be single use. Changing a needle or cannula and using the same syringe may support transmission of pathogens or viruses. Fluid infusion and administration should be single use.[74] Single-dose vials should be used whenever possible and clearly dedicated to a single patient. If multiple-dose vials are used, they must be stored appropriately according to manufacturer recommendations and kept in immediate patient treatment areas. Bags or bottles of intravenous solution used as a common source for multiple patients is an unsafe practice and has been associated with outbreaks.[75]

Inappropriate use of one product among multiple patients has resulted in many large and harmful outbreaks. Examples include a hepatitis B outbreak in New York City in 2001 that correlated with the use of multiple-dose vials for injections and contaminated syringes left on the table where medications were prepared; a hepatitis C outbreak in a Nevada endoscopy clinic in 2007 due to reuse of the same syringe for propofol administration; and reuse of glucometers and insulin pens resulting in hepatitis B and C transmission.[75–78]

### Bioterrorism and Disaster Planning

A risk assessment of the clinic location and the community it services provides guidance for emergency preparedness plans. Factors to consider in planning are the socioeconomic level and vaccine status of the population, natural disasters the area may be prone to, and access routes to the clinic. Clinics associated with health systems should be included in the emergency plans of the health system. Independent clinics need to collaborate with a local hospital, public health department, and government agencies and have a generic screening form for infectious disease disasters. The plans should provide a process by which the facility can use mitigation strategies to become prepared to respond to and recover from all types of disasters. IPs should actively participate in the planning process.[79]

## SUMMARY

Outpatient services are continually increasing and changing with expansion of new technologies. Increased use of invasive devices and procedures provides new and challenging risks for infection. Risks associated with contaminated equipment can be decreased by knowledge and maintenance of aseptic technique and disinfection practices. The challenge to IPs and ambulatory staff is to remain updated and familiar with emerging technologies to increase the likelihood of preventing health care-associated infection and providing safe patient care. More patients with a high acuity of illness are now being seen in ambulatory instead of inpatient settings, and these patients often spend prolonged periods in waiting rooms, in close proximity to others. The risk of communicable disease transmission and the relatively high prevalence of some MDROs in health care and community settings necessitate standard and transmission-based precautions for all patient care settings, including ambulatory settings. The health care worker, patient, and family members of patients need to be provided education to support patient safety and minimize infection risk. The IP has unique challenges in providing the ambulatory clinic both infection prevention and regulatory strategies.

## REFERENCES

1. Smith PW, Bennett G, Bradley SF, et al. Infection prevention and control in long-term care facilities. Infect Control Hosp Epidemiol 2008;29:785–814.
2. Friedman C, Barnette M, Buck AS, et al. Requirement for infrastructure and essential activities of infection control and epidemiology in out-of-hospital settings: a consensus panel report. Infect Control Hosp Epidemiol 1999;20:695–705.
3. Jarvis WR. Infection control and changing health-care delivery systems. Emerg Infect Dis 2001;7:170–3.
4. Aronow WS. Clinical causes of death of 2372 older persons in a nursing home during 15-year follow-up. J Am Med Dir Assoc 2000;1:95–6.
5. Strausbaugh LJ, Joseph CL. The burden of infection in long-term care. Infect Control Hosp Epidemiol 2000;21:674–9.
6. Warren JW, Palumbo FB, Fitterman L, et al. Incidence and characteristics of antibiotic use in aged nursing home patients. J Am Geriatr Soc 1991;39:963–72.
7. Gurwitz JH, Field TS, Avorn J, et al. Incidence and preventability of adverse drug events in nursing homes. Am J Med 2000;109:87–94.
8. Stone ND, Ashraf MS, Calder J, et al. Surveillance definitions of infections in long-term care facilities: revisiting the McGeer criteria. Infect Control Hosp Epidemiol 2012;33:965–77.
9. Loeb M, Bentley DW, Bradley S, et al. Development of minimum criteria for the initiation of antibiotics in residents of long-term-care facilities: results of a consensus conference. Infect Control Hosp Epidemiol 2001;22:120–4.
10. Wang L, Lansing B, Symons K, et al. Infection rate and colonization with antibiotic-resistant organisms in skilled nursing facility residents with indwelling devices. Eur J Clin Microbiol Infect Dis 2012;31:1797–804.

11. Olsho LE, Bertrand RM, Edwards AS, et al. Does adherence to the Loeb minimum criteria reduce antibiotic prescribing rates in nursing homes? J Am Med Dir Assoc 2013;14:309.e1-7.

12. Mody L, Krein SL, Saint S, et al. A targeted infection prevention intervention in nursing home residents with indwelling devices: a randomized clinical trial. JAMA Intern Med 2015;175:714–23.

13. Evans ME, Kralovic SM, Simbartl LA, et al. Nationwide reduction of health care-associated methicillin-resistant Staphylococcus aureus infections in Veterans Affairs long-term care facilities. Am J Infect Control 2014;42:60–2.

14. Schora DM, Boehm S, Das S, et al. Impact of detection, education, research and decolonization without isolation in long-term care (DERAIL) on methicillin-resistant Staphylococcus aureus colonization and transmission at 3 long-term care facilities. Am J Infect Control 2014;42:S269–73.

15. Ho ML, Seto WH, Wong LC, et al. Effectiveness of multifaceted hand hygiene interventions in long-term care facilities in Hong Kong: a cluster-randomized controlled trial. Infect Control Hosp Epidemiol 2012;33:761–7.

16. Ho SS, Tse MM, Boost MV. Effect of an infection control programme on bacterial contamination of enteral feed in nursing homes. J Hosp Infect 2012;82:49–55.

17. Coleman EA. Falling through cracks: challenges and opportunities for improving transitional care for persons with continuous complex care needs. J Am Geriatr Soc 2003;51:549–55.

18. Epstein L, Edwards JR, Halpin AL, et al. Evaluation of a novel intervention to reduce unnecessary urine cultures in intensive care units at a Tertiary Care Hospital in Maryland, 2011-2014. Infect Control Hosp Epidemiol 2016;37(5): 606–9.

19. Aiello A, Malinis M, Knapp J, et al. Hand hygiene practices in nursing homes: does knowledge influence practice? Am J Infect Control 2009;37:164–7.

20. Centers for Disease Control and Prevention. Guideline for hand hygiene in health-care settings: recommendations of the Healthcare Infection Control Practices Advisory Committee and the HICPAC/SHEA/APIC/IDSA Hand Hygiene Task Force. MMWR Recomm Rep 2002;51:S3–40.

21. Pittet D, Allegranzi B, Boyce J. The World Health Organization guidelines on hand hygiene in health care and their consensus recommendations. Infect Control Hosp Epidemiol 2009;30:611–22.

22. Hocine MN, Temime L. Impact of hand hygiene on the infectious risk in nursing home residents: a systematic review. Am J Infect Control 2015. [Epub ahead of print].

23. Stone PW, Herzig CT, Pogorzelska-Maziarz M, et al. Understanding infection prevention and control in nursing homes: a qualitative study. Geriatr Nurs 2015;36(4): 267–72.

24. Schweizer ML, Reisinger HS, Ohl M, et al. Searching for an optimal hand hygiene bundle: a meta-analysis. Clin Infect Dis 2014;58(2):248–59.

25. Mody L, Saint S, Kaufman S, et al. Adoption of alcohol-based handrub by United States hospitals: a national survey. Infect Control Hosp Epidemiol 2008;29: 1177–80.

26. Pedersen LK, Held E, Johansen JD, et al. Less skin irritation from alcohol-based disinfectant than from detergent used for hand disinfection. Br J Dermatol 2005; 153:1142–6.

27. Mody L, McNeil SA, Sun R, et al. Introduction of a waterless alcohol-based hand rub in a long-term care facility. Infect Control Hosp Epidemiol 2003;24:165–71.

28. Pittet D, Sax H, Hugonnet S, et al. Cost implications of successful hand hygiene promotion. Infect Control Hosp Epidemiol 2004;25:264–6.

29. Roghmann MC, Johnson JK, Sorkin JD, et al. Transmission of methicillin-resistant Staphylococcus aureus (MRSA) to healthcare worker gowns and gloves during care of nursing home residents. Infect Control Hosp Epidemiol 2015;36(9): 1050–7.

30. Centers for Disease Control and Prevention Antibiotic Resistance Threats. 2013. Available at: http://www.cdc.gov/drugresistance/threat-report-2013/pdf/ar-threats-2013-508.pdf. Accessed June 14, 2016.

31. Dommeti P, Wang L, Flannery EL, et al. Patterns of ciprofloxacin-resistant gram-negative bacteria colonization in nursing home residents. Infect Control Hosp Epidemiol 2011;32:177–80.

32. Spencer RC. The emergence of epidemic, multiple-antibiotic-resistant *Stenotrophomonas (Xanthomonas) maltophilia* and *Burkholderia (Pseudomonas) cepacia*. J Hosp Infect 1995;30(Suppl):453–64.

33. Hayakawa K, Marchaim D, Bathina P, et al. Independent risk factors for the co-colonization of vancomycin-resistant *Enterococcus faecalis* and methicillin-resistant *Staphylococcus aureus* in the region most endemic for vancomycin-resistant *Staphylococcus aureus* isolation. Eur J Clin Microbiol Infect Dis 2013; 32(6):815–20.

34. Daneman N, Bronskill SE, Gruneir A, et al. Variability in antibiotic use across nursing homes and the risk of antibiotic-related adverse outcomes for individual residents. JAMA Intern Med 2015;175:1331–9.

35. Min L, Galecki A, Mody L. Functional disability and nursing resource use are predictive of antimicrobial resistance in nursing homes. J Am Geriatr Soc 2015;63:659–66.

36. Bradley SF. Issues in management of resistant bacteria in long-term care facilities. Infect Control Hosp Epidemiol 1999;20:362–6.

37. Hujer AM, Bether CR, Hujer KM, et al. Antibiotic resistance in the institutionalized elderly. Clin Lab Med 2004;24:343–61.

38. Goldrick BA. MRSA, VRE and VRSA: how do we control them in nursing homes? Am J Nurs 2004;104:50–1.

39. Muto CA, Jernigan JA, Ostrowsky BE, et al. SHEA guideline for preventing nosocomial transmission of multidrug-resistant strains of Staphylococcus aureus and enterococcus. Infect Control Hosp Epidemiol 2003;24:362–86.

40. Siegel JD, Rhinehart E, Jackson M, et al. Management of multi-drug resistant organisms in healthcare settings. 2006. Available at: http://www.cdc.gov/ncidod/dhqp/pdf/ar/MDROGuideline2006.pdf. Accessed June 14, 2016.

41. Bowler WA, Bresnahan J, Bradfish A, et al. An integrated approach to methicillin-resistant Staphylococcus aureus control in a rural, regional-referral healthcare setting. Infect Control Hosp Epidemiol 2010;31(3):269–75.

42. Siegel JD, Rhinehart E, Jackson M, et al. Guideline for isolation precautions: preventing transmission of infectious agents in healthcare settings. 2007. Available at: http://www.cdc.gov/ncidod.dhqp/pdf/isolation2007.pdf. Accessed June 14, 2016.

43. Mody L, Crnich C. Effects of excessive antibiotic use in nursing homes. JAMA Intern Med 2015;175:1339–41.

44. McKinnell JA, Miller LG, Eells SJ, et al. A systematic literature review and meta-analysis of factors associated with methicillin-resistant Staphylococcus aureus colonization at time of hospital or intensive care unit admission. Infect Control Hosp Epidemiol 2013;34:1077–86.

45. Kindschuh W, Russo D, Kariolis I, et al. Comparison of a hospital-wide antibiogram with that of an associated long-term care facility. J Am Geriatr Soc 2012; 60:798–800.
46. Troillet N, Carmeli Y, Samore MH, et al. Carriage of methicillin-resistant *Staphylococcus aureus* at hospital admission. Infect Control Hosp Epidemiol 1998;19: 181–5.
47. Latour K, Catry B, Broex E, et al. Indications for antimicrobial prescribing in European nursing homes: results from a point prevalence survey. Pharmacoepidemiol Drug Saf 2012;21:937–44.
48. Horan TC, Gaynes RP. Surveillance of nosocomial infections. In: Glen Mayhall C, editor. Hospital epidemiology and infection control. 3rd edition. Philadelphia: Lippincott Williams & Wilkins; 2004. p. 1661–702.
49. McGeer A, Campbell B, Emori TG, et al. Definitions of infection for surveillance in long-term care facilities. Am J Infect Control 1991;19:1–7.
50. Stevenson KB, Moore J, Colwell H, et al. Standardized infection surveillance in long-term care: interfacility comparisons from a regional cohort of facilities. Infect Control Hosp Epidemiol 2005;26:231–8.
51. Mody L, Bradley SF, Galecki A, et al. Conceptual model for reducing infections and antimicrobial resistance in skilled nursing facilities: focusing on residents with indwelling devices. Clin Infect Dis 2011;52:654–61.
52. Jones M, Nielson C, Gupta K, et al. Collateral benefit of screening patients for methicillin-resistant *Staphylococcus aureus* at hospital admission: isolation of patients with multidrug-resistant gram-negative bacteria. Am J Infect Control 2015; 43(1):31–4.
53. Gibson KE, McNamara SE, Cassone M, et al. Methicillin-resistant *Staphylococcus aureus*: site of acquisition and strain variation in high-risk nursing home residents with indwelling devices. Infect Control Hosp Epidemiol 2014;35(12): 1458–65.
54. Cassone M, McNamara SE, Perri MB, et al. Impact of intervention measures on MRSA clonal type and carriage site prevalence. MBio 2016;7(2).
55. Muder RR, Brennen C, Wagener MM, et al. Methicillin-resistant staphylococcal colonization and infection in a long-term care facility. Ann Intern Med 1991;114: 107–12.
56. Ramsey AH, Skonieczny P, Coolidge DT, et al. *Burkholderia cepacia* lower respiratory tract infection associated with exposure to a respiratory therapist. Infect Control Hosp Epidemiol 2001;22(7):423–6.
57. Embril JM, McLeod JA, AL-Barrak AM, et al. An outbreak of methicillin-resistant *Staphylococcus aureus* on a burn unit: potential role of contaminated hydrotherapy equipment. Burns 2001;27:681–8.
58. Centers for Disease Control and Prevention, Rutala W, Weber D. Guideline for disinfection and sterilization in healthcare facilities. Atlanta, GA: Infection Control Practices Advisory Committee (HICPAC); 2008.
59. Bardenheier BH, Shefer AM, Lu PJ, et al. Are standing order programs associated with influenza vaccination? - NNHS, 2004. J Am Med Dir Assoc 2010; 11(9):654–61.
60. Centers fro Disease Control and Prevention: Influenza vaccination information for health care workers. Missing reference on usefulness of flu vaccination in reducing mortality in NH residents and reducing absenteeism in HCWs. 2016. Available at: www.cdc.gov/flu/professionals/. Accessed June 14, 2016.
61. Advisory Committee on Immunization Practices, Centers for Disease Control and Prevention (CDC). Immunization of health-care personnel: recommendations of

the Advisory Committee on Immunization Practices (ACIP). MMWR Recomm Rep 2011;60(RR-7):1–45.

62. Roup BJ, Scaletta JM. How Maryland increased infection prevention and control activity in long-term care facilities, 2003-2008. Am J Infect Control 2011;39(4): 292–5.

63. Smith PW, Bennett G, Bradley S, et al. Society for Healthcare Epidemiology of America (SHEA); Association for Professionals in Infection Control and Epidemiology (APIC). SHEA/APIC guideline: infection prevention and control in the long-term care facility. Am J Infect Control 2008;36(7):504–35.

64. Cohen CC, Pogorzelska-Maziarz M, Herzig CT, et al. Infection prevention and control in nursing homes: a qualitative study of decision-making regarding isolation-based practices. BMJ Qual Saf 2015;24(10):630–6.

65. Travers J, Herzig CT, Pogorzelska-Maziarz M, et al. Perceived barriers to infection prevention and control for nursing home certified nursing assistants: a qualitative study. Geriatr Nurs 2015;36(5):355–60.

66. Jensen PA, Lambert LA, Iademarco MF, et al. Centers for disease control and prevention guidelines for preventing the transmission of Mycobacterium tuberculosis in healthcare settings. Atlanta (GA): Centers for Disease Control and Prevention; 2005.

67. Comprehensive guide to steam sterilization and sterility assurance in health care facilities. Arlington (VA): Association for the Advancement of Medical Instrumentation. 2015 edition.

68. Steam Sterilization—Update on The Joint Commission's Position. Available at: www.jointcommission.org/Library/WhatsNew/steam_sterilization.htm. Accessed June 14, 2016.

69. AAMI Standards and Recommended Practices. ST 91 flexible and semi-rigid endoscope processing in health care facilities; ST 79 comprehensive guide to steam sterilization and sterility assurance in health care facilities. 2015 edition.

70. Spaulding EH. Chemical disinfection of medical and surgical materials. In: Lawrence C, Block SS, editors. Disinfection sterilization and preservation. Philadelphia: Lea & Febiger; 1968. p. 517–31.

71. Ambulatory Health Care Accreditation Program. Chapter: National Patient Safety Goals. The Joint Commission on accreditation of Healthcare Organizations. 2010. Available at: www.jointcommission.org/assets/1/6/2016_NPSG_AHC.pdf. Accessed June 14, 2016.

72. Edwards JR, Peterson KD, Yi Mu, et al. National Healthcare Safety Network (NHSN) report: Data summary for 2006 through 2008, issued December 2009. Am J Infect Control 2009;37:783–805.

73. Needlestick Safety and Prevention Act (PL 106-430), 2000.

74. Centers for Disease Control and Prevention National Center for Emerging and Zoonotic Infectious Diseases, Division of Healthcare Quality Promotion Single-dose/Single-use Vial Position and Messages. CDC website. 2012. Available at: http://www.cdc.gov/injection safety/PDF/CDC-SDV-Position05022012.pdf. Accessed June 14, 2016.

75. Balter S, Layton M, Bornschlegel K, et al. Transmission of Hepatitis B and C Viruses in Outpatient Settings-New York, Oklahoma, and Nebraska, 2000-2002. MMWR Morb Mortal Wkly Rep 2003;52(38).

76. Hepatitis B outbreak in New York City, 2001. Infect Control Hosp Epidemiol 2005; 26:745–60.

77. Labus B, Sands L, Rowley P, et al. Acute hepatitis C virus infections attributed to unsafe injection practices at an endoscopy clinic—Nevada, 2007. MMWR Morb Mortal Wkly Rep 2008;57(19):513–44.

78. U.S. Food and Drug Administration alert. FDA: insulin pens and insulin cartridges must not be shared. Spring (MD): US Food and Drug Administration; 2009.

79. APIC Text of Infection Control and Epidemiology 4th Edition 2014 Volume III. Community-based infection prevention practices. Emergency management chapter 119 and chapter 120 infectious disease disasters: bioterrorism, emerging infections, and pandemics.

# Preventing Hospital-acquired Infections in Low-income and Middle-income Countries: Impact, Gaps, and Opportunities

Ana Cecilia Bardossy, MD[a], John Zervos, JD[b],
Marcus Zervos, MD[a,c],*

## KEYWORDS

- Infection control • Developing countries • Health care–associated infections
- Capacity building • Gaps and recommendations • Resources-limited settings

## KEY POINTS

- In low-income and middle-income countries (LMIC) health care–associated infections (HAIs) are a serious concern, with an estimated risk of up to 25% of hospitalized patients.
- Factors associated with HAIs, including prolonged hospital stay, disability, increased resistance to antimicrobial agents, increased costs, and excess deaths, are accentuated in those countries.
- The gaps are lack of infrastructure, paucity and inconsistency in surveillance, deficiency in trained personnel, and poverty-related factors such as basic sanitation.
- Building infection control capacity in LMIC is possible where strategies are tailored to the specific needs of LMIC.
- Strategies must start with simple and cost-effective measures, then expand to include more complicated measures. Resources should be prioritized.

## INTRODUCTION

Health care–associated infections (HAIs) are a serious problem for patient safety and affect hundreds of millions of patients worldwide.[1,2] In low-income and middle-income countries (LMIC) there are often unique and formidable challenges to implementing

Disclosure: None (A.C. Bardossy and J. Zervos); M. Zervos has received research grants from Pfizer, Cerexa, Cubist, Merck, Tetraphase, Paratek, and Rempex.
[a] Division of Infectious Disease, Henry Ford Health System, 2799 West Grand Boulevard, CFP 302, Detroit, MI 48202, USA; [b] Division of Infectious Disease, The Global Health Initiative, Henry Ford Health System, 2799 West Grand Boulevard, CFP 302, Detroit, MI 48202, USA; [c] Wayne State University School of Medicine, Detroit, MI, USA
* Corresponding author. Division of Infectious Disease, Henry Ford Health System, 2799 West Grand Boulevard, CFP 302, Detroit, MI 48202.
E-mail address: Mzervos1@hfhs.org

Infect Dis Clin N Am 30 (2016) 805–818
http://dx.doi.org/10.1016/j.idc.2016.04.006
0891-5520/16/$ – see front matter © 2016 Elsevier Inc. All rights reserved.

effective prevention programs. The World Health Organization (WHO) "Report on the Burden of Endemic Health Care-Associated Infection Worldwide" indicates that, in high-income countries (HIC; gross national income per capita ≥$12,736), HAI surveillance systems are in place at a national/subnational level. However, in low-income countries (gross national income ≤$1045) and some middle-income countries (gross national income >$1045 but <$12,736) the burden of HAIs remains largely unknown.[3,4]

The principal goal of an infection control (IC) program is to reduce the risk of HAIs between patients, health care workers, and the environment, leading to a reduction in HAI-related morbidity, mortality, and avoidable costs.[5] Because of limited resources, LMIC face significant and often insurmountable challenges to accomplish this goal. Therefore, optimal approaches must be tailored for LMIC and balance effectiveness and cost.

## HEALTH AND ECONOMIC IMPACT

The impact of HAIs is very high in LMIC. The often-cited factors associated with HAIs are accentuated in these countries and include prolonged hospital stay; disability; increased resistance of microorganisms to antimicrobial agents; increased costs for health care institutions, patients, and their families; and excess deaths.[2,3] In LMIC, although the magnitude and impact of the problem is more remarkable, there are few objective data on the financial burden, and this burden varies from country to country. The limitations in health care facilities, including infrastructure, patient load, and staff shortages, provide many challenges. Limitations in access to care, issues of sanitation, and poverty also complicate measures to control HAIs.

The WHO report on the burden of endemic HAIs worldwide in 2011 revealed that, in LMIC, the increased length of stay associated with HAIs (5–30 days) is greater than in HIC.[3] There is no information in this report on the risk of death attributable to HAIs, because most of the studies evaluated reported crude mortality without considering risk factors, confounders, or patients with HAIs compared with noninfected patients.[3] A study done in an intensive care unit (ICU) in northern India found that patients with ventilator-associated pneumonia (VAP) had longer hospital stays (21 days vs 11 days) and an attributable cost of US$5200.[6] A case-control study analyzing hospital-acquired bacteremia in a cardiothoracic unit in an Indian hospital found longer total hospital stay (mean, 22.9 days) and a significantly higher mortality (mean, 54%) with a cost of US$14.818 compared with controls.[7] In a study done in a medical ICU in Turkey, the mean length of stay was 4-fold higher for patients with VAP, and that the total costs were about 3 times higher than for patients without VAP.[8] Another study estimated that the length of stay caused by catheter-associated bloodstream infections (CLABSI) increased in 10 of 11 ICUs in Argentina, Brazil, and Mexico, varying from 1.23 days to 4.69 days.[9]

One study estimated an excess length of ICU stay of 1.59 days, and an increase of the risk of death by 15% caused by catheter-associated urinary tract infections (CAUTI).[10] The study, which was done in 29 ICUs in 10 developing countries, attributed the increased risk of death to confounding factors.[10] The International Nosocomial Infection Control Consortium (INICC) reported that device-associated infections increase length of stay 10 days, costs between US$5000 and US$12,000, and doubles the rate of mortality.[11]

## GAPS AND OPPORTUNITIES

International guidelines have been developed for identification of gaps and for the control of HAIs.[12,13] Many LMIC have attempted to implement IC programs with varying degrees of success, whereas other countries have no programs. For LMIC with programs, the central issue is that there is clear evidence that major deficits exist in the ability to support the essential resources, having properly trained personnel, and having the needed components of IC programs.[5] However, HAIs are preventable in LMIC, with at least one-third of HAIs thought to be preventable if key elements of IC are adequately followed.[5]

Because of a lack of IC infrastructure in most LMIC settings, information on rates of HAIs are not always available.[3] There is a paucity and inconsistency of available data on rates of infection and risk factors.[3] The difference between the risk factors for HAIs in HIC compared with those in LMIC is that, in addition to the known risk factors (eg, use of catheters or other procedures, prolonged hospitalization, admission to intensive care), low-income countries have heightened poverty-related determinants, such as lack of basic hygiene sanitation and limited resources for control efforts.[3] In addition, the lack of financial support, lack of sufficient staff in the units and working in IC, and insufficient equipment and supplies are described as risk factors in those settings.[3,14]

In a recent study done in 6 LMIC, an infection control assessment tool (ICAT) was used to identify gaps in IC practices. The investigators found several gaps and opportunities for improvement of IC practices in several areas, including need for hospital-wide IC programs and surveillance, antibiotic stewardship, written and posted guidelines and policies across a range of topics, surgical instrument sterilization procedures, and improved hand hygiene (HH).[15] The 6 sites completed 5 modules related to surgical site infection (SSI). Of 121 completed sections, scores of less than 50% of the recommended IC practices were received in 23 (19%) and scores from 50% to 75% were received in 43 (36%).[15] The investigators concluded that IC programs had various limitations in many sites and surveillance of HAIs was not consistently performed. Lack of administration of perioperative antibiotics, inadequate sterilization and disinfection of equipment, and paucity of HH were found.[15] Importantly, there was country-to-country variability based on the income level of the county; however, adherence to recommended IC practices in all countries was suboptimal.[15] Sites had various degrees of financial support for prevention of HAI with many locations, including middle-income countries, having no support.[15]

### Surveillance and Rates of Health Care–associated Infections

In LMIC the risk of HAI has been estimated to be up to 25% of hospitalized patients.[2] A survey done by WHO in 2010 showed that only 23 of 147 developing countries (16%) were reporting a functioning national surveillance system.[16] In a review of the burden of endemic HAIs in developing countries in 2011, the pooled prevalence of overall HAI was 15.5% per 100 patients in high-quality studies, and 8.5% in low-quality studies, which is much higher than in HIC.[14] SSIs were the most frequent hospital-wide HAI with a pooled incidence of 11.8% per 100 patients.[14] The investigators also reported that pooled HAI density in adult ICUs was 47.9% per 1000 patient-days, with high heterogeneity detected, and densities of specific types in 31 studies varied between 1.7 and 44.6 per 1000 catheter-days for CLABSI, 1.4 and 23.0 per 1000 urinary catheter-days for CAUTI, and 3.2 and 56.8 per 1000 ventilator-days for VAP.[14] The paucity of available data and some regions being poorly represented were noted in this study.[14] Data from medical-surgical ICUs in developing countries from the INICC showed rates of 8.9 per 1000 catheter-days for CLABSI, 19.8 per 1000 ventilator-days for VAP, and 6.6 per 1000 urinary catheter-days for CAUTI, with the CLABSI rate being 4.86 times higher, the VAP rate 5.5 times higher, and the CAUTI rate 1.9 times higher than the US Centers for Disease Control and Prevention (CDC) National Healthcare Safety Network rates.[11,17]

Hospitals that perform surveillance activities for HAIs have lower infection rates than those that do not.[18] These efforts have not only shown reductions in HAIs but also in antimicrobial-resistant organisms, and are critical for detection of emerging and reemerging pathogens.[18] However, there is significant variability in rates in sites between countries, settings, types of HAI studied, and the definitions and measures used for identification of infections.

## Antimicrobial Resistance Surveillance

With a global increase in the use of so-called last-resort antibiotics and the increasing concern for resistant organisms, surveillance for antimicrobial-resistant organisms is essential to control spread because many of these organisms originate in LMIC. The ultimate goal of surveillance is to formulate strategies and interventions to prevent infection and improve patient outcomes. High use of antibiotics in hospitals, the general population, and agriculture has resulted in resistant strains in bacteria because of selection pressure.[19] The increase in hospitalizations, high prevalence of hospital infections, and limitations in infection prevention cause further spread.[19] Measures to improve the knowledge and impact of the problem and consequences, and to create regulations for the rational use of antibiotics in both human and nonhuman use, are imperative.[19] Also critical are practical IC measures, development and expanded use of rapid diagnosis, point-of-care testing, bioinformatics, availability of cost-effective testing, improved laboratory capacity, and surveillance to detect trends and new organisms. There remains an urgency to develop new antibiotics, and to coordinate the actions worldwide.[19–21] There is clear and increasing evidence for global spread of antimicrobial-resistant bacteria. The decrease in infections caused by antibiotic-resistant bacteria at the source would have clear and measurable local and global health benefits.[20] Reasons for the burden of antibiotic resistance in LMIC should be evaluated as well as the relation to lack of quality laboratory support, outpatient use of antimicrobials, and transmission in the hospital setting. This information will be critical in the implementation and evaluation of cost-effective and feasible control measures.[22,23]

Surveillance for antimicrobial resistance is a critical component of an effective IC strategy. There are different models of surveillance around the world. For antimicrobial resistance, among the most important are the WHO Antimicrobial Resistance Surveillance sponsored by the WHO, the European Antimicrobial Resistance Surveillance Network sponsored by the European Centre for Disease Prevention and Control, and the Emerging Infections Program sponsored by the CDC.[24] The WHO and CDC have partnered with various countries and organizations, including the American Public Health Laboratories (APHL), to assess and build laboratory capacity.[25] APHL partnered to offer voluntary laboratory capacity assessments to international influenza laboratories involving the WHO Global Influenza Surveillance and Response System.[25] During the assessments, influenza experts observe laboratory operations, capturing information used to guide laboratories in capacity building, enhancing influenza surveillance, and achieve or maintain a National Influenza Centers designation.[25] To capture the information from the assessments and allow the assessor to identify strengths and determine recommendations for influenza laboratory practice improvement, APHL and CDC developed the International Influenza Laboratory Capacity Review Tool with a quantitative analysis.[25] The tool analyzes assessment data in a standardized manner, measures changes over time, and provides an objective way to aggregate data regionally, or globally, to understand specific gaps and training opportunities.[25] Since the program began in 2009, more than 35 countries have been assessed using the tool. The information generated from the tool and the quantitative analysis assist countries with demonstrating compliance with international health regulation expectations.[25]

The WHO recently issued a report on antimicrobial resistance surveillance, which provided an assessment of the current state of surveillance globally.[26] Data from 129 countries were obtained for a selected set of 9 bacteria–antibacterial drug combinations. Of these, 114 countries provided information regarding at least 1 of 9 bacteria–antibacterial drug combinations and only 22 countries contributed data on all 9 combinations.[26] Many countries had limited data and numerous gaps.[26] Gaps included lack of agreement on surveillance standards and the lack of structures for coordinating and sharing information. In addition, most data obtained belonged to proportions of resistant bacteria among tested isolates in hospital settings, without representing community-acquired and uncomplicated infections or measuring impact in the population.[26] The report showed increasing resistance to third-generation cephalosporins for *Escherichia coli*, *Klebsiella pneumoniae*, and *Neisseria gonorrhoeae*; increasing resistance to fluoroquinolones for *E coli*, nontyphoidal *Salmonella*, and *Shigella* species; increasing resistance to beta-lactam antibiotics for *Staphylococcus aureus*; and increasing resistance to penicillin for *Streptococcus pneumoniae*.[26]

### Health Care–associated Tuberculosis

With up to a third of the world population infected with tuberculosis (TB), all health care workers (HCWs) are at risk of latent TB infection (LTBI).[27,28] Risk seems particularly high when there is increased exposure combined with inadequate facilities for respiratory isolation, and lack of rapid diagnostic tools.[28,29] In a review comparing the risk of TB infection and disease in HIC and LMIC, the median prevalence of LTBI in HCWs was 63% in LMIC and 24% in HIC.[28] The median annual incidence of TB infection that was considered to be caused by health care exposure was 5.8% in LMIC and 1.1% in the HIC studied.[28] Rates of active TB in HCWs were also higher than in the general population in all countries, although findings were variable in HIC.[28] When evaluating the effectiveness of IC measures, Menzies and colleagues[28] concluded, even with limited available evidence, that it is possible for a reduction in the risk of TB infection in LMIC to be achieved with simple administrative controls, but they pointed out the need to evaluate these measures in those settings with larger and better-controlled studies.

The WHO guidelines separate IC measures into 3 levels: (1) administrative measures, including rapid diagnosis and triage of infective patients with TB, early isolation of patients, and prompt initiation of treatment; (2) personal respiratory protection, including the use of N95 mask by HCWs and fit testing program, the use of masks by patients when undergoing procedures, and the use of hooded positive pressure respirator; and (3) environmental measures, including maximizing ventilation, negative pressure rooms, monitoring ventilation systems, ultraviolet germicidal irradiation, and the use of high-efficiency particulate air.[30] The guidelines recommend a prioritization of administrative controls as the most important measures, because engineering and personal controls do not work in the absence of solid administrative measures.[30] Although engineering measures require resources, opening windows to increase natural ventilation and the use of fans to control the direction of airflow are examples of inexpensive measures that can be implemented. Personal measures are the most expensive and least effective measures, therefore should only be used in specialized settings and when all other IC measures have been implemented.[30]

For control of the spread of TB in health care settings, better use of isolation precautions and rapid diagnostic testing using nucleic acid amplification for TB screening of HCWs is needed.[31] Use of nucleic acid amplification has been shown to reduce nosocomial TB exposure in ICUs by decreasing the length of time to diagnosis and the nosocomial transmissible period.[31]

### Health Care–associated Infections After Natural Disasters and During Conflicts

A summary of recommendations concerning IC issues in disaster settings has been published.[32] Field hospitals vary in size and design. Some consist of a series of small tents, often with each providing a specific type of care. Others are either structured as large tents or organized within buildings that previously served other functions, such as churches or schools. Lack of running water is a common problem in most of these makeshift health care centers.[32] Despite the limitations, it is possible to implement basic techniques of HH, perioperative use and minimization of overuse of antibiotics, safe water and food, human waste, pest control, and HCW safety in disaster settings.[32] In conflict situations, the situation is exponentially made worse by the physical injury and even killing of health workers. IC becomes a low priority when medical institutions have been attacked and patients and health workers injured and killed.[33] In these settings infection prevention is a low priority.

## SUCCESSFUL HEALTH CARE–ASSOCIATED INFECTION INTERVENTIONS IN LOW-INCOME AND MIDDLE-INCOME COUNTRIES

### Examples of Successful Implementation of World Health Organization Hand Hygiene Guidelines

HH is a simple and highly effective measure for reducing the rate of HAIs.[34] The WHO guidelines for HH in health care, written by experts from both HIC and LMIC countries, provide appropriate recommendations for LMIC to improve practices and reduce transmission of pathogenic microorganisms to patients and HCWs.[35] These recommendations have been shown to be effective and low cost.[35]

In Vietnam, a cost-effectiveness study analyzed the impact of an HH program in ICUs.[36] The study used the steps recommended by the WHO, including upgrading HH facilities, training, surveillance, and feedback.[36] The team focused on improving compliance during the moments with lowest compliance. The study showed that HH compliance increased from 25.7% to 57.5% and the incidence of HAI decreased from 31.7% to 20.3% ($P<.001$) after the intervention. The cost-effectiveness was estimated at $1074 saved per HAI prevented.[36] In Colombia, a prospective study promoting HH using alcohol-based hand rub performed in 6 ICUs resulted in a CLABSI reduction.[37] The intervention consisted of introducing dispensers in the ICUs, twice-weekly replacement of bottles, simultaneous education in HH, and giving feedback about HAI rates to ICU teams.[37]

### Example of Successful Infection Control Strategy in Resources-limited Settings

In an infection prevention intervention of postoperative SSI in Peru, patients admitted to a surgical service of a 400-bed tertiary hospital were evaluated.[38] CDC definitions were used to define surgical site infections.[39] Patients were followed after hospital discharge to assess development of wound infection. In the intervention, 211 patients were followed over a 3-month period, of whom 192 (91%) underwent a surgical intervention. The mean age of surgical patients was $42.8 \pm 18.4$ years (18–88 years). The types of surgery were predominantly emergent (58.9%) and the remaining elective (41.2%). Duration of antibiotic prophylaxis was less than 24 hours perioperatively in 56% of patients. Cefazolin was most commonly used for perioperative prophylaxis (99.1%). Among surgical patients, 13.5% (n = 26) were colonized with *S aureus*. Only 4 of these isolates (2.1%) were methicillin-resistant *S aureus*. There were only 6 wound infections reported among the 158 patients available for follow-up (rate of

SSI of 3.8%) and only 1 with a positive culture growing *E coli*. None of the patients colonized by *S aureus* developed postoperative wound infections.[38] These results have important implications for infection prevention strategies in a resource-limited hospital setting. The study showed that with prolonged use of perioperative antibiotics in some patients, postoperative infection was uncommon. Hospital antimicrobial resistance should always be evaluated and considered for defining the hospital's antibiotic polices and national recommendations.

Successful interventions for reduction of HAI in LMIC have also included programs for CLABSI, VAP, and CAUTI. A consortium of 15 LMIC developed a successful strategy by focusing on education, performance feedback and outcome, and outcome and process surveillance.[40] The study took place in 86 ICUs and showed improved IC adherence and reduced CLABSI incidence by 54%.[40]

The implementation of a multidisciplinary approach for prevention of VAP in ICUs from 14 developing countries of 4 continents showed a 55.83% reduction in the VAP rate.[41] Measures included were a bundle of IC interventions, education, outcome and process surveillance, feedback of VAP rates, and performance feedback of IC practices.[41] In a medical ICU in Thailand, the implementation of an educational program including a self-study module with preintervention and postintervention assessments, lectures, fact sheets, and posters, directed to respiratory care practitioners and ICU nurses, generated sustained reductions in the incidence of VAP, duration of hospital stay, cost of antibiotic therapy, and cost of hospitalization.[42] This intervention was easy to implement and did not require the purchase of expensive technologies in an LMIC.[42]

In 57 adult ICUs in 15 developing countries, a multidimensional IC approach including the use of a bundle of IC interventions, education, outcome surveillance, process surveillance, feedback of CAUTI rates, and performance feedback of IC practices resulted in a CAUTI rate reduction from baseline of 37%.[43] These results were confirmed in similar studies from Turkey. In 10 cities in Turkey a similar strategy for CAUTI also showed a reduction in CAUTI incidence rates.[44] In a public hospital located in a resource-limited setting in Kenya, a low-cost and multifaceted intervention, including lectures, reminder signs, and infection prevention rounds, resulted in a reduction of CAUTI rates.[45] In Lebanon, a multidimensional inexpensive IC approach consisting of a bundle of IC interventions, education, surveillance of CAUTI rates, feedback on CAUTI rates, process surveillance, and performance feedback showed an 83% CAUTI rate reduction.[46] The implementation of an infection surveillance and prevention program at a university teaching hospital in Turkey was associated with a reduction in HAIs rates.[47]

## RECOMMENDATIONS
### Building Infection Control Capacity Through Partnerships

Capacity building refers to a broad set of strategies that have the aim of equipping an organization with the tools to address health issues.[48] Mutually beneficial partnerships (the sharing of resources and experience between more than 1 institution) are a powerful capacity building strategy that can be used to improve IC. However, partnership capacity building strategies cannot be sustainable and successful unless LMIC organizations are seen as active participants rather than passive recipients.[48] LMIC cannot implement IC practices designed for HIC, especially where international guidelines ignore social, economic, and cultural determinants unique to LMIC.

There is much rationale for capacity building partnerships between organizations that have common needs, and complimentary areas of experience, including shared health challenges, cost sharing, and complexity of problems.[49] For example, capacity building partnerships such as South-South (partnerships between developing countries) have been extremely successful.[49] These partnerships have resulted in interventions that are more suitable to LMIC settings. South-South partnerships also have the power to influence international guidelines to reflect LMIC interests.

Ministries of health have an essential role in building capacity by partnering with local hospitals to prevent HAIs and promote patient safety.[34] Ministries of health should evaluate the structure in facilities and laboratories for preventing HAI, and should also develop the necessary national policies and plans for strengthening the hospitals in HAI prevention.[50,51]

HIC also have a shared interest in building the capacity of neighboring countries because the organisms that cause these infections transcend borders. Recent history has provided many examples of the need to strengthen surveillance and hospital infection prevention capacity worldwide, including severe adult respiratory syndrome, H1N1 pandemic influenza, Ebola, and multiple organisms with antimicrobial resistance. However, to ensure approaches are adequately tailored to LMIC and sustainable, LMIC need to be in control and provide input to international tools and guidelines. HIC countries should assist LMIC by providing financial resources, technical assistance, and training.

### Identify Health Care–associated Gaps

Multiple tools have been developed for the assessment of IC. The US Agency for International Development has created an ICAT that provides an approach that is being used by IC teams for identifying and solving problems economically and practically in low-resource health care facilities.[13] ICAT recommendations can be found as modules and are summarized in **Box 1**.[13] A second set of tools is the infection prevention and control assessment tools (IPCAT) developed by the WHO.[12] IPCAT can be used by hospitals to assess, plan, organize, implement, and monitor an IC program. The tool gives a general overview, providing quantitative evaluation of the components of the infection prevention and control (IPC) program. Printed versions of the tool can be used; however, storing data electronically is recommended to calculate scores.[12]

---

**Box 1**
**ICAT modules**

1. Modules for the facility as a whole:
   a. Health facility information, IC program, isolation and standard precautions, employee health, pharmacy, tuberculosis precautions, waste management.

2. Modules administered once for specific services (if present in the facility):
   b. Labor and delivery, surgical antibiotic use and equipment reprocessing, surgical area practices, ICUs, microbiology laboratory.

3. Modules administered once where disinfection or sterilization takes place:
   a. Equipment and intravenous fluids, needles and syringes, sterile gloves.

4. Modules administered once for each clinical area (if relevant):
   a. General ward, HH, injections, airway suctioning, intravenous catheters, intravenous fluids and medications, urinary catheters.

*Data from* Strengthening Pharmaceutical Systems. Infection control assessment tool, 2nd edition: user manual. Submitted to the US Agency for International Development by the Strengthening Pharmaceutical Systems Program. Arlington (VA): Management Sciences for Health; 2009. Available at: http://projects.msh.org/projects/sps/SPS-Documents/loader.cfm?cs Module=security/getfile&pageid=43763. Accessed December 28, 2016.

## Designing and Sustaining Infection Control Programs and Interventions

When planning interventions, it is critical to consider behavioral, transcultural, and religious factors that may affect outcomes.[34] Culture plays an important role in successfully implementing IC strategies.[52] Borg and colleagues[52] describes how the cultural dimensions for analyzing behavioral differences within countries, such as power distance in the workplace, uncertainty avoidance, and masculinity, have been associated with key performance indicators relevant to IC. Anglo-Saxon and Scandinavian countries have specific characteristics in relation to those cultural dimensions, and interventions that take into consideration these characterizes show improvements of IPC strategies.[52] However, these same interventions are not necessary applicable to other countries.[52] Because there is a lack of information from LMIC in relation to the cultural dimensions and impact when doing interventions and addressing IC problems, it is a challenge to incorporate this perspective when confronting IC problems in LMIC and applying guidelines and recommendations from HIC.[52] Borg and colleagues[52] suggests that "successful IC strategies are likely to be those that are compatible with the cultural background where they are implemented."[53] Bono and colleagues[54] described how successful IC measures depend also on leadership roles, multidisciplinary teams, adherence to organizational policies, job satisfaction and commitment, innovation, communication, behavior change, and performance monitoring. In our own experience in South America, working consecutively in 2 different hospitals, IC was improved not by additional resources but when hospital leadership gave the IC team total decision-making power. The IC team was able to execute interventions and improve processes, resulting in achievement of targets.

## Addressing Gaps While Prioritizing Resources

**Box 2** provides a summary of recommendations for improving IC in LMIC. Efforts should first focus on minimal and inexpensive IC measures for ensuring success with limited resources, and then later medium-term and long-term solutions. Low-cost measures, such as educational programs on HH and prevention of device-associated infections, have shown cost-effectiveness[36,42,47,50] and should be the first things to be addressed.

When considering IC measures that are applicable to the setting and resources, it is always better to consider first the available national guidelines or international guidelines that address the LMIC settings and resources. Examples are the WHO guidelines for injection safety,[55] for HH,[35] and for the prevention of tuberculosis in health care facilities in resource-limited settings,[30] or the use of checklists such as the surgical safety checklist to reduce morbidity and mortality in a global population.[56] Guidelines, recommendations, and interventions known to be effective in HIC settings can be a starting point to prioritize and plan how and where measures should be implemented.

Surveillance of process (ie, adherence to surgical antibiotic prophylaxis guidelines, monitoring of device use, or compliance with a group of validated care processes known to prevent infection) should be prioritized more than outcome surveillance, because process surveillance is essential for identifying inappropriate and unsafe IC practices immediately in those settings. Outcome surveillance (ie, CAUTI, CLABSI, and VAP rates in ICU patients) is more expensive and time consuming and requires trained IC personnel, so it is recommended to be used only for high-risk patients, such as those exposed to device-associated infections.[57,58] Periodic point prevalence surveillance can be used to monitor the effectiveness of IC measures.[57] Surveillance should be prioritized to the highest risk units, infections, and patients.

---

**Box 2**
**LMIC guide to improving HAI: 3-phase prioritization approach, short term (low cost) to long term (high cost)**

*Phase 1*
- Identifying gaps in IC using tools available
- Designation of at least 1 IC practitioner and a physician epidemiologist
- IC committee
- Provision of support from the facility leaders and senior management to IC team
- HH campaign
- Cleaning and hospital environmental policies
- Education to staff in basic infection prevention measures

*Phase 2*
- Training in IC recommendations to IC nurse and physician epidemiologist
- Use of contact precautions with available resources for patients with high-risk infections
- Process surveillance
- Outcome surveillance only in high-risk patients
- Develop and implement bundles for prevention of most common HAIs
- Develop and implement IC policies

*Phase 3*
- Expand outcome surveillance to all patients
- Research in IC and epidemiology
- Antimicrobial stewardship program

---

## SUMMARY

The main objective of an IC program in LMIC is to reduce HAIs to the irreducible minimum through practical measures. These measures must be simple, cost-effective, and designed to suit the local needs and circumstances. LMIC should use evidence-based measures; set achievable goals; and a plan for short-term, medium-term, and long-term actions. LMIC can leverage guidelines and tools that have proved effective in LMIC and should model approaches after other successful LMIC IC interventions. LMIC should work with other LMIC partners to design novel approaches where innovation is needed and collaborate on research. More studies are necessary to evaluate the implementation of programs and policies that are possible in LMIC. HIC must have a shared interest in developing the capacity of neighboring countries and can serve an important role by providing training and resources.

## REFERENCES

1. Burke JP. Infection control – a problem for patient safety. N Engl J Med 2003; 348(7):651–6.
2. Pittet D, Allegranzi B, Storr J, et al. Infection control as a major World Health Organization priority for developing countries. J Hosp Infect 2008;68(4):285–92.

3. WHO. Report on the Burden of Endemic Health Care-Associated Infection World-wide. 2011. Available at: Available at: http://apps.who.int/iris/bitstream/10665/80135/1/9789241501507_eng.pdf. Accessed January 17, 2016.

4. The World Bank. Available at: http://data.worldbank.org/about/country-and-lending-groups. Accessed December 14, 2015.

5. Vandijck D, Cleemput I, Hellings J, et al. Infection prevention and control strategies in the era of limited resources and quality improvement: a perspective paper. Aust Crit Care 2013;26(4):154–7.

6. Mathai AS, Phillips A, Kaur P, et al. Incidence and attributable costs of ventilator-associated pneumonia (VAP) in a tertiary-level intensive care unit (ICU) in northern India. J Infect Public Health 2015;8(2):127–35.

7. Kothari A, Sagar V, Ahluwalia V, et al. Costs associated with hospital-acquired bacteraemia in an Indian hospital: a case-control study. J Hosp Infect 2009; 71(2):143–8.

8. Alp E, Kalin G, Coskun R, et al. Economic burden of ventilator-associated pneumonia in a developing country. J Hosp Infect 2012;81(2):128–30.

9. Barnett AG, Graves N, Rosenthal VD, et al. Excess length of stay due to central line-associated bloodstream infection in intensive care units in Argentina, Brazil, and Mexico. Infect Control Hosp Epidemiol 2010;31(11):1106–14.

10. Rosenthal VD, Dwivedy A, Calderon ME, et al. Time-dependent analysis of length of stay and mortality due to urinary tract infections in ten developing countries: INICC findings. J Infect 2011;62(2):136–41.

11. Rosenthal VD. Device-associated nosocomial infections in limited-resources countries: findings of the International Nosocomial Infection Control Consortium (INICC). Am J Infect Control 2008;36(10):S171.e7–12.

12. WHO. Core components for infection prevention and control programmes. Assessment tools for IPC programmes. 2011. Available at: http://www.wpro.who.int/hrh/about/nursing_midwifery/core_components_for_ipc.pdf. Accessed November 12, 2015.

13. Strengthening Pharmaceutical Systems. Infection control assessment tool, 2nd edition: user manual. Submitted to the U.S. Agency for International Development by the Strengthening Pharmaceutical Systems Program. Arlington (VA): Management Sciences for Health; 2009. Available at: http://projects.msh.org/projects/sps/SPS-Documents/loader.cfm?csModule=security/getfile&pageid=43763. Accessed December 28, 2016.

14. Allegranzi B, Bagheri Nejad S, Combescure C, et al. Burden of endemic health-care-associated infection in developing countries: systematic review and meta-analysis. Lancet 2011;377(9761):228–41.

15. Weinshel K, Dramowski A, Hajdu A, et al. Gap analysis of infection control practices in low- and middle-income countries. Infect Control Hosp Epidemiol 2015; 36(10):1208–14.

16. WHO. The burden of health care-associated infection worldwide. A summary. 2010. Available at: http://www.who.int/gpsc/country_work/summary_20100430_en.pdf. Accessed December 11, 2016.

17. Rosenthal VD, Maki DG, Mehta A, et al. International Nosocomial Infection Control Consortium report, data summary for 2002-2007, issued January 2008. Am J Infect Control 2008;36(9):627–37.

18. Zoutman DE, Ford BD. The relationship between hospital infection surveillance and control activities and antibiotic-resistance pathogen rates. Am J Infect Control 2005;33(1):1–5.

19. Laxminarayan R, Duse A, Wattal C, et al. Antibiotic resistance-the need for global solutions. Lancet Infect Dis 2013;13(12):1057–98.

20. Gilbert DN, Guidos RJ, Boucher HW, et al. The 10 x '20 initiative: pursuing a global commitment to develop 10 new antibacterial drugs by 2020. Clin Infect Dis 2010;50(8):1081–3.

21. Aiken AM, Allegranzi B, Scott JA, et al. Antibiotic resistance needs global solutions. Lancet 2014;14(7):550–1.

22. Alp E, Damani N. Healthcare-associated infections in intensive care units: epidemiology and infection control in low-middle income countries. J Infect Dev Ctries 2015;9(10):1040–5.

23. Lynch P, Pittet D, Borg MA, et al. Infection control in countries with limited resources. J Hosp Infect 2007;65(Suppl 2):148–50.

24. Perez F, Villegas MV. The role of surveillance systems in confronting the global crisis of antibiotic-resistant bacteria. Curr Opin Infect Dis 2015;28(4):375–83.

25. Building International Influenza Laboratory Capacity. Association of Public Health Laboratories. Available at: http://www.aphl.org/aphlprograms/infectious/influenza/Pages/Building-International-Influenza-Laboratory-Capacity.aspx. Accessed Dec 12, 2015.

26. WHO. Antimicrobial resistance. Global report on surveillance. 2014. Available at: http://apps.who.int/iris/bitstream/10665/112642/1/9789241564748_eng.pdf. Accessed November 25, 2015.

27. Agaya J, Nnadi CD, Odhiambo J, et al. Tuberculosis and latent tuberculosis infection among healthcare workers in Kisumu, Kenya. Trop Med Int Health 2015;20(12):1797–804.

28. Menzies D, Joshi R, Pai M. Risk of tuberculosis infection and disease associated with work in health care settings. Int J Tuberc Lung Dis 2007;11(6):593–605.

29. Jesudas CD, Thangakunam B. Tuberculosis risk in healthcare workers. Indian J Chest Dis Allied Sci 2013;55(3):149–54.

30. WHO. Guidelines for the prevention of tuberculosis in health care facilities in resource-limited settings. 1999. Available at: http://www.who.int/tb/publications/who_tb_99_269.pdf. Accessed December 29, 2015.

31. Wang JY, Lee MC, Chang JH, et al. *Mycobacterium tuberculosis* nucleic acid amplification tests reduce nosocomial tuberculosis exposure in intensive care units: a nationwide cohort study. Respirology 2015;20(8):1233–40.

32. Lichtenberg P, Miskin IN, Dickinson G, et al. Infection control in field hospitals after a natural disaster: lessons learned after the 2010 earthquake in Haiti. Infect Control Hosp Epidemiol 2010;31(9):951–7.

33. Heisler M, Baker E, McKay D. Attacks on health care in Syria — normalizing violations of medical neutrality? N Engl J Med 2015;373(26):2489–91.

34. Allegranzi B, Pittet D. Healthcare-associated infection in developing countries: simple solutions to meet complex challenges. Infect Control Hosp Epidemiol 2007;28(12):1323–7.

35. WHO. The WHO guidelines on hand hygiene. First Global Patient Safety Challenge Clean Care is Safer Care. 2009. Available at: http://apps.who.int/iris/bitstream/10665/44102/1/9789241597906_eng.pdf. Accessed December 21, 2015.

36. Thi Anh Thu L, Thi Hong Thoa V, Thi Van Trang D, et al. Cost-effectiveness of hand hygiene program on health care-associated infections in intensive care patients at a tertiary care hospital in Vietnam. Am J Infect Control 2015;43(12):e93–9.

37. Barrera L, Zingg W, Mendez F, et al. Effectiveness of a hand hygiene promotion strategy using alcohol-based handrub in 6 intensive care units in Colombia. Am J Infect Control 2011;39(8):633–9.

38. Hall AD, Moreno D, Angulo D, et al. Methicillin-resistant *Staphylococcus aureus* (MRSA) colonization in patients and healthcare workers at a tertiary acute care hospital in Lima, Peru. Abstract #1866 (poster). 23rd European Congress of Clinical Microbiology and Infectious Diseases (ECCMID). Berlin, Germany, April 27–30, 2013.

39. Mangram AJ, Horan TC, Pearson ML, et al. Guideline for the prevention of surgical site infection, 1999. Hospital Infection Control Practices Advisory Committee. Infect Control Hosp Epidemiol 1999;20(4):250–78.

40. Rosenthal VD, Maki DG, Rodrigues C, et al. Impact of International Nosocomial Infection Control Consortium (INICC) strategy on central line-associated bloodstream infection rates in the intensive care units of 15 developing countries. Infect Control Hosp Epidemiol 2010;31(12):1264–72.

41. Rosenthal VD, Rodrigues C, Alvarez-Moreno C, et al. Effectiveness of a multidimensional approach for prevention of ventilator-associated pneumonia in adult intensive care units from 14 developing countries of four continents: findings of the International Nosocomial Infection Control Consortium. Crit Care Med 2012;40(12):3121–8.

42. Apisarnthanarak A, Pinitchai U, Thongphubeth K, et al. Effectiveness of an educational program to reduce ventilator-associated pneumonia in a tertiary care center in Thailand: a 4-year study. Clin Infect Dis 2007;45(6):704–11.

43. Rosenthal VD, Todi SK, Alvarez-Moreno C, et al. Impact of a multidimensional infection control strategy on catheter-associated urinary tract infection rates in the adult intensive care units of 15 developing countries: findings of the International Nosocomial Infection Control Consortium (INICC). Infection 2012;40(5):517–26.

44. Leblebicioglu H, Ersoz G, Rosenthal VD, et al. Impact of a multidimensional infection control approach on catheter-associated urinary tract infection rates in adult intensive care units in 10 cities of Turkey: International Nosocomial Infection Control Consortium findings (INICC). Am J Infect Control 2013;41(10):855–91.

45. Tillekeratne LG, Linkin DR, Obino M, et al. A multifaceted intervention to reduce rates of catheter-associated urinary tract infections in a resource-limited setting. Am J Infect Control 2014;42(1):12–6.

46. Kanj SS, Zahreddine N, Rosenthal VD, et al. Impact of a multidimensional infection control approach on catheter-associated urinary tract infection rates in an adult intensive care unit in Lebanon: International Nosocomial Infection Control Consortium (INICC) findings. Int J Infect Dis 2013;17(9):e686–90.

47. Alp E, Altun D, Cevahir D, et al. Evaluation of the effectiveness of an infection control program in adult intensive care units: a report from a middle-income country. Am J Infect Control 2014;42(10):1056–61.

48. Crisp BR, Swerissen H, Duckett SJ. Four approaches to capacity building in health: Consequences for measurement and accountability. Health Promot Internation 2000;15(2):99–107.

49. Thorsteinsdóttir H. South–south collaboration in health biotechnology: growing partnerships amongst developing countries. Ottawa (Canada): IDRC; 2012.

50. Rosenthal VD. Central line-associated bloodstream infections in limited-resource countries: a review of the literature. Clin Infect Dis 2009;49(12):1899–907.

51. Padoveze MC, Fortaleza CM, Kiffer C, et al. Structure for prevention of health care-associated infections in Brazilian hospitals: a countrywide study. Am J Infect Control 2016;44(1):74–9.

52. Borg MA, Waisfisz B, Frank U. Quantitative assessment of organizational culture within hospitals and its relevance to infection prevention and control strategies. J Hosp Infect 2015;90(1):75–7.

53. Borg MA. Lowbury Lecture 2013. Cultural determinants of infection control behaviour: understanding drivers and implementing effective change. J Hosp Infect 2014;86(3):161–8.

54. De Bono S, Heling G, Borg MA. Organizational culture and its implications for infection prevention and control in healthcare institutions. J Hosp Infect 2014; 86(1):1–6.

55. WHO best practices for injections and related procedures toolkit. 2010. Available at: http://apps.who.int/iris/bitstream/10665/44298/1/9789241599252_eng.pdf. Accessed January 21, 2016.

56. Haynes AB, Weiser TG, Berry WR, et al. A surgical safety checklist to reduce morbidity and mortality in a global population. N Engl J Med 2009;360(5):491–9.

57. Damani N. Simple measures save lives: an approach to infection control in countries with limited resources. J Hosp Infect 2007;65(S2):151–4.

58. Lee TB, Montgomery OG, Marx J, et al. Recommended practices for surveillance: Association for Professionals in Infection Control and Epidemiology (APIC), Inc. Am J Infect Control 2007;35(7):427–40.

# Index

*Note:* Page numbers of article titles are in **boldface** type.

## A

Accreditation organizations, influence on IPP, 569–570
Acid fast bacillus (AFB), in ambulatory care centers, 796
*Acinetobacter sp.,* environmental transmission of, 622–624, 641
    outbreak investigations of, 664, 674–675
    water safety and, 699
Active surveillance, 579
    in nursing homes, 790, 792–793
Acuity-adaptable patient-care rooms, 719
Adenosine triphosphate (ATP) assays, in surface cleaning monitoring, 644–646
Adenovirus, outbreak investigations of, 664
Adherence, to hand hygiene, 596–598
    barriers to, 598–599
    improving, 600–601
Administrative assistant, as IPCC member, 571, 573
Agar slide cultures, in surface cleaning monitoring, 645
Air, as reservoir of infections, 715–716
Air conditioning systems, safe design of, 718–719
Airborne infection isolation room, 719–720
Airborne precautions, in ambulatory care centers, 796–797
    in nursing homes, 791–792
Alcohol, for patient-care item disinfection, 619
Alcohol-based hand rub, in hand hygiene, 593–594, 596, 598–600
    for nursing homes, 789–790
Alternative health care settings, infection control in, **785–804**
    ambulatory care centers as, 569, 796–799. See also *Ambulatory care centers.*
    background on, 785
    key points of, 785
    nursing homes as, 786–796. See also *Nursing homes (NHs).*
Ambulatory care centers. See also *specific service or type.*
    infection control in, 796–799
        bioterrorism and, 798–799
        communicable disease and, 796–797
        disaster planning and, 798–799
        environmental hygiene for, 797
        isolation management for, 796–797
        safe injection practices, 798
        scope of, 796
        surgical, special interventions for, 797–798
    infection risks in, 569
Ammonium compounds, quaternary, for patient-care item disinfection, 620
Animal bites, immunization for, 735

Infect Dis Clin N Am 30 (2016) 819–851
http://dx.doi.org/10.1016/S0891-5520(16)30057-5
0891-5520/16/$ – see front matter

id.theclinics.com

Animal (*continued*)
  postexposure prophylaxis for, 746–747
Anthrax, immunization for, 735
Antibiotic-resistant bacteria. See also *specific antibiotic or bacteria.*
  as health care facility issue, 631
  in developing countries, 808–809
  in nursing homes, 790–791
  informatics identification of, 765–766
  national initiatives for, 773
  public health consequences of, 771–773
Antibiotics, stewardship for, **771–784**. See also *Antimicrobial stewardship.*
    informatics in, 765–766
  susceptibility patterns of, in outbreaks, 670, 765–766
Antimicrobial soap, in hand hygiene, 593
Antimicrobial stewardship, **771–784**
  definition of, 773
  economics of, 581, 774, 779–780
  goals of, 773–774
  improved use in, national initiatives for, 773
  in nursing homes, 792–793
  infection control and, 776–780
    device-associated infection prevention in, 778
    disease-based stewardship, 777–778
    drug-based stewardship, 776–777
    implementation barriers to, 778–779
    maintenance of programs, 778–779
    making business care for, 779
    measuring impact of, 779–780
    multidisciplinary bundles in, 777–778
    team members for, 776
  informatics in, 765–766
  key points of, 771
  misuse impact in, 772–773
  overuse impact in, 772–773
  resistance impact on public health, 771–772. See also *Antibiotic-resistant bacteria.*
    multidrugs in. See *Multidrug-resistant organisms (MDROs).*
  summary of, 780–781
  team members for, 774–776
    clinical pharmacist as, 775
    health care epidemiologist as, 775
    hospital administration as, 776
    infection preventionist as, 775–776
    infectious disease physician as, 774–775
    information technology as, 775
    microbiology laboratory as, 775
    pharmacy and therapeutics committee as, 776
  use impact in, 772–773
    in developing countries, 808–809
Aseptic techniques, in ambulatory surgical centers, 797–798
*Aspergillus sp.,* outbreak investigations of, 664, 676–677
ATP (adenosine triphosphate) assays, in surface cleaning monitoring, 644–646

Autocratic management style, 574–575
Automated technologies, for surveillance, 579
      fully or semi-, 761


B

*Bacillus atrophaeus,* 631
Bacteria. See also *specific bacteria.*
    EOC as source of, 715–716
    HCP exposures to. See *Occupational health.*
    resistance to antibiotics, 631. See also *Antibiotic-resistant bacteria.*
Bacterial colonization, in channel scopes, 629–630
    in nursing homes, 790–791
Bacterial DNA, in outbreaks, 671
Behavioral performance/practice, in hand hygiene, 600
Biofilms, in endoscope reprocessing, 621
Bioterroism/bioterrorism agents, ambulatory surgical centers and, 797–798
    as health care facility issue, 631
Biotyping, of outbreaks, 670
Bites, immunization for, animal, 735
      postexposure prophylaxis for, animal, 746–747
          human, 746
Blades, laryngoscope, HAIs linked to, 630–631
        storage issues of, 629
Bleach, for environmental surface disinfection, 648
Bloodborne pathogens, 568
    in nursing homes, 791–792
    occupational health regulations for, 731
Bloodstream infections, from central lines. See *Central line–associated bloodstream infections (CLABSI).*
    from laryngoscope blades, 630–631
Budget, IPCC preparation of, 575–577
    reductions in, 583
Building capacity through partnerships, in developing countries, 811–812
Building water distribution systems, LD pneumonia related to, 701
    safety plans for, 703–705
Bundles, multidisciplinary, in antimicrobial stewardship, 777–778
        in developing countries, 811
      treatment protocol, in nursing homes infection prevention programs, 787–789
*Burkholderia cepacia,* outbreak investigations of, 664
Business case, for antimicrobial stewardship, 779
Business plan, for IPCC, 581–583


C

*Campylobacter fetus,* outbreak investigations of, 665
*Candida sp.,* outbreak investigations of, 664
Capacity building, through partnerships, in developing countries, 811–812
Capital expenses, in IPCC budget, 576–577
Carbapenem-resistant *Enterobacteriaceae* (CRE), antimicrobial stewardship for, 772–773
    as health care facility issue, 610, 621–622

Carbapenem-resistant (*continued*)
    environmental transmission of, 630–631
    outbreak investigations of, 675–676
Case definition, for outbreak investigations, 662–663
Catheter–associated infections (CAUTIs), antimicrobial stewardship for, 778
    as targeted HAI, 569–570, 578
    in developing countries, 806–807, 811
    in nursing homes, 787
    informatics surveillance of, 762–764
CAUTIs. See *Catheter–associated infections (CAUTIs)*.
CDC. See *Centers for Disease Control and Prevention (CDC)*.
Ceilings, safe designs of, 721
Centers for Disease Control and Prevention (CDC), guidelines for disinfection and
    sterilization of medical devices, 610, 621
    HAIs prevalence surveys by, 567–568
    hand hygiene guidelines/indications of, 593–595, 600
    health care reform consultations, 569
    immunization recommendations of, 731
    occupational health regulations of, 731, 735, 750
    on antibiotic resistance, 790
    on antimicrobial stewardship, 772
    on environmental hygiene, 642, 645, 648, 693
    on safe design of health care facilities, 721
    surveillance recommendations of, 577, 810
Centers for Medicare and Medicaid Services (CMS), health care reform consultations,
    568–570
    on surgical equipment infection control, 798
Central line–associated bloodstream infections (CLABSI), antimicrobial stewardship for,
    778
    as targeted HAI, 569–570, 578
    in developing countries, 807, 811
    informatics surveillance of, 761–762
Channel scopes, disinfection and sterilization of, immersion vs. perfusion for, 629–630
Charlson's Comorbidity Score, 790
Chemical agents, for environmental surface disinfection, 648–649
    for patient-care item sterilization, 613–617
Chemoprophylaxis, postexposure, for HCP, 735–747, 750. See also *Postexposure
    prophylaxis (PEP)*.
CLABSI. See *Central line–associated bloodstream infections (CLABSI)*.
Cleaning, vs. cleanliness, 650–651
Cleaning surfaces, in health care facilities, 642–648
    ambulatory surgical centers as, 797–798
    cleanliness vs., 650–651
    evaluation and monitoring of, 642–644
        benefits and challenges of, 646–648, 650
        objectivity in, 651
    importance of, 642
    improvement strategies for, 643–644, 649–650
    methods for, 644–646
        agar slide cultures as, 645
        ATP assays as, 644–646

basic cultures as, 645
covert direct practice observation as, 645
fluorescent markers as, 644, 646–647
overview of, 644–645
Cleanliness, in environmental hygiene, improving, 655
by evaluating emerging interventions, 655
measuring, 654
vs. cleaning, 650–651
Clinical criteria, for evaluating evidence strength for environmental sources of infection, 714–715
in surveillance data, 577–578
Clinical pharmacist, antimicrobial stewardship role of, 775
*Clostridium difficile,* antimicrobial stewardship for, 772–774, 778
as targeted infection, 569–570, 578
environmental transmission of, 622–624, 641, 649, 714
in nursing homes, 791
informatics surveillance of, 760–762, 764
outbreak investigation of, 671, 678
CMS. See *Centers for Medicare and Medicaid Services (CMS).*
Combined surveillance methodologies, 578
Communicable disease, electronic reporting of, 766
HCP-to-patient transmission of, 750
in ambulatory care centers, 569, 796
Communication, importance of, during outbreak investigations, 670
Compliance, with hand hygiene, 596–598
barriers to, 598–599
improving, 600–601
Computer science, for surveillance, 579, 761. See also *Informatics.*
in hand hygiene monitoring, 601
Concurrent surveillance, 576–577
Conflicts, HAI prevention during, in developing countries, 810
Conjunctivitis, in HCP, work restrictions for, 748
Conservation, as water management priority, 696
Construction, of health care facilities, for patient safely and infection prevention, **713–728.**
See also *Design of health care facilities.*
Consultative management style, 574–575
Contact dermatitis, in hand hygiene, 599
Contact precautions, in nursing homes, 791
Containment methods, for construction and renovation, of health care facilities, 718–719
Contaminants, in drinking water, 690–691
in EOC, 713–715
Contaminated surfaces, in health care facilities, cleaning of, 642–648
decontamination of. See *Surface decontamination.*
disinfecting of, 648–651
epidemiology of, 639–641
Core value statement, of IPPs, 571
Coronavirus, as targeted infection, 631, 640
Cost-effectiveness analysis, of infection control and prevention programs, 581–583
Costs, of infection prevention and control, 581–583, 779–780
in developing countries, 805–806
Cough etiquette, in ambulatory care centers, 796–797

Counseling, as postexposure prophylaxis, in HCP, 736–737
Covert direct practice observation, in surface cleaning monitoring, 645
Creeping outbreak, of LD pneumonia, 702–703
Critical items, disinfection and sterilization of, 613–617
Cultural dimensions, of infection control programs, in developing countries, 813
Cultures, in active surveillance, 579, 790
    in surface cleaning monitoring, agar slide, 645
        basic, 645
Cystoscopes, disinfection and sterilization of, 629–630
Cytomegalovirus, in HCP, work restrictions for, 748


    D

Daily use, defined, as antimicrobial stewardship metric, 779–780
Data, informatics software implementation consideration of, device data challenges in, 767
        microbiology data challenges in, 767
        validation challenges as, 767–768
Data programmer and analyst, as IPCC member, 571–573
Data sources, for surveillance, active, 579
        concurrent or retroactive, 577–578
        in nursing homes, 787
        informatics and, 761
Data validation, in surveillance, 760–761
    informatics software challenges with, 767–768
Days of therapy (DOTs), as antimicrobial stewardship metric, 779–780
Decontamination, of rooms. See *Room decontamination.*
    of surfaces. See *Surface decontamination.*
Decorative water features, in health care facilities, as transmission risk, 695, 717
Defined daily use, as antimicrobial stewardship metric, 779–780
Democratic management style, 574–575
Denominators, in hospital rate of infection, 578–579
Dental clinics, infection prevention programs in, 796
Dental unit waterlines, infection risks from, 694
Dermatitis, contact, in hand hygiene, 599
Design of health care facilities, for patient safely and infection prevention, **713–728**
        evidence strength for environmental sources of infection, criteria for evaluating,
            714–715
        future directions for, 721–722
            informing future guidelines development in, 721–722
            trends in, 721
        in developing countries, 810, 813
        introduction to, 713–714
        key points of, 713
        resources for, 722
        summary discussion of, 722
        supportive strategies and elements for, 718–721
            air conditioning and, 718–719
            airborne infection isolation room as, 719–720
            ceilings as, 721
            containment methods as, 718–719
            FGI guidelines as, 717–718

finishes as, 720–721
floors as, 721
furnishings as, 720–721
handwashing stations as, 716–717, 720
heating and, 718–719
patient-care rooms in, 719–720
protective environment room as, 720
surfaces as, 720–721
toilets as, 720
ventilation and, 718–719
walls as, 721
waste disposal, human, 720
transmission risks and, 715–716
air as reservoir of infections, 715–716
decorative water features in, 695, 717
handwashing stations in, 716–717
inpatient rooms, surfaces, and finishes in, 717–718
water as reservoir of infections, 716
Developing countries, preventing HAIs in, **805–818**
gaps and opportunities of, 806–810
after natural disasters, 810
during conflicts, 810
health care-associated tuberculosis as, 809–810
identification of, 807, 812
resource support as, 807
surveillance and rates of HAIs as, 807–808
surveillance of antimicrobial resistance as, 808–809
health and economic impact of, 806
introduction to, 805–806
key points of, 805
recommendations for, 811–814
building capacity through partnerships as, 811–812
designing sustainable programs and interventions as, 813
identification of gaps as, 807, 812
successful interventions for, 810–811
hand hygiene guidelines as, 810
infection control strategy in resource-limited settings as, 810–811
summary of, 814
Device data, informatics software challenges with, 767
Device-associated infection prevention, antimicrobial stewardship for, 778
Device-associated infections. See also *specific device*.
informatics reduction of, 765
rate calculation of, 579
Diabetic therapy, safe injection practices for, 798
Dialysis, infection risks from, 569, 693
Dialysis centers, infection prevention programs in, 796
Diarrheal diseases, in HCP, work restrictions for, 748
Diphtheria, in HCP, postexposure prophylaxis for, 745
work restrictions for, 748
Direct observation, of hand hygiene compliance, 597–598, 601
Disaster planning, by ambulatory surgical centers, 797–798

Disaster (*continued*)
    in developing countries, 810
Discharge cleaning, thoroughness of, 647
Disease-based antimicrobial stewardship, 777–778
Disinfection, in health care facilities, **609–637**
        agents and methods for, 618–621. See also *High-level disinfection (HLD); Low-level disinfection (LLD).*
            for surfaces, 648–649
        ambulatory surgical centers as, 569, 797–798
        of patient-care items, 610–613, 622–624
        of surfaces, 648–651
            challenges of measuring, 650–651
            chemicals for, 648–649
            environmental, 610–613, 622–624
            improving to decrease contamination, 643–644
            technologies to augment, 649–650
                no-touch as, 649
                self-disinfecting surfaces as, 649–650
Disinfection and sterilization, in health care facilities, **609–637**. See also *Disinfection; Sterilization.*
        ambulatory surgical centers as, 569, 797–798
        current issues in, 618, 620–631
            antibiotic-resistant bacteria as, 631
            bioterrorism agents as, 631
            carbapenem-resistant *Enterobacteriaceae* infection as, 610, 621–622
            cystoscopes as, 629–630
            duodenoscopes as, 610, 621–622
            emerging pathogens as, 631
            endoscope reprocessing as, 609–610, 618, 620
            environment role in transmission as, 622–627
            gastroscopes as, 609–610, 618, 621–622
            human papilloma virus as, 624, 628
            hydrogen peroxide mist system for probes as, 628–629
            immersion vs. perfusion of channel scopes as, 629–630
            laryngoscopes as, 630–631
            patient risk from failures of, 621, 624, 628
            reuse of single-use devices as, 629, 797–798
            storage of semicritical items as, 613, 629
        introduction to, 609–610
        key points of, 609
        of critical items, 613–617
        of noncritical items, 612, 617–620
        of semicritical items, 611–617
        rational approach to, 610–613
        summary of, 631
Disposable wipes, for environmental surface disinfection, 649
Distribution, as water management priority, 692–696. See also *Water distribution.*
DNA, bacterial, in outbreaks, 671
DNA microarray hybridization, of outbreaks, 671
Dose optimization, for drugs, in antimicrobial stewardship, 773–774
Drinking water, treatment of, 690

Droplet precautions, in nursing homes, 791
Drug selection, in antimicrobial stewardship, 773–774
Drug-based antimicrobial stewardship, 776–777
Duodenoscopes, disinfection and sterilization of, 610, 621–622
Duration of drug therapy, in antimicrobial stewardship, 773–774
      mean, as metric of, 779–780
   in developing countries, 810–811


**E**

E coli O157:H7, outbreak investigations of, 665
Ebola, as targeted infection, 568, 631
Economics, of antimicrobial stewardship, 581, 774, 778–780
   of HAIs in developing countries, 806
   of infection prevention and control, 581–583
Ectoparasites, postexposure prophylaxis for, 747
Elective behavior, in hand hygiene, 600
Electronic communicable disease reporting, 766
Electronic medical records, surveillance and, 579
Emergency supply, as water management priority, 696
Employee health programs. See also Occupational health.
   in nursing homes, 794
Endocavity disinfection, as challenge, 618, 621–622
   trophon for, 628–629
Endoscope reprocessing, for disinfection and sterilization. See also specific scope.
      as health care facility issue, 609–610, 618, 620
      immersion vs. perfusion in, 629–630
      steps for, 618, 620
Endoscopy suites, as high-risk setting for outbreaks, 679–680
Enterobacter sp., carbapenem-resistant. See Carbapenem-resistant Enterobacteriaceae (CRE).
   outbreak investigations of, 665, 678
   water safety and, 700
Enterococcus faecalis, outbreak investigations of, 665
Enterococcus sp., antibiotic-resistant. See Vancomycin-resistant Enterococcus (VRE).
Enterovirus D68, 631
Environment of care (EOC). See also Hospital environment.
   as infection source, criteria evaluating strength of evidence for, 714–716
      designs for prevention of, 716–721
      future design trends for, 721
         informing for development guidelines, 721–722
Environmental hygiene, in health care facilities, **639–660**
      ambulatory care centers as, 797
      ambulatory surgical centers as, 797–798
      cleaning surfaces in, 642–648
         cleanliness vs., 650–651
         evaluation and monitoring of, 642–644
            benefits and challenges of, 646–648, 650
            objectivity in, 651
         importance of, 642
         improvement strategies for, 643–644, 649–650

Environmental (*continued*)
        methods for, 644–646
     contaminated surfaces in, cleaning of, 642–648
        disinfecting of, 648–651
        epidemiology of, 641
     disinfecting surfaces in, 648–651
        challenges of, 650–651
        chemicals for, 648–649
        improving to decrease contamination, 643–644
        technologies to augment, 649–650
     hand hygiene and, 651–653
     horizontal healthcare hygienic practice in, 640–641
     introduction to, 639–641
     key points of, 639
     research opportunities and challenges for, 653–655
        improving cleanliness as, 655
          by evaluating emerging interventions, 655
        measuring cleanliness as, 654
        proposed hygienic practice agenda as, 654
        study design improvements as, 653–654
        understanding transmission events and patient room surfaces as, 654
     term descriptions for, 640, 650–651
Environmental Protection Agency (EPA), 620, 695–696, 716
Environmental rounds, 642
   in nursing homes, 795
Environmental services (EVS) personnel, role in surface cleaning, 642–643, 647–648
Environmental surfaces, in health care facilities. See also *Surface entries.*
     as transmission risk, 717–718
     cleaning of, 642–651
     contaminated, 639–651
     disinfection methods for, 610–613, 622–624
     safe designs for, 720–721
     self-disinfecting, 649–650
     sterilization methods for, 610–611, 613, 622–624
EOC. See *Environment of care (EOC); Hospital environment.*
EPA (Environmental Protection Agency), 620, 695–696, 716
Epidemiologist, health care, antimicrobial stewardship role of, 775
   hospital physician. See *Hospital physician epidemiologist.*
   national. See *Centers for Disease Control and Prevention (CDC).*
Epidemiology, business analyses framework for, 582–583
   of contaminated surfaces, in health care facilities, 639–641
   of HAIs, 568
     in developing countries, 805–806
*Escherichia coli,* outbreak investigations of, 665
   water safety and, 700
ESKAPE pathogens, 772
Ethylene oxide (ETO), for patient-care item sterilization, 613, 616, 622, 630
Evidence-based practice, for disinfection and sterilization, in ambulatory surgical centers, 797–798
     of patient-care items, 622
EVS (environmental services) personnel, role in surface cleaning, 642–643, 647–648

Expenses, in IPCC budget, 576–577

Exposure risk, calculation of, 578–579

Exposure risk factor analysis, in outbreak investigations, 664–669

Exposures, in HCP, postexposure prophylaxis for, 735–747, 750. See also *Postexposure prophylaxis (PEP).*

pre-exposure interventions for, 731, 733–735. See also *Pre-exposure interventions.*

in patients, after failure of disinfection and sterilization, investigation protocol for, 624, 628

building designs and, 714


F

Fabrics, furniture, safe designs of, 720–721

Failure, in disinfection and sterilization, of patient-care items, 621

patient risk with, 622, 624

protocol for exposure investigation after, 624, 628

FDA. See *Food and Drug Administration (FD).*

First aid, as postexposure prophylaxis, in HCP, 736

Fiscal analysis, as IPCC role, 583

Floors, safe designs of, 721

Fluid administration, safe practices for, 798

Fluorescent markers, in surface cleaning monitoring, 644, 646–647

Focused surveillance, 578

Food and Drug Administration (FD), on disinfection and sterilization of medical devices, 610, 621–622, 628–629

Food preparation, infection risks from, 693

Funding, for IPCC, 581–583

Fungus, EOC as source of, 714–715

outbreak in health care settings, 676–677

Furnishings, safe designs of, 720–721


G

Gastroscopes, disinfection and sterilization of, 609–610, 618, 621–622

Genotyping, of outbreaks, 670–671

GlideRite rigid stylets, 631

GlideScope video laryngoscope system, portable, 630–631

Gloves, for HCP, in nursing homes, 790

in hand hygiene, 599

Glutaraldehyde, for patient-care item sterilization, 614, 624, 628, 630

Government agencies. See also *specific agency or department.*

influence on IPP, 568–570

in developing countries, 812–814

Gowns, for HCP, in nursing homes, 790

Group A streptococcus, in HCP, work restrictions for, 749


H

HAI identification, antibiotic-resistant bacteria and, informatics for, 765–766

as outbreak source, 662–664

in developing countries, 807, 812

HAIs. See *Health care-associated infections (HAIs)*.
Hand antisepsis, in hand hygiene, 593
Hand hygiene (HH), **591–607**
    adherence to, 596–598
      barriers to, 598–599
      improving, 600–601
    alcohol-based hand rubs, 593–594, 596, 598–600
    as targeted strategy, 569–570
    CDC guidelines/indications for, 593–595
    definition of, 593
    environmental hygiene and, 651–653
    evolution of guidelines for, 593–594
    HAIs prevention with, 591–592, 601–602
    handwashing stations and, 720
    human skin and skin flora in, 592–593
    in developing countries, 810
    introduction to, 591
    key points of, 591
    summary of, 602–603
    terms for, 592–593
Hand hygiene events, monitoring of, 598
Hand rub, in hand hygiene, alcohol-based, 593–594, 596, 598–600
      for nursing homes, 789–790
    surgical, 593
Handles, of laryngoscopes, HAIs linked to, 630–631
Handwashing, in hand hygiene, 592–593
Handwashing stations, in health care facilities, as transmission risk, 716–717
    safe designs of, 720
HAV. See *Hepatitis A (HAV)*.
HBV. See *Hepatitis B (HBV)*.
HCP. See *Health care personnel (HCP)*.
HCV. See *Hepatitis C (HCV)*.
Health care epidemiologist, antimicrobial stewardship role of, 775
Health care facilities/settings, alternative, **785–804**. See also *Alternative health care settings*.
    designing for patient safely and infection prevention, **713–728**. See also *Design of health care facilities*.
    disinfection and sterilization in, **609–637**. See also *Disinfection and sterilization*.
    environmental hygiene of, **639–660**. See also *Environmental hygiene*.
    future design trends for, 721
      informing for development guidelines, 721–722
    infection control in. See *Infection control program*.
    infection prevention in. See *Infection prevention program (IPP)*.
    occupational health for, 730. See also *Occupational health*.
Health care personnel (HCP), as infection source, 714
    as outbreak source, 672
    cleaning patient-care items, 622
    hand hygiene education for, 600
    in developing countries, education strategies for, 813–814
    in nursing homes, infection prevention education for, 795
    occupational health for, **729–757**. See also *Occupational health*.

professional role of, in hand hygiene, 599–600
    protection of, as IPP goal, 568
Health care practices, optimal, reimbursement and, 568–569, 582–583
Health care reform, for nursing homes, 787, 795–796
    paradigm shift in infection programs, 569
Health care workers. See *Health care personnel (HCP).*
Health care-associated infections (HAIs), environmental transmission of. See also *Health care facilities/settings.*
        epidemiology of, 639–641
        hygiene prevention of, **639–660**. See also *Environmental hygiene.*
        reducing, 622–624. See also *Disinfection; Sterilization.*
    hand hygiene prevention of, 591–592, 601–602
    identification of. See *HAI identification.*
    in low-income and middle-income countries, **805–818**. See also *Developing countries.*
    most common types of, 568
    prevalence surveys of, 567–568
    prevention programs for. See *Infection control program; Infection prevention program (IPP).*
    surveillance of. See *Surveillance entries.*
    targeted categories of, 569–570
    water-based. See *Water safety.*
Health status, HAIs impact on, in developing countries, 806, 812
Heater-cooler devices, infection risks from, 694
Heating systems, safe design of, 718–719
Hemodialysis, infection risks from, 569, 693
Hemodialysis centers, infection prevention programs in, 796
HEPA (high-efficiency particulate air) filters, 720
Hepatitis A (HAV), in HCP, immunization for, 735
        postexposure prophylaxis for, 745–746
        work restrictions for, 748
    outbreak investigations of, 665
Hepatitis B (HBV), in HCP, immunity proof for, 733
        immunization for, 731, 733–734
            special use of, 733–735
        postexposure prophylaxis for, 739–740
        work restrictions for, 748
    outbreak investigations of, 666, 798
Hepatitis C (HCV), in HCP, work restrictions for, 748
    outbreak investigations of, 666
Herpes simplex, in HCP, work restrictions for, 748
Herpes virus, outbreak investigations of, 666
HH. See *Hand hygiene (HH).*
High-efficiency particulate air (HEPA) filters, 720
High-level disinfection (HLD), agents and methods for, 613–617
    of patient-care items and environmental surfaces, 610–611, 613, 617–618, 621–622, 628, 630–631. See also *Ultraviolet (UV) light.*
High-risk settings, for infection outbreaks, 678–680
HIV. See *Human immunodeficiency virus (HIV).*
Hospital administration, antimicrobial stewardship role of, 776
Hospital environment. See also *Environment entries.*
    as infection source, criteria evaluating strength of evidence for, 714–715

Hospital (*continued*)
  as outbreak source, 672
  role in transmission, 622–627
Hospital physician epidemiologist, as IPCC member, 571–573
  environmental monitoring role of, 648
  primary responsibilities of, 573
Hospital rate of infection, 570, 578
  calculation of, 578–579
Hospital-acquired conditions (HACs), as infection reduction target, 569
  economic impact of, 581–582
    in developing countries, 805–806
  value-based purchasing and, 582–583
Hospital-acquired infections. See *Health care-associated infections (HAIs)*.
HP. See *Hydrogen peroxide entries*.
Human bites, postexposure prophylaxis for, 746
Human immunodeficiency virus (HIV), postexposure prophylaxis for, 739, 741
  work restrictions for, 748
Human papilloma virus, as health care facility issue, 624, 628
  environmental transmission of, 631, 649
Human skin, hand hygiene and, 592–593
Human waste disposal, in design of health care facilities, 720
HVAC systems, safe design of, 718–719, 721
Hydrogen peroxide (HP) gas plasma, for patient-care item disinfection, improved, 619
  for patient-care item sterilization, 613–614, 616
    improved, 615
    ozone and, 617
    vaporized, 616
Hydrogen peroxide mist system for probes, 628–629
Hydrogen peroxide (HP) systems, for environmental surface disinfection, 648
  for laryngoscope disinfection, 630
  for room decontamination, 624
    advantages vs. disadvantages of, 624, 627
    clinical trials on, 624–626
    UV light vs., 624
Hydrotherapy, infection risks from, 693
Hygienic practice, continuum of, 651–652
  elements of, 651–652
  horizontal healthcare, 640–641
  interventions for, 651, 653
    evaluation cleanliness based on, 655
    sequential, 601
  research agenda for, 654
Hypothesis analysis, of risk factors, for outbreaks, 663


I

ICAT (infection prevention and control assessment tools), for developing countries, 812
Ice machines, infection risks from, 693, 716
ICRA (infection control risk assessment), 715, 718, 722
Immersion of channel scopes, for disinfection and sterilization, 629–630
Immunity, proof of, in HCP, 731, 733

Immunizations, as pre-exposure intervention, for HCP, contraindications to, 735
        immunity proof vs., 731, 733
        recommendations for, 731–732, 734
        special use, 734–735
Immunocompromised personnel, immunizations for, 733
Incident report, for postexposure prophylaxis, in HCP, 736
Infection control program, antimicrobial stewardship in, **771–784**. See also *Antimicrobial stewardship.*
    as team member, 776–780
    in health care facilities. See also *Infection prevention program (IPP).*
        alternative settings for, **785–804**
        building a successful, **567–589**
    in low-income and middle-income countries, **805–818**. See also *Developing countries.*
    informatics in, **759–770**. See also *Informatics.*
        background on, 759–760
        efficacy of, 759–760
        implementing software for, 766–768
        infection prevention and, 759, 764–766
        infection surveillance and, 759–764
        key points of, 759
        public health and, 766
        summary of, 768
        term description for, 759
Infection control risk assessment (ICRA), 715, 718, 722
Infection control risk mitigation recommendations (ICRMR), 718
Infection precautions. See *Isolation precautions.*
Infection prevention and control assessment tools (ICAT), for developing countries, 812
Infection prevention and control committee (IPCC), in health care facilities, authority of, 571
        budget preparation by, 575–577
        key members of, 571–575
        management styles effect on, 574–575
        meeting management strategies for, 574, 576
        multidisciplinary members of, 571, 581
        primary responsibilities of, 572
        review of surveillance findings, 571–572
Infection prevention program (IPP), in health care facilities, alternative settings of, **785–804**.
    See also *Alternative health care settings.*
        ambulatory care centers as, 569, 796–799
        background on, 785, 799
        nursing homes as, 786–796
    antimicrobials in, **771–784**. See also *Antibiotics; Antimicrobial entries.*
    designing for patient safety, **713–728**. See also *Design of health care facilities.*
    disinfection and sterilization in, **609–637**. See also *Disinfection; Sterilization.*
    environmental hygiene of, **639–660**. See also *Environmental hygiene.*
    hand hygiene in, **591–607**. See also *Hand hygiene (HH).*
    informatics in, **759–770**. See also *Informatics.*
    *Legionella pneumophilia* and, **689–712**. See also *Legionella pneumophilia; Water entries.*
    occupational health in, **729–757**. See also *Occupational health.*
    of low-income and middle-income countries, **805–818**. See also *Developing countries.*

Infection (*continued*)

    outbreak investigations in, 579–580, **661–687**. See also *Outbreaks.*

    successful for HAIs prevention, **567–589**. See also *Health care-associated infections (HAIs).*

    components of, 570–572

       budget as, 575–577, 583

       business plan as, 581–583

       committee as, 571–572

       mission, vision, and values as, 570–571

       outbreak investigations as, 579–580, 661

       quality improvement as, 581

       surveillance as, 576–579

       team members as, 572–575

    current initiatives for, 568–569

    economics and, 581–583, 774, 779–780

       in developing countries, 805–806

    evolution of regulation and requirements for, 567–570

    in alternative health care settings, **785–804**. See also *Alternative health care settings.*

    key points of, 567

    major goals of, 568

    summary of, 583

    team for, committee in, 571–572

       key members of, 572–575

    team meeting management in, 574–576

    team members for, 572–575

       administrative assistant as, 571, 573

       data programmer and analyst, 571–573

       hospital physician epidemiologist as, 571–573

       infection prevention staffing as, 571, 574–575

       infection preventionist as, 571, 573–574, 581

       medical director of infection prevention as, 571–573

Infection prevention staffing, as IPCC member, 571, 574–575

Infection preventionist (IP), activities reported by, 577

    electronic via informatics, 766

  antimicrobial stewardship role of, 775–776. See also *Antimicrobial stewardship.*

  as IPCC member, 571, 573–574, 581

  ICRA developed by, 715

  in nursing homes, 794–795

  management styles of, 574–575

  nursing home role of, 786–796

  primary responsibilities of, 574

Infection rate, in developing countries, 807–808

  in hospital, 570, 578

    calculation of, 578–579

  in nursing homes, 792–793

Infection risk, as high, in nursing homes, 793

  from critical items for patient-care, 613

  from water uses, 692–694

  in hospital environment, criteria for evaluating, 714–715

    of outbreaks, 672–674

nosocomial, 568, 806. See also *Health care-associated infections (HAIs)*.
Infectious diseases physician, antimicrobial stewardship role of, 774–775
Influenza, immunity proof for, 733
   immunization for, 731, 733–734
      special use of, 733–735
   in developing countries, 808
   postexposure prophylaxis for, 747, 750
Informatics, in infection control, **759–770**
      background on, 759–760
      efficacy of, 759–760
      implementing software for, 766–768
      infection prevention and, 759, 764–766
         admission recognition of MDROs, 764–765
         antibiotic stewardship, 765–766
         identification of inappropriate precautions, 765
         reduction of device use, 765
      infection surveillance and, 759–764
         data sources for, 761
         fully automated vs. semiautomated, 761
         outbreak detection with, 764, 766
         subjective vs. objective, 579, 760–761
      key points of, 759
      medical, for surveillance, 579
      metric enhancement with, 761–764
         for *C difficile,* 760–762, 764
         for catheter-associated urinary tract infections, 762–764
         for central line–associated bloodstream infections, 761–762
         for multidrug-resistant organisms, 762, 764
         for surgical site infections, 762–763
         for ventilator-associated pneumonia, 762–763
      public health and, 766
      summary of, 768
      term description for, 759
Informatics software, implementing, 766–768
      data validation in, 767–768
      device data challenges in, 767
      general considerations for, 766
      microbiology data challenges in, 767
Information technology. See also *Computer science.*
   antimicrobial stewardship role of, 775
Inherent behavior, in hand hygiene, 600
Injection practices, safe, in ambulatory care centers, 798
      in nursing homes, 791
Instrument asepsis, in ambulatory surgical centers, 797–798
Instrument design, in endoscope reprocessing, 621
Intensive care unit (ICU), designs for patient safety and infection prevention, 716, 720–721
   hand hygiene in, 598, 600–601
   in developing countries, 806, 810–811, 813
Intravenous therapy, safe practices for, 798
Iodophors, for patient-care item disinfection, 620
IP. See *Infection preventionist (IP).*

IPCC. See *Infection prevention and control committee (IPCC)*.
IPP. See *Infection prevention program (IPP)*.
Isolation precautions, in ambulatory care centers, 796–797
    in nursing homes, 791–792
    inappropriate, informatics identification of, 765
Isolation room, for airborne infection, 719–720, 796


**K**

*Klebsiella pneumoniae,* outbreak investigations of, 666
    water safety and, 700


**L**

Labor expenses, in IPCC budget, 576–577
Laboratory, microbiology, antimicrobial stewardship role of, 775
Laboratory tests, for outbreaks, in health care settings, 670–671
Laryngoscope blades, HAIs linked to, 630
    storage issues of, 629
Laryngoscopes, disinfection and sterilization of, 630–631
LD pneumonia, building water distribution systems and, 701
    description of, 697
    unapparent or creeping outbreak of, 702–703
Leak testing, of endoscopes, for disinfection and sterilization, 618
*Legionella pneumophilia,* water safety and, in health care, **689–712**
        building water safety plans for, 703–705
            decision points for, 703–704
            infections prevention plan in, 704–705
            stakeholders in, 704–705
            team approach to, 703–704
        future of, 706
        introduction to, 690–691
        key points of, 689
        outbreak investigations of, 666, 673–674
        pathogens and, 690–703
            transmission routes of, 690–691
        pneumonia and, building water distribution systems in, 701
            description of, 697
            unapparent or creeping outbreak in, 702–703
        summary of, 706
        water distribution systems and, 690–691
        water management priorities for, 691–696
            conservation as, 696
            distribution and quality as, 692
            emergency security as, 696
            safety as, 692–696
        water uses and infection risks of, 692–694
        water-based HAIs and, 696–703
            *Acinetobacter sp.* as, 699
            *E coli* as, 700
            *Enterobacteriaceae sp.* as, 700

*Klebsiella sp.* as, 700
*Legionella sp.* as, 696–698, 701–703
*Mycobacterium sp.* as, 698
NTM as, 690–691, 698
other gram-negative pathogens as, 700
*Pseudomonas aeruginosa* as, 690–691, 699
scope of, 696–697
*Stenotrophomonas maltophilia* as, 699
Legislation, on health care reform, effect on infection programs, 569
Level of care, in nursing home settings, information transfer during transitions of, 788–789
*Listeria monocytogenes,* outbreak investigations of, 667
Low-income and middle-income countries (LMIC), preventing HAIs in, **805–818**. See also *Developing countries.*
Low-level disinfection (LLD), of patient-care items and environmental surfaces, 610, 612–613


**M**

Management strategies, for IPCC meetings, 574, 576
Management styles, in IPCC meetings, 574–575
McGrath video laryngoscope system, 630
MDROs. See *Multidrug-resistant organisms (MDROs).*
Measles, in HCP. See also *Rubella.*
    immunity proof for, 733
    immunization for, 731, 733–734
        special use of, 733–735
    postexposure prophylaxis for, 745
    work restrictions for, 748
Mechanical (no-touch) methods, for environmental surface disinfection, 649
    for room decontamination, 623
Medical director of infection prevention, as IPCC member, 571–573
    primary responsibilities of, 573
Medical informatics, for surveillance, 579. See also *Informatics.*
Medication preparation, infection risks from, 693
Medication therapies, optimizing patient outcomes with, 773–774. See also *Antimicrobial stewardship.*
Meningococcal infections, in HCP, immunization for, 731, 733–734
        special use of, 733–735
    postexposure prophylaxis for, 741–742
    work restrictions for, 748
Methicillin-resistant *Staphylococcus aureus* (MRSA), antimicrobial stewardship and, 772
    as targeted infection, 569–570
    environmental transmission of, 622–624, 641, 644
    in HCP, work restrictions for, 749
    in nursing homes, 787—791
    outbreak investigations of, 676
Microbiology, of outbreaks, in health care settings, 670
Microbiology data, informatics software challenges with, 767
Microbiology laboratory, antimicrobial stewardship role of, 775
Microorganisms. See *Pathogens.*
Middle-income countries, preventing HAIs in, **805–818**. See also *Developing countries.*

Ministries of Health, in developing countries, 812
Miscellaneous expenses, in IPCC budget, 576–577
Mission statement, of IPPs, 570
Mist system for probes, hydrogen peroxide, 628–629
Mold, outbreak in health care settings, 676–677
Molecular testing, of outbreaks, 670
MRSA. See *Methicillin-resistant Staphylococcus aureus (MRSA).*
Multidisciplinary bundles, in antimicrobial stewardship, 777–778
Multidisciplinary team, for antimicrobial stewardship, 774–776
    for infection prevention and control, 571, 581
Multidrug-resistant organisms (MDROs), antimicrobial stewardship for, 772–773
    as targeted infection, 570, 578, 621, 631
    economic impact of, 581–582, 774
    environmental transmission of, 622–623, 641, 714
    in nursing homes, 768–788, 790–794
    informatics recognition during admission, 764–765
    informatics surveillance of, 762, 764
    rate calculation of, 579
Multilocus sequence typing (MST), of outbreaks, 671
Mumps, in HCP, immunity proof for, 733
        immunization for, 731, 733–734
            special use of, 733–735
        work restrictions for, 749
*Mycobacterium chelonea,* 631
*Mycobacterium terrae,* 628–629
*Mycobacterium tuberculosis,* 631
    in HCP, work restrictions for, 749
    outbreak investigations of, 667
    water safety and, 698


    **N**

National Healthcare Safety Network (NHSN), antimicrobial stewardship and, 780
    as surveillance data source, 573, 578
Natural disasters, HAI prevention after, in developing countries, 810
Needlestick injuries. See also *Safe injection practices.*
    postexposure prophylaxis for, 731, 737–739
    reduction methods for, 738
Negative pressure room, in ambulatory care centers, 796
Neonatal intensive care unit (NICU), as high-risk setting for outbreaks, 678–679
NHs. See *Nursing homes (NHs).*
Noncritical items, disinfection and sterilization of, 612, 617–620
Nonpotable water (process water), safety issues of, 692, 695–696, 716
Nontuberculous mycobacteria (NTM), outbreak investigations of, 667, 674
    water safety and, 690–691, 698
Norovirus, as targeted infection, 631
Nosocomial infections, 568, 806. See also *Health care-associated infections (HAIs).*
No-touch (mechanical) methods, for environmental surface disinfection, 649
    for room decontamination, 623
Numerators, in hospital rate of infection, 579
Nursing homes (NHs), infection prevention programs in, 786–796

CAUTIs in, 787
components of, 787
employee health programs and, 794
environmental hygiene for, 794
environmental rounds for, 795
evolution of, 786
functions of, 787
hand hygiene for, 787, 789–790
infection preventionist role in, 794–795
information transfer during care transitions, 788–789
isolation precautions for, 791–792
MDROs and, 768–788, 790–794
MRSA in, 787—791
outbreak management for, 791–793
oversight of, 787–788, 795–796
protocol bundles for, 787–789
rehabilitation services and, 793–794
resident health programs and, 794
resources for, 787–788
safe injection practices for, 791
staff education on, 795
surveillance for, 792–793

**O**

Occupational health, infection prevention in, **729–757**
components of, 731–732
definitions for, 730–732
health care personnel covered by, 730
health care settings included in, 730
ill health care personnel evaluations for, 748–750
in developing countries, 809–810
in nursing homes, 794
introduction to, 729–730
key points of, 729, 732
postexposure prophylaxis for, 732, 735–747, 750
animal bites, 746–747
counseling in, 736–737
diphtheria, 745
ectoparasites, 747
general guidelines of, 735–736
hepatitis A, 745–746
hepatitis B, 739–740
human bites, 746
human immunodeficiency virus, 739, 741
influenza, 747, 750
measles, 745
meningococcal infections, invasive, 741–742
pertussis, 743–744
protocol for, 736
rabies, 746–747

Occupational (*continued*)
  sharps injuries in, 731, 737–739
  syphilis, 747
  tetanus, 744
  varicella, 742–743
  pre-exposure interventions for, immunizations as, 731, 733–735
    contraindications to, 735
    immunity proof vs., 731, 733
    recommendations for, 731, 734
    special use, 734–735
  screening as, 731–732
  professional guidelines for, 731
  scope of programs, 731
  work restrictions for health care personnel, 732, 748–750
Occupational Health and Safety Administration (OSHA), 731
Occupational health services (OHSs), 730–731
Occupational therapy (OT), in nursing homes, infection prevention for, 793–794
OPA (ortho-phthalaldehyde), for patient-care item sterilization, 614, 624, 628
Optical mapping, of outbreaks, 671
Ortho-phthalaldehyde (OPA), for patient-care item sterilization, 614, 624, 628
Outbreaks, in health care settings, **661–687**
  approach to, 662–670
  definitions of, 662–663
  delay in identification of, 662
  diagnosis verification for, 662–663
  high-risk settings for, 678–680
    endoscopy suites as, 679–680
    NICU as, 678–679
    transplant units as, 680
  hospital unit closures due to, 662
  hypothesis analysis of risk factors for, 663
    specific organism exposures in, 664–669
  impact on patients, 662
  informatics detection of, 764, 766
  introduction to, 661–662
  investigations of, case definition for, 662–663
    communication importance during, 670
    exposure risk factor analysis in, 664–669
    laboratory and testing in, 670–671
    primary components in, 579–580, 662–663, 670
    source identification in, 662–664
  key points of, 661
  LD pneumonia as, 702–703
  measures to stop, 663, 670
  nursing homes as, 793
  of SARS, 662, 677
  organisms in, 674–678
    *Acinetobacter sp. as,* 664, 674–675
    adenovirus as, 664
    *Aspergillus sp.* as, 664, 676–677
    *C difficile* as, 671, 678

*Campylobacter fetus.* as, 665
*Candida sp..* as, 664
carbapenem-resistant *Enterobacteriaceae* as, 675–676
coronaviruses as, 677
*E coli.* as, 665
*Enterobacter sp. as,* 665, 678
exposure risk analysis of, 664–669
fungus as, 676–677
gastrointestinal infections as, 665, 668, 678
hepatitis A, B, and C as, 665–666, 798
herpes virus as, 666
influenza A and B as, 677
*Klebsiella pneumoniae as,* 666
*Legionella sp. as,* 666, 673–674
*Listeria monocytogenes . as,* 667
MERS as, 677
mold as, 676–677
MRSA as, 676
*Mycobacterium tuberculosis. as,* 667
nontuberculous mycobacteria as, 667, 674
pertussis as, 677–678
*Pseudomonas sp. as,* 667, 675
*Ralstonia pickettii as,* 667
respiratory infections as, 662, 666, 677
rotovirus as, 662
*S aureus* as, 668–669, 671, 676
*Salmonella sp. as,* 667
SARS as, 662, 677
*Serratia marcescens as,* 668
*Streptococcus pyogenes as,* 669
varicella as, 669
*Yersinia enterocolitica as,* 669
pseudo-outbreaks vs., 670
sources of, 672–674
health care personnel as, 672
hospital environment as, 672
identification of, 662–664
waterborne, 672–674
summary of, 680
Outcome measures, of aseptic practices, in ambulatory surgical centers, 797–798
Outpatient settings, for health care. See *Ambulatory care centers; specific service or type.*
Oversight committee, for infection control, in nursing homes, 787–788, 795–796
for nursing homes, 787–788, 795–796

**P**

Parasite infestations, postexposure prophylaxis for, 747
Partnerships, for capacity building, in developing countries, 811–812
Pathogens. See also *specific microorganism.*
bloodborne, 568
in nursing homes, 791–792

Pathogens (*continued*)
    occupational health regulations for, 731
  emerging, as health care facility issue, 631
  EOC as source of, 714–716
  ESKAPE, 772
  outbreak investigations of, 663
    exposure risk analysis of, 664–669
    organisms in, 674–678
  resistance to antimicrobials. See *Antibiotic-resistant bacteria.*
  water-based. See *Waterborne pathogens.*
Patient outcomes, with medication therapies, strategies for optimizing, 773–774. See also *Antimicrobial stewardship.*
Patient risk, from disinfection and sterilization failures, as health care facility issue, 621–622, 624
    protocol for exposure investigation after, 624, 628
Patient role, in hand hygiene, 600
Patient safety, designing health care facilities for, **713–728**. See also *Design of health care facilities.*
Patient safety initiatives, as IPP goal, 568
Patient-care items, disinfection and sterilization of, critical items, 613–617
    in ambulatory surgical centers, 797–798
    noncritical items, 612, 617–620
    semicritical items, 611–617
  disinfection methods for, 610–613
  sterilization methods for, 610–611, 613
Patient-care rooms, as infection transmission risk, 717–718
  cleaning of. See *Discharge cleaning; Room decontamination.*
  safe design of, 719–720, 796
PE (protective environment) room, 720
PEP. See *Postexposure prophylaxis (PEP).*
Peracetic acid, for environmental surface disinfection, 648
  for patient-care item sterilization, 615
Peracetic acid/HP, for environmental surface disinfection, 648
  for patient-care item disinfection, 620
  for patient-care item sterilization, 614
Performance feedback, in hand hygiene, 600–601
Perfusion of channel scopes, for disinfection and sterilization, 629–630
Pertussis, in HCP, immunity proof for, 733
    immunization for, 731, 733–734
      special use of, 733–735
    postexposure prophylaxis for, 743–744
    work restrictions for, 749
PFGE (pulse field gel electrophoresis), for outbreaks, 671
Phage typing, of outbreaks, 670
Pharmacist, clinical, antimicrobial stewardship role of, 775
Pharmacy. See also *Medication therapies.*
  infection risks from, 693
Pharmacy and therapeutics (P & T) committee, antimicrobial stewardship role of, 776
Phenolics, for patient-care item disinfection, 620
Physical Self Maintenance Score (PSMS), 790
Physical therapy (PT), in nursing homes, infection prevention for, 793–794

Physician epidemiologist. See *Hospital physician epidemiologist.*
Physicians, hand hygiene in, 599, 601
Plain soap, in hand hygiene, 592–593
Plasmid typing, of outbreaks, 670
Pneumonia. See *LD pneumonia; Ventilator-associated pneumonia (VAP).*
Poliomyelitis, immunization for, 735
Polymerase chain reaction (PCR), for outbreaks, 671
Postexposure prophylaxis (PEP), for HCP, 732, 735–747, 750
        animal bites, 746–747
        counseling in, 736–737
        diphtheria, 745
        ectoparasites, 747
        general guidelines of, 735–736
        hepatitis A, 745–746
        hepatitis B, 739–740
        human bites, 746
        human immunodeficiency virus, 739, 741
        illness evaluation and, 750
        influenza, 747, 750
        meningococcal infections, invasive, 741–742
        pertussis, 743–744
        protocol for management, 736
        rabies, 746–747
        sharps injuries in, 737–739
        syphilis, 747
        tetanus, 744
        varicella, 742–743
        work restrictions and, 748–750
Precautions, infection, in ambulatory care centers, 796–797
        in nursing homes, 791–792
        inappropriate, informatics identification of, 765
Pre-exposure interventions, for HCP, 731, 733–735
        immunizations as, 731, 733–735
            contraindications to, 735
            immunity proof vs., 731, 733
            recommendations for, 731, 734
            special use, 734–735
        screening as, 731–732
Pregnant personnel, immunizations for, 734–735
Prevalence surveys, of HAIs, 567–568
Probes, hydrogen peroxide mist system for, 628–629
Process education, on disinfection and sterilization, in ambulatory surgical centers, 797–798
        of patient-care items, 622
Process (nonpotable) water, safety issues of, 692, 695–696, 716
Product consumption evaluation, in hand hygiene compliance, 597–598, 601
Product education, in hand hygiene, 600
Professional role, of NCP, in hand hygiene, 599–600
Professional societies, business analyses framework of, 582–583
        immunization recommendations of, 731
        influence on IPP, 568

Professional (*continued*)
    occupational health recommendations of, 735
    on ambulatory surgical center programs, 797–798
    on antibiotic resistance, 790–791
    on designing health care facilities, 717–722
    support of automated surveillance technologies, 579
Protection, of health care workers, as IPP goal, 568
Protective environment (PE) room, 720
Protocol bundles, in developing countries, 811
    in nursing homes infection prevention programs, 787–789
*Pseudomonas sp.,* environmental transmission of, 641
    outbreak investigations of, 667, 675
    water safety and, 690–691, 699
Pseudo-outbreaks, in health care settings, 670
PSMS (Physical Self Maintenance Score), 790
PT (physical therapy), in nursing homes, infection prevention for, 793–794
Public health, informatics and, 766
Public water utilities, 690
Pulse field gel electrophoresis (PFGE), for outbreaks, 671

**Q**

Quality, as water management priority, 692–696
Quality improvement, as infection preventionist role, 581
Quaternary ammonium compounds, for patient-care item disinfection, 620

**R**

Rabies, immunization for, 735
    postexposure prophylaxis for, 746–747
Radiofrequency tracking, in hand hygiene compliance, 598
*Ralstonia pickettii,* outbreak investigations of, 667
Random amplification of polymorphic DNA (RAPD), of outbreaks, 671
Rate of infection. See *Infection rate.*
Rational approach, to health care facilities disinfection and sterilization, 610–613
Regulatory bodies. See *Government agencies.*
Rehabilitation services, in nursing homes, infection prevention for, 793–794
Reimbursement, as regulatory leverage, 568–570
    value-based purchasing and, 582–583
Renovation, of health care facilities, for patient safely and infection prevention, **713–728**.
    See also *Design of health care facilities.*
Reporting, of postexposure prophylaxis, for HCP, 736
    of surveillance data, electronic via informatics, 577, 766
        voluntary vs. regulatory, 568–570
Reprocessing, of scopes. See *Endoscope reprocessing.*
Resident health programs, in nursing homes, 794
Resources, for infection control programs, design of health care facilities and, 722
    in developing countries, as limited, 807
        building capacity through partnerships, 811–812
        identification of, 807, 812
        prioritization of, 813–814

successful interventions despite, 810–811
successful examples of, 810–811
in nursing homes, 787–788
Respiratory equipment, infection risks from, 694
Respiratory hygiene, in ambulatory care centers, 796–797
Respiratory tract infections, in developing countries, 812
Legionella pneumophilia as, **689–712**. See also LD pneumonia.
outbreaks of, in health care settings, 662, 666, 677
tuberculosis as. See Mycobacterium tuberculosis.
ventilator-related. See Ventilator-associated pneumonia (VAP).
viral, in HCP, work restrictions for, 749
Restriction fragment length polymorphisms (RFLP), of outbreaks, 671
Retrospective surveillance, 577–578
Reuse, of single-use devices, 629, 798
of single-use instruments, in ambulatory surgical centers, 797–798
Ribotyping, of outbreaks, 671
Risk factors, hypothesis analysis of, for outbreaks, 663
Risk of infection. See Infection risk; Patient risk.
RNA probe, for outbreaks, 671
Room decontamination, advantages vs. disadvantages of, 624, 627
clinical trials on, 624–626
comparison of methods for, 624
effectiveness in reducing HAIs, 622–623
hydrogen peroxide systems for, 624
in ambulatory surgical centers, 797–798
no-touch (mechanical) methods for, 623
ultraviolet light for, 623–624
Rooms. See Patient-care rooms; specific design.
Route selection, for drugs, in antimicrobial stewardship, 773–774
Rubella, in HCP, immunity proof for, 733
immunization for, 731, 733–734
special use of, 733–735
work restrictions for, 749


S

Safe injection practices, in ambulatory care centers, 798
in nursing homes, 791
Safety, as water management priority, 692–696. See also Water safety.
of patients. See Patient safety initiatives.
Safety margin, in disinfection and sterilization, 621, 624, 628
Salmonella sp., outbreak investigations of, 667
Scopes, reprocessing of. See Endoscope reprocessing.
Screening, pre-exposure, of HCP, 731–732
in developing countries, 809–810
Security, as water management priority, 696
Self-disinfecting surfaces, 649–650
Self-protection behavior, in hand hygiene, 599
Semicritical items, disinfection and sterilization of, 611–617
storage issues of, 613, 629
SENIC (Study on the Efficacy of Nosocomial Infection Control), 568, 571, 575

Sequential interventions, for hand hygiene improvement, 601
Serotyping, of outbreaks, 670
Serratia marcescens, outbreak investigations of, 668
Sharps injuries. See also Safe injection practices.
    postexposure prophylaxis for, 731, 737–739
    reduction methods for, 738
SHEA. See Society for Healthcare Epidemiology of America (SHEA).
Single locus sequence typing (SLST), of outbreaks, 671
Single-occupancy patient-care rooms, 719–720
Single-use devices, reuse of, 629, 798
Single-use instruments, in ambulatory surgical centers, 797–798
Sink accessibility, in hand hygiene, 598
Skin flora, hand hygiene and, 592–593
Smallpox, immunization for, 735
Soap, in hand hygiene, antimicrobial, 593
        plain, 592–593
Society for Healthcare Epidemiology of America (SHEA), business analyses framework of, 582–583
    influence on IPP, 568
Sodium hypochlorite, for patient-care item disinfection, 619
Source of outbreaks, in health care settings, 672–674
        health care personnel as, 672
        hospital environment as, 672
        identification of, 662–664
        waterborne, 672–674
Sporicidal agents, for environmental surface disinfection, 648
SSIs. See Surgical site infections (SSIs).
Stakeholders, in water safety plans, 704–705
Standard precautions, in nursing homes, 791
Standardized infection rate, 578–579
Staphylococcus aureus, antibiotic-resistant. See Methicillin-resistant Staphylococcus aureus (MRSA).
    antimicrobial stewardship for, 778
    hand hygiene and, 591
    in developing countries, 811
    outbreak investigations of, 668–669, 671, 676
Steam, for patient-care item sterilization, 616
Stenotrophomonas maltophilia, water safety and, 699
Sterilization, in health care facilities, **609–637**. See also Disinfection and sterilization.
        agents and methods for, 613–617
        ambulatory surgical centers as, 797–798
        of patient-care items and environmental surfaces, 610–611, 613, 622–624
Storage, of semicritical items, as infection issue, 613, 629
Streptococcus, group A, in HCP, work restrictions for, 749
Streptococcus pyogenes, outbreak investigations of, 669
Study on the Efficacy of Nosocomial Infection Control (SENIC), 568, 571, 575
Surface decontamination, in health care facilities, advantages vs. disadvantages of, 624, 627
        clinical trials on, 624–626
        comparisons of methods for, 624
        disinfection methods for, 610–613

improving, 622–624
effectiveness in reducing HAIs, 622–623
sterilization methods for, 610–611, 613
improving, 622–624
Surface finish, as transmission risk, 717–718
safe designs of, 720–721
Surgical hand rub, in hand hygiene, 593
Surgical instruments, disinfection and sterilization of, in ambulatory surgical centers, 797–798
Surgical scrub, in hand hygiene, 593
Surgical site infections (SSIs), as targeted HAI, 569–570, 578
in ambulatory care centers, 797
informatics surveillance of, 762–763
rate calculation of, 579
Surveillance, automated technologies for, 579
fully or semi-, 761
concurrent, 578
data sources for, active, 579
concurrent or retroactive, 577–578
informatics and, 761
definition of, 576–577, 760
in developing countries, gaps and opportunities for, 807–808
of antimicrobial resistance, 808–809
in nursing homes, 790, 792–793
methodologies for, 578–579
priorities for, 578
retrospective, 577–578
subjective vs. objective, 760–761
syndromic, informatics for, 766
Surveillance activities, reported by infection preventionist, 577, 766
Surveillance data, IPCC review of, 571–572
reporting of, electronic via informatics, 577, 766
voluntary vs. regulatory, 568–570
Syndromic surveillance, informatics for, 766
Syphilis, postexposure prophylaxis for, 747


T

Targeted surveillance, 578
TB. See Tuberculosis (TB).
Tdap. See Pertussis.
TDC (thoroughness of disinfection cleaning) score, 642–643
Team approach, to infection prevention and control, 571, 581
to water safety plans, 703–704
Technologies, automated, for surveillance, 579
fully or semi-, 761
in hand hygiene compliance, 597–598, 601
information, 579. See also Computer science.
antimicrobial stewardship role of, 775
to augment disinfection of surfaces, 649–650
Tetanus, immunization for, 735

Tetanus (*continued*)
    postexposure prophylaxis for, 744
The Joint Commission (TJC), hospital accreditation standards of, 568–570
    on disinfection and sterilization of medical devices, 629
    on isolation precautions, in ambulatory care centers, 797
    on safe design of health care facilities, 718
    surveillance recommendations of, 577
Thoroughness of discharge cleaning, 647
Thoroughness of disinfection cleaning (TDC) score, 642–643
Time savings, with alcohol-based hand rub, 596, 598–599
TJC. See *The Joint Commission (TJC)*.
Toilets, in design of health care facilities, 720
Total house surveillance, 578
Transmission role, of hands. See *Hand hygiene (HH)*.
    of health care environment, 622–627. See also *Environmental hygiene*.
    of health care personnel, 750
Transmission routes, of waterborne pathogens, 690–691
Transmission-based precautions, in nursing homes, 791–792
Transplant units, as high-risk setting for outbreaks, 680
Treatment protocol bundles, in developing countries, 811
    in nursing homes infection prevention programs, 787–789
Trophon, for endocavity disinfection, 628–629
Tuberculosis (TB). See also *Mycobacterium tuberculosis*.
    in developing countries, prevention of, 809–810
    in HCP, work restrictions for, 749


U

Ultraviolet (UV) light, for environmental surface disinfection, 649
    for room decontamination, 623–624
        advantages vs. disadvantages of, 624, 627
        clinical trials of, 624–626
        HP systems vs., 624
Unapparent outbreak, of LD pneumonia, 702–703
Universal patient-care rooms, 719


V

Vaccinia, immunization for, 735
Validation, of data, in surveillance, 760–761
        informatics software challenges with, 767–768
Value statement, core, of IPPs, 571
Value-based purchasing, and HACs, 582–583
Vancomycin-resistant *Enterococcus* (VRE), antimicrobial stewardship and, 772
    environmental transmission of, 622–624, 630–631, 641, 644
    in nursing homes, 790–791
VAP. See *Ventilator-associated pneumonia (VAP)*.
Varicella, in HCP, immunity proof for, 733
        immunization for, 731, 733–734
            special use of, 733–735
        postexposure prophylaxis for, 742–743

work restrictions for, 749
outbreak investigations of, 669
Ventilation systems, safe design of, 718–719
Ventilator-associated pneumonia (VAP), as targeted HAI, 569, 578
    in developing countries, 806–807, 811, 813
    informatics surveillance of, 762–763
Video laryngoscope systems, portable GlideScope, 630–631
Video surveillance, in hand hygiene compliance, 598, 601
Viruses. See also *specific virus.*
    as health care facility issue, 624, 628–629, 631
        surrogate microbes of, 631
    as targeted infection, 593, 631, 640
    environmental transmission of, 622–624
    HCP exposures. See also *Occupational health.*
        work restrictions for, 749
    outbreak investigations of, 662, 664, 666, 677
Vision statement, of IPPs, 570
Visual audits/monitoring, of environment, 642–643
    of hand hygiene compliance, 597–598, 601
    of surface cleaning, 645
VRE. See *Vancomycin-resistant Enterococcus (VRE).*


**W**

Walls, safe designs of, 721
Water, as reservoir of infections, 690–691, 716
Water conservation, as priority, 696
Water distribution, as priority, 692–696
    balance between scald prevention and microbial control, 694–695
    construction activities and, 695, 716
    decorative water features and, 695, 717
    disinfectant residual and, 692–694
    leaking pipes/condensation and, 695
    nonpotable water (process water) and, 692, 695–696, 716
    stagnation in pipes and, 692, 716
    thermostatic mixing valves/anti-scald devices and, 695
    water temperature and, 694
Water distribution systems, in health care facilities, as pathogen reservoir, 714–716
    building safety plans for, 703–705
    LD pneumonia related to, 701
Water management priorities, for health care facilities, 691–696
    conservation as, 696
    distribution and quality as, 692
    safety as, 692–696
    security as, 696
Water quality, as priority, 692–696
Water safety, as priority, 692–696
    balance between scald prevention and microbial control and, 694–695
    construction activities and, 695
    decorative water features and, 695, 717
    disinfectant residual and, 692–694

Water (*continued*)
    leaking pipes/condensation and, 695
    nonpotable water (process water) and, 692, 695–696, 716
    stagnation in pipes and, 692, 716
    thermostatic mixing valves/anti-scald devices and, 695
    water temperature and, 694
  *Legionella pneumophilia* and, **689–712**. See also *Legionella pneumophilia*.
    outbreak investigations of, 666, 673–674
Water safety plans, building, 703–705
    decision points for, 703–704
    *Legionella* prevention plans in, 704–705
    stakeholders in, 704–705
    team approach to, 703–704
Water security, as priority, 696
Water supply, emergency, as priority, 696
Water uses, in health care, infection risks of, 692–694
Water utility systems, 690, 716
Waterborne pathogens, categorized by transmission routes, 690–691, 716
  in health care facilities, 716
    safety initiatives for. See *Water safety*.
    strength of evidence for, 714–715
  in outbreaks, 672–674
WGS (whole genomic sequencing), of outbreaks, 671
WHO. See *World Heathcare Organization (WHO)*.
Whole genomic sequencing (WGS), of outbreaks, 671
Whole surveillance, 578
Wipes, disposable, for environmental surface disinfection, 649
Wireless sensors, in hand hygiene compliance, 598, 601
Work restrictions, post-exposure, for HCP, 732, 748–750
        of conjunctivitis, 748
        of cytomegalovirus, 748
        of diarrheal diseases, 748
        of diphtheria, 748
        of group A streptococcus, 749
        of hepatitis A, 748
        of hepatitis B, 748
        of hepatitis C, 748
        of herpes simplex, 748
        of HIV, 748
        of measles, 748
        of meningococcal infections, 748
        of MRSA, 749
        of mumps, 749
        of pertussis, 749
        of rubella, 749
        of tuberculosis, 749
        of varicella, 749
        of viral respiratory tract infections, 749
        of zoster, 749
World Heathcare Organization (WHO), hand hygiene guidelines/indications of, 600, 651, 789

on alternative health care settings, 787
on HAIs in developing countries, 806, 808–810, 812

**Y**

*Yersinia enterocolitica,* outbreak investigations of, 669

**Z**

Zero rates, of HAIs, 570
Zoster, in HCP, work restrictions for, 749

# *Moving?*

## Make sure your subscription moves with you!

To notify us of your new address, find your **Clinics Account Number** (located on your mailing label above your name), and contact customer service at:

**Email: journalscustomerservice-usa@elsevier.com**

**800-654-2452** (subscribers in the U.S. & Canada)
**314-447-8871** (subscribers outside of the U.S. & Canada)

Fax number: 314-447-8029

**Elsevier Health Sciences Division**
**Subscription Customer Service**
**3251 Riverport Lane**
**Maryland Heights, MO 63043**

*To ensure uninterrupted delivery of your subscription, please notify us at least 4 weeks in advance of move.

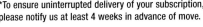
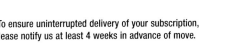

ELSEVIER

Edwards Brothers Malloy
Ann Arbor MI. USA
August 28, 2017